P9-DXO-894

ALSO AVAILABLE

The New Atkins for a New You

THE *NEW* ATKINS FOR A NEW YOU COOKBOOK

200 SIMPLE and DELICIOUS Low-Carb Recipes in 30 Minutes or Less

Colette Heimowitz

Photography by Mark Ferri

A TOUCHSTONE BOOK
Published by Simon & Schuster
New York London Toronto Sydney New Delhi

Touchstone
A Division of Simon & Schuster, Inc.
1230 Avenue of the Americas
New York, NY 10020

The information and recipes contained in this publication are intended to provide helpful and informative material useful for those following the Atkins Diet and for anyone preparing meals following a low-carbohydrate dietary approach. While the publisher, the author, and Atkins Nutritionals, Inc., have used their best efforts in preparing this book they make no representations or warranties as to the completeness or accuracy of its contents, and specifically disclaim any and all warranties of any kind, expressed or implied. The information and recipes contained herein may not be suitable for every reader, as each individual reader's general health and condition will differ. Each reader should consult his or her medical or health care professional before adopting a low-carbohydrate diet. The publisher, author, and Atkins Nutritionals, Inc., specifically disclaim all responsibility, liability, loss, or risk, personal or otherwise, which may be incurred as a result, directly or indirectly, of the use and application of any of the contents of this book.

First Touchstone trade paperback edition December 2011

Designed by Ruth Lee-Mui

Manufactured in the United States of America

1 3 5 7 9 10 8 6 4 2

Library of Congress Cataloging-in-Publication Data

Heimowitz, Colette.
The new Atkins for a new you cookbook : 200 simple and delicious low-carb recipes in 30 minutes or less / Colette Heimowitz ; photography by Mark Ferri.
p. cm.—(A Touchstone book)
Summary: "A follow-up to the *New York Times* bestseller *The New Atkins for a New You*—a complementary cookbook offering 200 quick, tasty, original recipes to support a healthy low-carb lifestyle. The 2010 bestseller *The New Atkins for a New You* introduced a whole new way to do the classic Atkins diet, offering a more flexible, more effective, and easier to maintain low-carb lifestyle—and dieters all over the world ate it up! After fourteen printings, more than thirty weeks on the New York Times bestseller list, and nearly half a million copies in print, sales are still going strong. But the #1 request among Atkins followers: more Atkins-friendly recipes. Now, *The New Atkins for a New You Cookbook* delivers—it's the first recipe book to reflect the innovative, modern Atkins program, featuring 200 original Atkins-friendly recipes that are quick, simple, accessible, and delicious. The book features color photographs of dozens of recipes, and simple instructions for making Atkins-friendly breakfasts, lunches, dinners, and desserts to keep anyone satisfied and on track. • Soups and Stews: including Hungarian Goulash and Thai Coconut-Shrimp Soup • Pizzas and Sandwiches: like tasty Paninis or Chicken Teriyaki Burgers • Vegetables and Sides: including 30 low-carb recipes for all your favorite veggie dishes • Poultry, Meat, and Seafood: more than 50 innovative ways to prepare these Atkins-friendly staples • Breakfast options: go beyond scrambled eggs with low-carb versions of muffins, scones, even smoothies. • Dessert: more than 35 decadent, delicious, and totally Atkins-friendly treats. With *The New Atkins for a New You Cookbook*, dieters will have all the ammunition they need to maintain the low-carb lifestyle for years to come"—Provided by publisher.
Includes bibliographical references and index.
1. Reducing diets. 2. Low-carbohydrate diet—Recipes. 3. Cookbooks. I. Title.
RM222.2.H3458 2011
641.5'6383—dc23 2011030663

ISBN 978-1-4516-6084-5
ISBN 978-1-4516-6085-2 (ebook)

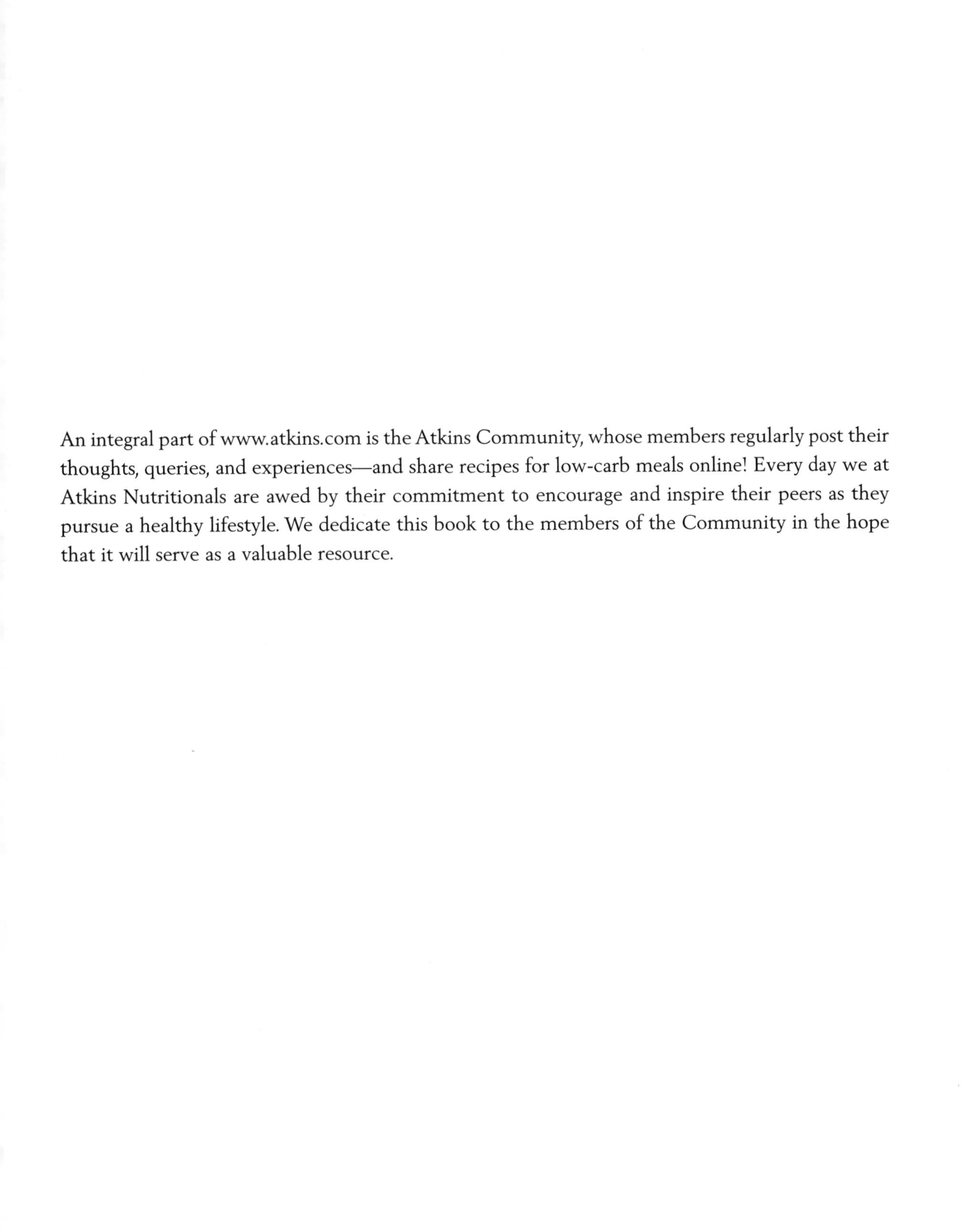

An integral part of www.atkins.com is the Atkins Community, whose members regularly post their thoughts, queries, and experiences—and share recipes for low-carb meals online! Every day we at Atkins Nutritionals are awed by their commitment to encourage and inspire their peers as they pursue a healthy lifestyle. We dedicate this book to the members of the Community in the hope that it will serve as a valuable resource.

CONTENTS

WHY A NEW ATKINS COOKBOOK?

Can you really eat delicious food morning, noon, and night—including a couple of snacks—and still shed pounds? If Mushroom-Herb-Stuffed Chicken Breasts, Beef and Asian Vegetable Stir-Fry, Chinese Sweet-and-Sour Pork, Yogurt-Marinated Butterflied Leg of Lamb, and Roasted Ginger-Tamari Salmon Steaks define delicious, the answer is a resounding yes. But those are just a few main dishes. How about sides of Garlicky Spinach and Feta Salad in Tomato Halves, Roasted Asparagus and Red Peppers with Dijon and Thyme, Spaghetti Squash with Cinnamon-Spice Butter, and Sweet Potato Pancakes? For your sweet tooth—admit it, we all have one—contemplate Pistachio-Chocolate Truffles, Pineapple Upside-Down Cake, and Crustless Ginger Cheesecake with Lime–Sour Cream Topping. Yum! Believe it or not, you can enjoy all these scrumptious dishes as you slim down, and continue to savor them as you maintain your trim new figure.

The more than two hundred recipes in *The New Atkins for a New You Cookbook* cover the gamut from on-the-run breakfasts to hearty main dishes and surprising salad combos to low-carb pizza (yes, pizza!), satisfying snacks, and desserts that only sound sinful. In many cases, we offer variations on the basic recipe.

THE WEIGHT GAME

Whether you're an old hand at Atkins, are just starting out, or are exploring whether a low-carb lifestyle is for you, you'll undoubtedly agree that gaining weight is easy and losing weight is difficult. But the reality is that maintaining one's goal weight is the *real* challenge. Studies show that only 5 percent of people who slim down can maintain their loss for a year or more. Most weight loss diets simply aren't sustainable. Why? It comes down to the food. Very few people can put up with nagging hunger and tasteless meals indefinitely. The Atkins Diet is different. First, the food is both appealing and filling. Second, as you move through the four progressively liberal phases while learning new eating habits, this slimming diet gradually morphs into a permanent lifestyle.

In the bestselling *The New Atkins for a New You*, Drs. Eric C. Westman, Steven D. Phinney, and Jeff S. Volek introduced a more flexible, personalized approach to the Atkins Diet. A key premise is that food must be both physiologically and emotionally satisfying. If meals consistently leave you craving more or fail to satisfy the complex psychological needs associated with food, sooner or later you'll revert to your old, familiar way of eating—and those pounds and inches will return. Although a number of Atkins cookbooks have been published, this companion volume to *The New Atkins for a New You* is the first that incorporates this more flexible attitude toward low-carb eating.

FOOD AND ME

As an Italian American, I grew up eating high-carb fare, but because I was a runner, I was never overweight. My parents and aunts and uncles weren't so fortunate. Many of my siblings and relatives have also developed type 2 diabetes. My interest in pursuing a career in nutrition arose from my family's health history and my desire to learn how to help people everywhere adopt a healthy lifestyle.

About twenty-five years ago I began working as a clinical nutritionist, and ten years later I joined Dr. Atkins's Manhattan practice. I quickly realized that boredom with food often led to noncompliance with any weight loss program. That meant I had two challenges if I wanted to enable my patients to get the results they craved. I needed to show them how to control their carbohydrate intake and get the right amount of protein and fat, as well as fiber and other micronutrients. However, I also had to create meal plans that offered enough taste and culinary variety to make it compliance easy. When I moved from the Atkins Center for Complementary Medicine to Atkins Nutritionals, I was able to communicate with a much larger group of people about their food habits via www.atkins.com, Atkins books, and other publications.

Like most of you, I love to eat. I also enjoy cooking, although I have little time during the week to spend in the kitchen. And while my son is now out of the house, I recall all too well the juggling act of parenting, working, and preparing meals. For a long time I've wanted to create a low-carb cookbook, but I also wanted to help busy people get great low-carb meals on the table in minimal time and with minimal effort.

THE LIFESTYLE FACTOR

Food must do more than satiate and soothe; it must also fit your lifestyle. No weight loss program works if preparing suitable food is so complex and time-intensive that we simply can't fit it into our busy lives. Cost is clearly another factor. With work, family, and community responsibilities—to say nothing of commuting to work and chauffeuring kids to various after-school activities—meal preparation has been relegated to the back burner in many a household. Even if you're single, childless, or are an empty nester, you may prefer spend your precious free time at the gym, taking a walk, working in your garden, or watching your latest Netflix DVD rather than slaving in the kitchen.

No wonder people increasingly rely on eating out, getting takeout, or heating up packaged foods in a microwave oven. The result, not surprisingly, is that most Americans are overfed and simultaneously deprived of vitamins, minerals, and other micronutrients. Statistics that chart the increase in fast-food consumption and the decline in the institution of the family dinner over the last several decades correspond closely to stats on an increasingly overweight population.

TIME IS OF THE ESSENCE

The need for tasty meals you can get to the table ASAP has not been lost on other cookbook authors, the producers of the Food Network and other cooking shows, and the people behind websites. Of the thousands of recipes found in popular magazines, or online, many are easy to prepare. The trouble is, the vast majority of these recipes are high in carbs or, at best, disregard carb content.

Food manufacturers have also responded to the needs of time-starved shoppers with countless convenience products. Some of these are a blessing for Atkins followers: roasted peppers or marinated artichoke hearts, to name just two, are savory low-carb condiments you'd likely never make from scratch. Frozen veggies are a godsend with little loss of vitamins, minerals, and antioxidants. Other time-savers may involve a trade-off, whether in cost or in nutrition. Bagged prewashed salad greens cost three times what an equivalent head of lettuce does. Chicken tenders are significantly pricier than a cut-up broiler-fryer. Peeled and cubed pumpkin or sliced bell peppers encased in plastic lose precious nutrients as they vegetate in the produce aisle. And, of course, many convenience foods—most barbecue sauces and many prepared entrées are prime examples—are full of sugar and highly refined grains, the empty carbs you want to avoid.

ATKINS TO THE RESCUE

Fortunately, you can follow the Atkins Diet and still have time for the other important things in your life. In keeping with the premise of *The New Atkins for a New You*—that you can customize the Atkins program to your preferences and lifestyle—this cookbook is your guide to getting tasty low-carb meals on the table (or in your backpack) pronto. Other than the offerings on the Atkins website, no other recipes are specifically developed, tested, and nutritionally analyzed to be in full compliance with the New Atkins Diet. These brand-new recipes complement the almost one thousand ones already at www.atkins.com, though occasionally we'll refer you to an existing recipe, such as a classic sauce or Atkins Cuisine Bread, on the website.

TELLING IT STRAIGHT

Just as *The New Atkins for a New You* dispelled certain misconceptions by presenting the research that validates the effectiveness and safety of the diet, this book overturns another set of culinary assumptions. Specifically:

- *Atkins is all about eating meat.* Although adequate protein is important to control your weight, so are those nutrient powerhouses known as vegetables. For proof, see Chapter 6, "Salads and Dressings," and Chapter 7, "Vegetables and Other Sides." Then check out Chapter 12, "Vegetarian Entrées."
- *Atkins-acceptable foods are budget busters.* Not true. Check out our poultry recipes, along with those for less costly cuts of meat such as pork butt and skirt steak. Vegetable protein sources are also on the menu. Repeat after me: Atkins is not just about steak and lobster!
- *Choices are limited.* No way! If you're worried that you'll be eating the same boring things day after day, scan the Recipe Phase Chart on page 261. You'll be amazed and tantalized by the variety of ingredients and combinations to tickle your taste buds. And by the way, breakfast on Atkins is far more than eggs, eggs, and more eggs, as you'll find in Chapter 3.

- *It takes hours to prepare low-carb meals.* Again, untrue. The active time required for these recipes is never more than 30 minutes. Other dishes that require marinating, baking, chilling, or roasting—what's called passive time—are usually more suitable for the weekend.
- *Low-carb cooking is complicated.* I'll be frank. If I can cook these recipes, so can you. If you know how to broil a burger, sauté onions, steam asparagus, and roast a chicken, you're already well on your way to making low-carb meals. Or if the only appliances you use are your fridge and microwave oven, as you master the basic techniques employed in the recipes in this book you'll soon develop a comfortable familiarity with your range.
- *You need to order lots of special ingredients to cook low carb.* You'll find virtually all your staple ingredients in the supermarket: produce, chicken, fish, poultry, cheese, and other dairy products. One-stop shopping is a major time-saver. We'll tell you where to find the few exceptions to this rule, such as a low-carb thickener that's a boon for making sauces.
- *You have to cook one meal for yourself and another for the rest of the family.* Wrong again. None of these recipes scream "for weight loss only," although you might want to prepare a side of rice, potatoes, or another starch for your perennially thin partner or growing kids.
- *Atkins ignores ethnic cuisines.* Just check out our recipes for Summer Rolls, Baba Ghanoush, Hungarian Goulash, Veal Marsala, Shrimp Diablo, and Thai Chicken Curry and you'll see that dishes inspired by far-flung lands find a place on the Atkins table.

I promise you that any such misconceptions will evaporate as you immerse yourself in these recipes. I hope not only that you will get low-carb meals on the table faster and more easily but also that you'll also experience a sense of mastery as you prepare nutritious meals for yourself and your loved ones. Eating tasty food, feeling good about yourself, and improving your health. What more could you want?

—Colette Heimowitz, M.Sc.

Chapter 1

A BRIEF LOOK AT THE NEW ATKINS DIET

In a nutshell, the New Atkins Diet adheres to the underlying principles that Dr. Robert C. Atkins set forth four decades ago but includes modifications that allow for greater flexibility. Some of these subtle but substantial shifts are simply the result of a greater understanding of human metabolism and food science. For example, now that we understand that fiber doesn't significantly impact blood sugar levels, it means that you can eat lots more high-fiber veggies than Dr. Atkins originally allowed.

As the sales of *The New Atkins for a New You* evidence, even forty years after Dr. Atkins introduced his diet, interest in his low-carb diet remains high. Moreover, many individuals who don't follow the program per se do watch their carbs. (If you're one of those people, this book's for you, too.) People also increasingly understand that going on *any* quickie diet to lose 10, 20, or even 100 pounds and then returning to their earlier way of eating won't result in permanent weight management. Only by adopting lifestyle changes, including a regular exercise program, is it possible to maintain weight loss.

Meanwhile, there's also greater understanding on the part of the medical, nutrition, and research communities that the causes of obesity are more nuanced than once assumed. Most health professionals have slowly but surely come to understand that being overweight is not just a matter of overconsuming calories. It's now widely acknowledged that it's not just the quantity but also the quality of the food we eat that has played a major role in the obesity epidemic of the last several decades.

THE MEANING OF THE WORD *DIET*

Atkins is a diet in the primary sense of the word: a way of eating. It's also a healthy way of eating. A large body of scientific research now associates heavy intake of sugar, white flour, and other refined carbohydrates with an increased risk for high triglyceride levels, low HDL ("good") cholesterol levels, and elevated blood pressure. These markers play a large role in increasing the risk of developing heart disease, type 2 diabetes, and other disease conditions. In fact, more than sixty studies support the principles upon which the Atkins Diet rests. We'll look at what's new about Atkins shortly, but first let's look at how burning fat, including your own body fat, for energy continues to be the governing principle of the Atkins Diet.

ATKINS BASICS

If this is your first exposure to the Atkins Diet, here's a quick snapshot of how it works. Your body burns both carbohydrate and fat—both, along with protein, known as macronutrients—as fuel for energy. Most people instinctively understand what fat and protein are and which foods contain them, but carbohydrates are a bit more elusive. They're found not just in grains, cereals, pasta, bread and other baked goods, and potatoes, but also in leafy greens and other vegetables, fruits, nuts and seeds, legumes, and dairy products. (Most of these foods also contain fat and/or protein as well.) As long as you eat the typical high-carb American diet, your body never gets much of a chance to burn its fat stores for energy.

SWITCHING TO FAT BURNING

Just as a Prius can run on either its electric battery or gasoline, your body can use either fat or carbohydrate as fuel. When you sufficiently reduce the total amount of carbs you consume and focus on vegetables and other such fiber-rich foods as nuts, seeds, and berries, your body shifts to burning primarily fat, including the stores of fat on your belly, hips, thighs, or buttocks. Adequate protein, which makes you feel full, as does fiber, is also essential. The result of eating this way: unwanted pounds and inches melt away.

When you reduce your carb intake and your body is running on a mostly fat metabolism, it's fine to have olive oil, avocados, olives, and other natural fats (as opposed to the chemically altered trans fats found in hydrogenated and partially hydrogenated oils). That's why our recipes call for butter, not margarine (some margarines still contain trace amounts of trans fats) or shortening. Natural fats also contribute to feeling pleasantly full. When you do Atkins, you watch your carbs but don't have to count calories. (The nutritional data that accompany each recipe do include calories. Note that grams of carbohydrates, protein, fat, and fiber have been rounded off to the nearest whole number.) With such satisfying meals and equally tasty snacks, most people find they aren't overly hungry when mealtime rolls around, enabling them to control their appetite—and ultimately their weight.

NO MORE BLOOD SUGAR ROLLER COASTER

As legions of failed dieters know, when your appetite is stimulated, it's very hard to ignore the messages your brain (and tummy) are beaming out. That's where blood sugar control comes in. When you moderate your carb intake, eat high-fiber, nutrient-dense carbs, consume sufficient protein (which is satiating), and have a meal or snack every three or four waking hours, your blood sugar stays on an even keel—and with it your appetite. In contrast, when you skimp on fat and protein and fill up on carbohydrates—which quickly convert to glucose (sugar) in your bloodstream—your blood sugar level rises quickly. Then a few hours later, it plummets as you run low on fuel, making you hungry, jittery, or sleepy—and craving another fix of high-carb foods. We call this the blood sugar roller coaster. It's almost impossible to control your appetite when your blood sugar is careening up and down. Doing Atkins almost immediately puts the blood sugar roller coaster out of business.

A FOUR-PHASE PROGRAM

The Atkins Diet is designed to allow you to transition from a relatively restrictive eating program to an increasingly liberal one. The first two

WHAT ARE NET CARBS?

The only carbs that matter when you do Atkins are Net Carbs, aka digestible carbs or non-impact carbs. In whole foods, such as vegetables, fruits, or cheese, you simply subtract the number of grams of dietary fiber in the food from the total number of carbohydrate grams to get the grams of Net Carbs. Why discount fiber? Although it's considered a carbohydrate, fiber doesn't impact your blood sugar level the way most carbohydrates do. Let's do the numbers: ½ cup of steamed green beans contains 4.9 grams of carbs, of which 2.0 grams are fiber, so subtract 2.0 from 4.9 and you get 2.9 grams of Net Carbs. Here's an even more dramatic example: 1 cup of romaine lettuce contains 1.4 grams of carbs, but more than half the carbs (1.0 gram) are fiber, for a Net Carb count of 0.4 gram. With packaged foods, simply check the Nutrition Facts panel and again subtract fiber grams from total carb grams to get the Net Carbs. Low-carb products, such as sugar-free chocolate, may use sugar alcohols as sweeteners. Moderate portions of sugar alcohols, including glycerin, don't impact blood sugar, and therefore their grams can also be subtracted from the total number of carb grams.

phases are designed for weight loss; the third is initially for weight loss and then becomes a dress rehearsal for Phase 4, which is all about weight maintenance. By gradually introducing more grams of carbohydrate while simultaneously broadening the array of carbohydrate foods, you stay in control of your intake, learn to identify foods you have trouble eating in moderation, and ultimately segue into a permanent, sustainable way of eating—a diet for life. Let's take a brief look at the four phases.

- *Phase 1, Induction,* which kick-starts weight loss, is where people usually begin. Induction lasts a minimum of two weeks, but it's perfectly safe to remain here for weeks or even months if you have lots of weight to lose. You'll consume 20 grams of Net Carbs daily (see "What Are Net Carbs?" above), primarily from leafy greens and other non-starchy vegetables. You'll also be eating eggs, poultry, fish and shellfish, meat, cream, aged or firm cheese, and olive oil and other natural fats. (After two weeks, you can introduce nuts and seeds, but remain at 20 grams of Net Carbs.) This phase excludes any form of sugar, fruit and fruit juice (other than lemon and lime juice), flour and other grains, and starchy vegetables.
- *Phase 2, Ongoing Weight Loss,* or OWL, is where you'll shed most of your excess pounds, eventually finding your tolerance level for consuming carbs while continuing to lose weight. You gradually increase your daily Net Carb intake, first to 25 grams, and then in 5-gram increments as long as weight loss proceeds. At the same time, you add back more carbohydrate foods in small portions, usually in this order: nuts and seeds; berries and other low-glycemic-impact fruit, such as most melons (but not watermelon); cottage cheese, ricotta, and most other fresh cheeses along with plain whole-milk yogurt; and finally lentils and other legumes. Most people stay in this phase until they're about 10 pounds from their goal weight.
- *Phase 3, Pre-Maintenance,* broadens your carb choices to include small portions of additional fruits, starchy vegetables, and finally whole grains. You'll continue to increase your daily carb intake, this time in 10-gram increments,

until weight loss stalls. This is good news, because it lets you know your carb threshold. When you reach it, drop back 5 or 10 grams a day and stay at that level until you reach your goal weight. Remain in Phase 3 for a month, as you practice holding your weight stable.

- *Phase 4, Lifetime Maintenance*, is not so much a phase as a lifetime way of eating. Continue to eat the way you did in Phase 3 and avoid added sugar (as opposed to the integral sugars in fruit, dairy, and vegetables), white flour, and refined grains, and you'll maintain your new weight. If you do start to regain after a vacation or a period of indulgence, drop back to Phase 2 before gaining more than 5 pounds and remain there until you get on track.

For more on how to do Atkins and complete lists of acceptable foods for each phase, log on to www.atkins.com or read *The New Atkins for a New You*.

WHAT'S NEW ABOUT ATKINS?

Some of the changes that define the New Atkins Diet, such as permitting caffeinated beverages—caffeine has been shown to modestly benefit fat burning—are fairly small. Coffee or tea can now also count toward two of your eight daily cups of water. But there are several more substantial updates. Overall, the objective is to make the program simpler, more versatile, and sustainable for a lifetime. Some changes relate to eating out, but others take place right in your kitchen.

- *Vegetables are key.* Even in the initial phase, we encourage you to eat lots of high-fiber "foundation vegetables." These include salad greens, tomatoes, green beans, asparagus, and more than seventy other non-starchy vegetables. (Most people can eat the remaining vegetables, such as sweet potatoes and most other root vegetables, winter squash, and even potatoes in moderation, as they approach their goal weight.) We recommend that you eat at least 12–15 grams of Net Carbs (see page 3) in the form of foundation vegetables each day, which translates to at least five servings of salad and cooked vegetables.
- *Transition easily.* Previously, people sometimes got trapped in Phase 1 of Atkins, afraid to start adding back carbohydrate foods and stalling weight loss. It can be tempting to lose all one's excess weight in this phase, but this doesn't allow you to explore your limits and capabilities. Instead, by moving through the phases of the program, you internalize new eating habits. The New Atkins puts much more emphasis on the natural transition from one phase to another. Recipes indicate the phases for which they are appropriate and often offer suggestions about how to modify them for an earlier phase. By gradually transitioning to a sustainable way of eating, you significantly increase your chances of being able to find the right weight for you—and stay there.
- *Customize to suit your needs.* Each of us has a unique body and metabolism. You may be able to consume more (or less) carbs or greater (or less) variety in carb foods than your spouse, daughter, or best friend. Watch your response to foods and recalibrate accordingly. You can also decide to start in Phase 2 or Phase 3 if you prefer to swap slower weight loss for more food choices. Or if you're already at a good weight and are interested in following a low-carb program for health reasons, simply start in

Phase 3. We advise vegetarians to start in Phase 2 at 30 grams of Net Carbs, so nuts, seeds, legumes, fresh cheese, and yogurt are on the menu from the get-go. Vegans, too, can start in Phase 2, but at 50 grams of Net Carbs to allow larger portions of nut, legume, and grain dishes.

- *Variety is the spice of life.* Dissatisfaction with a short list of acceptable foods and the resultant boredom torpedo most weight loss diets. On a typical calorie-restricted diet, the day comes when you simply cannot consume one more tasteless low-fat meal. Before you know it, you're "sneaking" some of your favorite forbidden foods. It's usually all downhill from there, as you abandon a way of eating that denies the perfectly normal desire to savor food. Because nuts, eggs, butter, cream, olive oil, and even chocolate and ice cream (made without added sugar, of course), and other satisfying foods are permitted on Atkins, you're far more likely to stay the course.

RECIPE CODING

Our recipes cover the gamut from on-the-run breakfasts to hearty main dishes and surprising salad combos to low-carb pizza (yes, pizza!), satisfying snacks, and desserts that only sound sinful. In many cases, we offer variations on the basic recipe. Each complete recipe provides full nutritionals per serving and is coded to indicate which of the four Atkins phases for which it's appropriate. In general, three factors determine phase coding, and each one can override the others:

- The number of grams of Net Carbs
- Whether the recipe is a main dish or side dish, appetizer, snack, or dessert
- The ingredients in the recipe

PHASE 1 RECIPES

- Main dishes generally contain no more than 7 grams of Net Carbs per serving.
- Appetizers, soups, sides, snacks, and desserts generally contain no more than 3 grams of Net Carbs per serving.
- Omit fruit or fruit juices (other than lemon or lime juice), fresh cheeses, yogurt or milk (reduced-carb dairy beverages and plain unsweetened soy milk, almond milk, and coconut milk beverage are acceptable), nuts, seeds, starchy vegetables, grains, legumes, and pasta.
- Alcohol is acceptable only if it has been heated or used in a marinade and discarded.

PHASE 2 RECIPES

- Main dishes generally contain no more than 12 grams of Net Carbs per serving.
- Appetizers, soups, sides, snacks, and desserts generally contain no more than 9 grams of Net Carbs per serving.
- In addition to Phase 1 foods, recipes can include nuts, seeds, berries, and a few other low-glycemic-impact fruits; all cheeses; unflavored, unsweetened whole-milk yogurt; tomato or tomato-vegetable (V-8, for example) juice; and legumes.

PHASES 3 AND 4 RECIPES

- Main dishes generally contain no more than 18–20 grams of Net Carbs per serving.
- Appetizers, soups, sides, snacks, and desserts generally contain no more than 12 grams of Net Carbs per serving.
- Recipes may include ingredients restricted in earlier phases, but not added sugars or white flour and other highly refined grains.

Note: Personal tolerances for carbohydrates in general and specific ingredients vary greatly.

Also please refer to the Recipe Phase Chart on page 261, which lists the phases for which each recipe is suitable, as well as whether it is more appropriate time-wise to make on a weekday or over the weekend. In a few cases, a recipe not coded for an earlier phase can be modified, for example, with a smaller portion or swapping out or eliminating one ingredient. Such exceptions are indicated with an asterisk (*).

In keeping with greater flexibility, you may also choose to eat a dish coded for a higher phase even if the carb count is higher than advised if the ingredients are acceptable for the phase you're in. For example, a side salad with lots of foundation vegetables might be more than 3 grams of Net Carbs per serving. As long as you stay within the total number of grams for the day, there's no reason why you couldn't have that salad with an entrée low in carbs such as a grilled chicken breast or broiled fish. Or simply have a smaller portion.

If you stay longer than two weeks in Phase 1, you can add nuts and seeds in Week 3. This means that you can have recipes coded for Phase 2 that include nuts or seeds but otherwise meet the other requirements for Phase 1. Such recipes are indicated in the Recipe Phase Chart.

RECIPES AND BEYOND

The New Atkins for a New You Cookbook is far more than just a collection of mouthwatering low-carb recipes. It's also packed with a wealth of helpful information to speed meal preparation and make you feel more in control and confident in the kitchen. That's why Chapter 2, "The New Atkins Kitchen: Ingredients and Equipment," provides information on the most common low-carb ingredients and a list of staple foods you should always have in your pantry, freezer, and fridge so you never get caught with "nothing to eat." You'll learn how to be a savvy low-carb shopper, including how to read food labels, along with time-saving meal-prep techniques and the few essential pieces of equipment that will enable you to cook just about anything. The Glossary (page 253) explains terms you may not be familiar with that appear in recipes.

Each recipe lists the active and total amount of time needed and is coded as a weekday (30 minutes or less total time) or weekend (more than 30 minutes total time) meal. Recipe headnotes offer shortcuts to shave off precious minutes, perhaps by substituting cooked shredded chicken from a salad bar instead of poaching a chicken breast, swapping one ingredient for another, or cross-referencing other dishes that would work well as accompaniments. Multiple tips range from how to pit olives and safely defrost frozen foods to how to fold up a burrito and freeze leftover egg whites.

I hope I've given you a small taste of the luscious delights and practical advice to come in the following pages. I'm excited to share with you these luxurious dishes you can enjoy on the Atkins Diet. The food is so good and so satisfying that you might even forget that you're on a diet! Here's to enjoying both the journey of great food that's easy to prepare and the destination of a permanently slimmer, healthier, more energetic you.

Chapter 2

THE NEW ATKINS KITCHEN: INGREDIENTS AND EQUIPMENT

Ready to get cooking? Before you turn to the recipes and turn on the oven, take the time to get your kitchen in order. This is where you'll learn what ingredients and tools to have on hand and how to use them to create delicious results.

THE ATKINS PANTRY

Naturally you'll have to purchase specific ingredients once you decide to make certain recipes, but stock your fridge, freezer, and cupboards with the following Atkins-friendly foods and you'll always be able to put together a tasty low-carb meal. Although most of these foods are suitable for Phase 1, they'll stand you in equally good stead in later phases. Here's what to add to your shopping list.

FOR THE FRIDGE

- Butter (salted for dressing vegetables; unsalted for baking and making desserts)
- Eggs
- Cheese
- Cream, half-and-half, sour cream
- Mayonnaise (regular, not low fat)
- Tofu
- Salad fixings and other vegetables
- Nuts and seeds
- Olives
- Lemons and/or limes
- Fresh berries

FOR THE FREEZER

- Hamburger patties, lamb chops, and/or pork chops
- Shrimp
- Chicken breasts or thighs in individual resealable plastic bags for quick defrosting
- Frozen vegetables
- Frozen berries

FOR THE PANTRY

- Virgin olive oil (for cooking), extra-virgin olive oil (for dressing salads and vegetables), and canola oil
- Tuna or salmon in cans or vacuum bags
- Canned sardines, crabmeat, and clams
- Canned tomatoes, perhaps some seasoned with Italian or Mexican flavorings
- Marinated artichoke hearts
- Marinated roasted red peppers
- Peanut butter and/or other nut butters
- Canned lentils, garbanzos, and other legumes
- Granular sugar substitute (sucralose)
- Unsweetened cocoa powder

- Unsweetened baking chocolate
- Atkins Cuisine All Purpose Baking Mix (order at www.atkins.com)

LOW-CARB CONDIMENTS

Although you don't need exotic ingredients to trim carbs, you might want to stock up on a few other items. If you have a collection of condiments on hand, you can take a basic recipe for pan-seared chicken, for example, and make it Italian, Chinese, Thai, or Mexican. Or toss a few items together and dress up a simple steak with an elegant sauce. Among the items you might want to keep on hand (note that not all of them are suitable for Phase 1):

- *Mustard.* Dijon mustard has a sophisticated bite that adds punch to salad dressings and sausages, but check out coarse-grain Dijon (sometimes called country Dijon) or flavored mustards without honey or sugar.
- *Vinegar.* Red wine vinegar is the most versatile for cooking; others vary in sourness and pungency. Rice and cider vinegars are comparatively mild; balsamic vinegar can be quite sweet (and higher in carbs). White wine vinegar is lighter than red wine vinegar, as is Champagne vinegar; sherry vinegar has elements of red wine vinegar but with a touch of sweetness.
- *No-sugar-added jams.* Melt these in the microwave or on the stove for a quick sauce. Raspberry, cherry, peach, and apricot work well with savory dishes, making them more versatile than strawberry or grape.
- *Tubes of pastes.* Tomato paste, olive paste, garlic paste, basil pesto (and other herbs), and even anchovy paste in tubes keep indefinitely in the fridge—simply cap the tube.
- *Jars of chopped garlic and ginger.* Fresh varieties of these two foods are always preferable, but we understand that sometimes you need to compromise a little. If you don't have time to peel and chop, using these shortcut ingredients is better than heading for the drive-through.
- *Herbs.* Fresh herbs have a purer, cleaner flavor, but if the thought of prepping one more ingredient gives you hives, reach for dried ones. Crumble them between your fingertips before you add them to the recipe. This releases their volatile oils and heightens their flavors. You'll need about one-third as much of a dried herb as a fresh one.
- *Sauces and syrups.* Ketchup, barbecue sauce, and maple syrup are used in a variety of recipes to add flavor and sweetness. Look for low-carb and sugar-free (or no-added-sugar) counterparts. If you're going to be trying some of our Asian-inspired recipes, make sure to have dark (toasted) sesame oil on hand. It and many other Asian condiments, including fish sauce (nam pla or nuoc mam), are now available in almost every supermarket. On the other hand, sugar-free hoisin sauce may be more difficult to find. Steel's Sugar-Free Rocky Mountain Hoisin Sauce can be ordered from multiple online sources. The only low-carb teriyaki sauce we have found is Seal Sama Teriyaki Sauce. If you can't find it locally, order it from www.carbsmart.com.

One last thing: don't forget to have a few avocados ripening on the counter.

TIP TIME

THE ART OF COMPROMISE

Cleaning and chopping vegetables in advance can streamline meal preparations for busy weeknights and simplify packing lunches to tote to work or school. That said, there's a trade-off between saving time and losing nutrients. If you do opt to prep veggies ahead, plan to use them within the next day or two. The longer they languish in the crisper, the more nutrients they'll lose.

SPECIALTY PRODUCTS

Tortillas. You can find La Tortilla Factory's Smart & Delicious Original Low Carb High Fiber Tortillas at Super Walmart and most other well-stocked supermarkets. Tumaro's Low in Carbs Multigrain Gourmet Tortillas are also widely available. Smaller low-carb tortillas should be no more than 3–4 grams of Net Carbs each, and larger ones no more than 7. However, other so-called low-carb tortillas can be considerably higher.

Pitas, wraps, and other flatbreads. Toufayan Bakeries low-carb pita bread, which has 7 grams Net Carbs, is widely available (to find a store near you, to to www.toufayan.com/locator.php). Another option is Flatout's Light line, which clocks in at 6–8 grams of Net Carbs per flatbread, making them acceptable in Phases 3 and 4 (go to www.flatoutbread.com/find-a-store/where-we-are).

CAREFUL SHOPPING

As you stroll through the aisles of the supermarket, familiarize yourself with the Nutrition Facts panels and ingredient lists that are required on all packaged foods. A quick glance at the label will give you carbohydrate and fiber counts. Once you've established that the Net Carbs (total grams of carbohydrates minus fiber grams, as well as those of any sugar alcohols) are acceptable, scan the ingredients list. Pass up anything with sugar, high-fructose corn syrup, starch (such as modified potato starch or cornstarch), refined flour, or hydrogenated or partially hydrogenated oils (trans fats).

MENU PLANNING

I'm not a big fan of the "If it's Monday, it must be meatloaf" school of meal planning—there are so many recipes to try and flavors to enjoy that I prefer a looser approach. Instead, I recommend planning menus based on seasonality of foods, budgeting, and schedules.

Just because you can buy asparagus in October and raspberries in January doesn't necessarily mean you should. Out-of-season produce tends to be bland—it's often picked before it's ripe because ripe foods are more perishable. Depending on where you live, produce may have been trucked across the country or imported. Either can be a rigorous, nutrient-destroying trip. Out-of-season food tends to be much more costly as well—part of its price reflects its scarce supply, but you're also paying for the shipping and storing costs.

Foods bought in season, especially those that are grown locally, have a rich, pure flavor that their out-of-season peers can't match. You'd expect them to taste better, but they're also usually less expensive, and easier to prepare. Doing as little as possible to them is the best way to let their flavors shine through. Complex sauces hide their tastes, and because they are so fresh and ripe, you don't need to do a lot to bring out their flavors. Consider tomatoes, for example. The best way to serve a fresh-from-the-garden one in August probably isn't the way you'd choose to prepare it in the depths of winter.

As you select dishes, pay attention to colors, textures, and flavors. Sole Meunière and Roasted Cauliflower would taste fine together, but they're both pale, and on the same plate they'd lack visual appeal. Opt for a more colorful side dish—there are plenty of green options, as well as red and orange ones.

Some meats and vegetables are more perishable than others. Leafy and high-moisture foods spoil quickly, especially once they've been cut or peeled. Whole peppers may last for five or so days, but cut one into strips and you reduce the storage time to a day or two. Fresh sausages and fish don't last as long as other cuts or types of protein. If you do your shopping once a week or so and these items are on your list, plan to use them within two or three days.

Finally, take your schedule and lifestyle into account. If weeknights are hectic, pick one new dish and round out the meal with simpler ones. Unless you have willing helpers for cleaning and chopping vegetables, you'll be hard pressed to get dinner on the table in 30 minutes or so if two of the recipes you plan to make require 15 minutes of prep. Unless you have two ovens, don't choose two dishes that call for different temperatures (unless you know that one dish is forgiving and will be okay if cooked at a lower or higher temp than recommended).

Roasts, soups, stews, meatloaf, and other foods with high yields are terrific weekend projects (assuming your weekends have more discretionary time than your weekdays). If you're roasting a chicken, consider putting a second one in the oven at the same time. By planning for leftovers, you'll have options for lunches as well as quick suppers. Extra veggies can be tossed into a soup or stir-fry at the last minute, or puréed in broth for a quick soup.

BASIC COOKING TECHNIQUES

Cooking methods divide into two categories, dry heat and moist heat. The former includes roasting, baking, searing, sautéing, pan-frying, stir-frying, deep-frying, grilling, and broiling; moist heat methods include boiling, simmering, braising, blanching, stewing, poaching, and steaming. (For more on each these cooking methods, see the Glossary on page 253). Even within these categories, the actual techniques can vary. Baked chicken, for example, is often covered with a sauce or foil to keep the meat from drying out. Cakes and cookies, on the other hand, are almost never covered while baking.

MAKING A FEW MODIFICATIONS

With few exceptions, there isn't a great deal of difference between low-carb cooking and traditional cooking. It's more a matter of choosing the right ingredients and developing the right habits so that you can sauté foods without resorting to breading and other high-carb coatings, and can thicken stews without flouring meat before browning it. A few small changes are in order:

* To thicken sauces and stews, you can purée vegetables, or use cream, butter, or Dixie Carb Counters Thick-It-Up low-carb thickener, which can be ordered from www.dixiediner.com.
* Instead of using milk when making sauces, use heavy cream, half-and-half, plain unsweetened soy milk, or unsweetened coconut milk. Or dilute heavy cream with water. For shakes and smoothies, experiment with plain unsweetened soy milk, plain unsweetened almond milk, or plain unsweetened coconut milk beverage.
* Rather than soy sauce, which is made in large part from fermented wheat, use tamari, which is made only from soy.
* In lieu of conventional bread crumbs for breading poultry or fish, make bread crumbs from Atkins Cuisine Bread (recipe at www.atkins.com) or use almond meal (almond flour), which can be found in natural foods stores, Trader Joe's, and the baking section of most well-stocked supermarkets. You can also make your own in a food processor. Do small batches and pulse only until it resembles corn meal; overprocess and you'll wind up with almond butter!
* Instead of white flour, recipes use Atkins Cuisine All Purpose Baking Mix, often in combination with almond meal, whole-wheat flour, or whole-wheat pastry flour.
* Rather than regular shredded coconut, which is full of sugar, use unsweetened shredded coconut.
* Instead of conventional pasta, use tofu shirataki noodles (okay in Phase 1) and low-carb pasta (Phase 2 and beyond, depending upon carb count).

HOW TO READ A RECIPE

Whether you've been cooking for decades or are only just beginning to navigate your kitchen, reading a recipe properly is the key to success. You're less likely to make mistakes if you assemble and prepare the ingredients before you start cooking. That way you won't be halfway through a recipe only to realize you're missing a critical ingredient.

You probably know how to measure, but did you know that there's a difference between "½ cup chopped walnuts" and "½ cup walnuts, chopped"? In the first example, you should chop walnuts and then measure ½ cup of them. In the second example, you should measure ½ cup of walnuts and then chop them. The easy way to remember is to look for a comma separating the ingredient from any preparation instructions—and to use common sense. Anything listed before the comma should be done before you measure, anything after should be done post-measuring. We try to write our recipes so you can use foods as you purchase them—a head of broccoli, a bunch of kale, two onions. And common sense tells you that it's pretty hard to fit a head of broccoli into a measuring cup and have it indicate an amount with any degree of accuracy.

The active time in our recipes includes all the preparation, as well as the hands-on cooking such as stirring, basting, and turning foods over.

Total time includes everything from marinating to chilling, heating the oven to the proper temperature, and cooking that doesn't need much monitoring.

Although we recommend chopping or otherwise preparing all the ingredients first, you may find that with experience, you can prep the ingredients for one step and get it cooking, and then begin working on ingredients used later. You might be able to reduce the total time of a recipe by doing this, but be sure to read through the recipe at least once so you know what's coming up and don't get taken by surprise.

Even seasoned cooks may not be aware of the differences between chopping, dicing, and mincing, for example. If you come across a term in a recipe with which you're unfamiliar, refer to the Glossary (page 253) for the definition.

THE RIGHT STUFF

When it comes to outfitting your kitchen, the latest isn't always the greatest. Whether you need a particular appliance or gadget depends largely on the type of cooking you do. That said, there are some items that all kitchens need:

- *Mixing bowls.* It's most useful to have a number of different sizes. Stainless steel, glass, or ceramic are preferable to plastic bowls.
- *Whisks* should have a fairly small diameter (2 or so inches) and be flexible. They're terrific not just for beating egg whites and light batters but also for sifting or mixing dry ingredients (particularly for incorporating baking soda or powder throughout flour).
- *Wooden spoons* serve many purposes. Have two or three spoons with ½-inch-diameter handles.
- *Forks* are useful for mixing light dough and batters; they can be used to serve low-carb pasta or noodles, too.
- *Silicone spatulas* are ideal for getting into corners of pans, where spoons are often too round to fit, as well as for folding together ingredients and for scraping every last bit of batter out of a mixing bowl.
- *Metal spatulas and pancake turners* are similar, although spatulas tend to be longer and narrower; they may or may not have slots in them. Be sure to have at least one that has a thin blade to slide under delicate foods such as fish fillets.
- *Slotted spoons* are terrific for lifting cooked foods out of a sauce that needs to be reduced further or out of poaching liquids.
- *Handheld electric mixers* are fine for many applications, from mixing batters and cookie dough to whipping egg whites and cream.
- *Stand mixers* are larger and have larger motors than hand mixers, so they can handle heavy, stiff dough with ease and knead bread dough.
- *Blenders*, with their tall, narrow shape, tight-fitting lids, and elevated blades, do a good job puréeing or liquefying ingredients.
- *Stick or immersion blenders* are ideal for making smoothies and puréeing small amounts of liquid.
- *Food processors* excel at chopping and grating foods and at kneading bread dough or mixing piecrust. They can also purée mixtures, but liquids may leak.
- *Mini food processors* are handy for chopping small amounts of ginger or garlic, or for making herb pastes.
- *A coffee grinder* is ideal for grinding spices, but it must be cleaned carefully. Wash the

lid in hot soapy water, and clean the grinding mechanism by whirling a slice of white bread. It will absorb the oils and any bits of coffee or spice; repeat this until the bread crumbs are perfectly white, with no flecks of coffee or spice in them. Better yet, use a dedicated grinder for spices.

- *Cutting boards.* You'll need at least two. Use one board (preferably of wood) for meats, poultry, and fish, and another for vegetables, fruit, and so on. Wash with hot water and detergent after each use. You can put plastic boards in the dishwasher.
- *Knives.* There are several different types that you'll find useful. Paring knives are small (3- to 4-inch blades) and are designed for peeling vegetables, especially garlic and onions. Chef's knives are best for chopping foods; they come in 6-, 8-, and 10-inch lengths. A boning knife has a very flexible blade for easy maneuvering; a utility knife is a bit stiffer. Serrated knives cut bread as well as soft foods such as tomatoes.
- *Graters.* A four-sided box grater is sturdy and versatile for grating cheese, chocolate, and other foods, but can be difficult to clean. Flat graters are easy to clean, but you'll need several, from fine to coarse holes. A Microplane grater, basically a woodworking tool for shaving wood, quickly zests citrus fruit and finely grates Parmesan and other hard cheeses.
- *Liquid measures* are made of glass, plastic, or metal; they're identifiable by their spouts. Plastic ones can crack or melt; with metal ones, it can be difficult to ascertain correct measurements. Although glass can break, most liquid measures are made of very thick glass and can withstand a great deal of abuse. You'll want 1-, 2-, and 4-cup measures.
- *Dry measures* are flat across the top, so you can spoon in dry ingredients and then draw a knife across the top to level them. They come in nesting sets.
- *Measuring spoons.* Believe it or not, a tablespoon is not always a tablespoon—an inexpensive, flimsy measuring spoon may hold considerably less than what it's touted to. Having two sets on hand is a good idea because invariably the spoon you need will have just been used for something else.
- *Vegetable peelers* have either fixed blades that work when drawn toward the body or swivel blades designed to be moved away from the body. You're less likely to cut yourself with a swivel blade.
- *Colanders.* Buy one that's larger than you think you'll need—when you're pouring boiling water, you want to catch all the pasta or vegetables you're draining. Stainless-steel ones are virtually indestructible, but heavy-duty plastic ones don't heat up.
- *Sieves* are made of mesh. A small one with fine mesh is convenient for straining out seeds when juicing citrus fruits; a 4- to 6-inch-diameter one can be used to make purées, drain liquid from canned foods, and sift dry ingredients.
- *Thermometers.* An instant-read thermometer is preferable to the old-fashioned meat thermometer, which has a large pointed shaft that allows a considerable amount of juices to escape during the cooking process. An instant-read thermometer, used at the end of cooking, has a very thin shaft that makes only a small puncture in the food when inserted. An oven

thermometer doesn't check the doneness of food, but it is a wise (and low-cost) investment, because an oven may be off by as much as 25°F, which can affect the cooking time and the level of browning of baked foods. If you know that your oven only gets to 310°F when you set it for 350°F, you'll know you must set it at a higher temperature.

- *Tongs* are ideal for lifting foods out of liquids and for flipping small foods such as chops or chicken parts quickly and easily without splashing hot fat, as a spatula might. Spring-loaded tongs, which snap open after you press them closed, are preferable to scissors-style ones.

CONSIDER THE COOKWARE

I don't recommend that you buy a matching set of pots and pans. Different weights and materials are better for different cooking techniques. The best utensil will depend on what you're cooking and what end result you want. Some materials are superb at distributing heat evenly across the pan. Others are better at heating rapidly. Sometimes you need a dark surface to encourage browning and other times you need a metal that won't react with acidic ingredients.

Here is a list of the most common cooking utensil materials with their advantages and disadvantages:

- *Stainless steel* is extremely durable, nonreactive, and easy to maintain. But it conducts heat poorly and unevenly, so better-quality stainless cookware comes with aluminum or copper bottoms, often sandwiched between steel. Foods cooked in solid stainless can scorch where the burners touch the metal.
- *Aluminum* conducts heat better than stainless steel, but it reacts with eggs and with lemon juice, red wine, and other acids. Aluminum is acceptable for boiling or simmering stocks and for cooking pasta.
- *Anodized aluminum*, such as Calphalon or Magnalite, is completely different from regular aluminum. Often quite pricey, it's heavy, has a nonreactive coating, and conducts heat very well. These pans are terrific for searing, braising, and stewing, as well as for making sauces.
- *Cast iron* pans conduct heat wonderfully, and like anodized aluminum retain it well. They're inexpensive and durable, although they must be seasoned to make them nonreactive and nonstick. Cast iron is very, very heavy, but it's wonderful for frying as well as for braising, searing, and stewing.
- *Enameled cast iron*, such as Le Creuset, conducts heat well without hot spots and is nonreactive. Foods will stick to it, however, and it is extremely heavy. It should be treated with care, too, lest the enamel chip.

A POT AND PAN PORTFOLIO

You'll be doing much of your range cooking in skillets, sauté pans, and omelet pans. All three types are fairly shallow—rarely more than two or three inches deep. Sauté pans and some skillets have straight sides, which work well for pan-searing because they keep fat from spattering, and they contain liquids with fewer spills if you're making something such as Chicken Marsala. But if the sides are too high, it can be difficult to turn or stir the food. Other skillets and omelet pans have sloping sides, which makes it very easy to flip or fold omelets and other foods.

All three types of pans typically range from 6 inches or so to more than 12 inches in diameter. A medium skillet is 10 or so inches; large ones are 12 inches. (Still larger pans are too big for most home ranges.) Ideally, you want to have skillets in a variety of sizes, weights, and finishes. Nonstick surfaces are a wise choice for cooking eggs and making crêpes. Dark metals such as anodized aluminum and cast iron are ideal for pan-searing meats; be sure the handle is heatproof if you'll be finishing a dish in the oven. Stainless steel and other shiny or paler metals are fine for sautéing vegetables.

Saucepans have one long handle (large or heavy ones may have a loop on the opposite side to help with lifting). They're fairly deep and almost always come with lids. A medium saucepan contains 3 quarts, a good size for cooking vegetables, grains, or small batches of soup. Large saucepans start at 5 or so quarts, which is large enough to hold a 4- to 5-pound pot roast or chicken. These should be heavy enough that sauces don't stick when simmered over low to medium-low heat. Dutch ovens are quite similar to saucepans, but they usually have two loop handles opposite each other. They may be oval or round in shape, and are often made of porcelain-coated cast iron.

For more on cookware, including bakeware such as baking sheets, jelly roll pans, muffin tins, and loaf pans, refer to the Glossary. Information on cooking techniques appears within relevant chapters, as well as in the Glossary.

And now for the recipes!

Chapter 3

BREAKFAST AND BRUNCH DISHES

The cliché that breakfast is the most important meal of the day is particularly true on the Atkins Diet. If you start the day with a low-carb breakfast, you'll continue to burn primarily fat, including your own body fat, for energy. But eat the typical sweet and starchy American fare and you'll be setting yourself up for cravings for more high-carb foods by midmorning. The ideal breakfast provides protein—aim for at least 16 grams of protein at breakfast and other meals—and beneficial fats, along with some complex carbohydrates, a combo that keeps your energy level up for hours. Sweetened cereal, doughnuts, and bagels washed down with OJ just don't cut it.

But does breakfast on Atkins mean having eggs morning after morning? No way, as you'll find in this chapter—notwithstanding several delectable recipes for frittatas, omelets, and even steak with eggs. The possibilities range from turkey hash to protein shakes—and yes, even French toast, pancakes, muffins, muesli, and granola. The recipes in this chapter complement the impressive array of other breakfast recipes in the www.atkins.com database. So, for example, you'll find a delicious Western Omelet in this book, but there are numerous other omelets online.

THE BASICS OF LOW-CARB BAKING

Traditionally prepared quick breads, pancakes, waffles, muffins, biscuits, and scones are high in white flour and/or sugar. Compounding their high carb content are the ridiculously oversized portions found in most bakeries. A typical muffin or cupcake tin yields muffins that are about 2 inches high by 2½ inches in diameter.

A bakery muffin is usually at least twice as large. Instead of white flour, most of the baked goods in this chapter, including Lemon–Poppy Seed Bread, Ginger-Spice Muffins, Cheddar-Dill Scones, and Peanut-Strawberry Breakfast Bars, combine Atkins Cuisine All Purpose Baking Mix and a small amount of whole-wheat flour, meaning they are coded for Phases 3 and 4.

The baking mix includes soy flour, wheat protein, and other low-carb ingredients. Our recipe developers and tasters have discovered that this combination produces the best taste and texture, albeit with a small trade-off in additional carbs. However, in several cases, we've provided the option of omitting the whole-wheat flour, making the recipe acceptable for Phase 2.

None of our baked goods recipes take more than 30 minutes of active time, so you can be busy with something else while they bake, filling your kitchen with their delicious aroma. Nor do they require kneading or special equipment. Most are better if mixed by hand rather than an electric mixer, and most are versatile enough to be baked in a variety of pans. If your kitchen lacks a loaf pan, for example, just spoon the batter into a muffin tin, square baking pan, or even a skillet. Adjust the cooking times—check muffins after 15 minutes, or breads baked in a baking pan or skillet after about 30 minutes.

If you're cooking for yourself or a small household, don't worry about the high yields for the muffin, scone, and quick bread recipes. They freeze well: simply wrap extra muffins in a layer of foil and then stash in a freezer bag. Or slice leftover bread and layer it between sheets of waxed paper before wrapping in foil and packing in a freezer bag. Thaw frozen breads at room temperature, or pop them in a toaster or toaster oven. You'll find those extra portions a lifesaver on busy weekday mornings.

EATING AND COOKING EGGS

Eating eggs was once mistakenly thought to promote high cholesterol, but extensive research reveals no link between egg consumption and heart disease. Eggs are almost carb-free, and they're true nutritional powerhouses. They provide all nine of the essential amino acids that are the building blocks of protein, as well as generous amounts of vitamins A, B, and D, and such minerals as calcium, magnesium, zinc, phosphorus, and iron. In fact, the only nutrient eggs don't contain is vitamin C. Nutritionally enhanced eggs contain amounts of omega-3 fatty acids comparable to those in such cold-water fish as salmon.

That said, techniques such as omelet folding or flipping fried eggs require practice. Even if your first attempts aren't lovely to look at, they'll still taste fine. Selecting the proper pan is important. Nonstick pans are ideal, but don't assume that "nonstick" must mean coated with Teflon or another material. Pans used for cooking eggs should also distribute heat evenly. With inexpensive nonstick skillets, the pan bottom usually stays hottest where the stove burner touches it rather than distributing the heat. Well-seasoned cast iron is both nonstick and heavy enough to distribute heat evenly; it makes an ideal egg-cooking pan. Keep the heat under eggs fairly low—medium is about the highest it should be—with the exception of omelets. Higher temperatures make for tough yolks and rubbery whites.

You'll note that unsalted butter is called for in our baked goods. Salt is used as a preservative, so unsalted butter is apt to be fresher and have a "cleaner" flavor, but you can use salted butter if that all you have in the fridge.

Now let's get down to those yummy recipes that will start your day right.

French Toast

Phases 2, 3, 4

PER SERVING:
Net Carbs: 5 grams
Total Carbs: 9 grams
Fiber: 4 grams
Protein: 17 grams
Fat: 21 grams
Calories: 290

Makes: 4 servings
Active Time: 10 minutes
Total Time: 10 minutes

We've used Atkins Cuisine Bread (recipe at www.atkins.com), upon which our nutritionals are based, or use Lemon–Poppy Seed Bread (page 21).

¼ cup heavy cream
2 large eggs
1 tablespoon granular sugar substitute
1 teaspoon pure vanilla extract
Pinch salt
8 slices Atkins Cuisine Bread (see note above)
2 tablespoons butter

1. Whisk cream, eggs, sugar substitute, vanilla, and salt in a shallow bowl. Dip bread into mixture; let soak for 10 seconds per side.
2. Melt butter a large skillet over medium heat. Add bread; cook until golden brown, about 3 minutes per side. Serve with a low-carb topping.

Variation: Baked French Toast

Phases 2, 3, 4

Heat oven to 425°F; mist a small baking sheet with olive oil cooking spray. Prepare as above, but cut each slice of bread in half to make 16 pieces. Dip bread in egg mixture; transfer to baking sheet. Bake until light golden brown, about 10 minutes; turn broiler to high. Broil until deep golden brown, about 2 minutes per side.

TIP TIME

SPEED CLEANUP

To keep cooking spray off the counter or sink, simply hold the baking pan in front of the open dishwasher (assuming dishes aren't clean) and mist away.

WEEKDAY

Spicy Pecan Pancakes*

Phases 2, 3, 4

Keep cooked pancakes warm in a 200°F oven while continuing to cook more batches, and serve them as soon as possible.

PER SERVING:
Net Carbs: 5 grams
Total Carbs: 8 grams
Fiber: 3 grams
Protein: 13 grams
Fat: 19 grams
Calories: 250

Makes: 5 (2-pancake) servings
Active Time: 30 minutes
Total Time: 35 minutes

- Olive oil cooking spray
- ¾ cup Atkins Cuisine All Purpose Baking Mix
- 1 tablespoon granular sugar substitute
- ½ teaspoon baking powder
- ¼ teaspoon salt
- 2 large eggs
- ¾ cup plain unsweetened soy milk
- 2 tablespoons melted unsalted butter
- 1 teaspoon pure vanilla extract
- ½ teaspoon ground cinnamon
- ¼ teaspoon ground nutmeg
- ¼ cup chopped toasted pecans

1. Combine baking mix, sugar substitute, baking powder, and salt in a large bowl. In another large bowl, whisk together eggs, soy milk, butter, and vanilla. Pour egg mixture into dry mixture; stir until combined, and then add cinnamon, nutmeg, and pecans. Stir again and let stand 5 minutes.
2. Mist a 12-inch nonstick skillet with cooking spray and heat over medium-high heat. Scooping from the bottom, pour 1 heaping tablespoon of batter into pan; use the back of the spoon to spread into a 4-inch circle. Repeat 3 times; cook until small bubbles form at edges of pancakes and bottoms are golden brown, about 3 minutes. Flip; cook until browned on reverse side, about 2 minutes. Repeat with remaining batter.
3. Serve with sugar-free pancake syrup or another low-carb topping.

TIP TIME

MEASURE METICULOUSLY

Too much baking powder can impart a metallic taste and cause baked goods to rise too quickly, making them fall later. Too little baking powder and the pancakes will be dense and gummy.

*See photo on color page 1

Ginger-Spice Muffins

Phases 3, 4

PER SERVING:
Net Carbs: 7 grams
Total Carbs: 10 grams
Fiber: 3 grams
Protein: 9 grams
Fat: 4 grams
Calories: 100

Makes: 12 (1-muffin) servings
Active Time: 10 minutes
Total Time: 25 minutes

Club soda helps muffins rise. Use 4 teaspoons pumpkin pie spice mix if you don't have all the spices called for. To make the muffins suitable for Phase 2, use 2 cups of baking mix and omit the whole-wheat flour; each muffin will contain 5 grams of Net Carbs.

- Olive oil cooking spray
- 1½ cups Atkins Cuisine All Purpose Baking Mix
- ½ cup whole-wheat flour
- ½ cup granular sugar substitute
- 1 tablespoon baking powder
- 2 teaspoons ground ginger
- 1½ teaspoons ground cinnamon
- ½ teaspoon ground nutmeg
- Pinch ground cloves
- ¼ teaspoon salt
- 2 large eggs
- 1 tablespoon canola oil
- 2 teaspoons pure vanilla extract
- 1 cup club soda

1. Heat oven to 350°F. Mist a 12-cup muffin tin with cooking spray.
2. Combine baking mix, flour, sugar substitute, baking powder, ginger, cinnamon, nutmeg, cloves, and salt in a large bowl. Combine eggs, oil, and vanilla in a medium bowl. Add egg mixture to baking mix mixture; stir until just combined. Stir in club soda. Spoon batter into muffin tin.
3. Bake until a toothpick inserted into the center of a muffin comes out clean, about 15 minutes. Serve warm, or cool on a wire rack. If desired, top muffins with sugar-free pancake syrup mixed with softened butter or the Cherry-Walnut Butter for Hot Wheat Cereal (page 28).

TIP TIME

WHISK TO BLEND

For best results, mix dry ingredients thoroughly with a whisk to be sure the baking powder and salt are thoroughly blended into the flour before adding the wet ingredients. Once you mix in the wet ingredients, don't waste any time getting the batter into the oven.

Lemon-Poppy Seed Bread

Phases 3, 4

Because of their high oil content, poppy seeds should be stored in the fridge to prevent them from going rancid. To make this recipe suitable for Phase 2, use 2 cups of baking mix and omit the whole-wheat flour. Each serving will contain 3 grams of Net Carbs.

PER SERVING:
Net Carbs: 5 grams
Total Carbs: 7 grams
Fiber: 2 grams
Protein: 7 grams
Fat: 10 grams
Calories: 140

Makes: 18 servings
Active Time: 25 minutes
Total Time: 1 hour 15 minutes

WEEKEND

- Olive oil cooking spray
- ½ cup plain unsweetened soy milk
- ¼ cup poppy seeds
- 1½ cups Atkins Cuisine All Purpose Baking Mix
- ½ cup whole-wheat flour
- ½ cup granular sugar substitute
- 1½ teaspoons baking powder
- 1 teaspoon baking soda
- ½ teaspoon ground cinnamon
- ½ teaspoon ground nutmeg
- ¼ teaspoon salt
- ½ cup (1 stick) unsalted butter, melted and cooled
- 2 large eggs
- ¾ cup sour cream
- 3 tablespoons freshly grated lemon zest
- 1 teaspoon pure lemon extract
- 1 teaspoon pure vanilla extract

1. Heat oven to 375°F. Mist a 5-by-9-inch loaf pan with cooking spray.
2. Combine soy milk and poppy seeds in a small bowl and soak for 15 minutes.
3. Meanwhile, combine baking mix, flour, sugar substitute, baking powder, baking soda, cinnamon, nutmeg, and salt in a large bowl. Combine butter, eggs, sour cream, lemon zest, lemon and vanilla extracts, and poppy seed mixture in another large bowl. Add to baking mix mixture; stir to combine. Pour batter into pan.
4. Bake until a toothpick inserted in the center comes out clean, 45 to 50 minutes. Cool in pan for 5 minutes; remove from pan, and cool on a wire rack before cutting into 18 slices.

Cheddar-Dill Scones

Phases 3, 4

PER SERVING:
Net Carbs: 7 grams
Total Carbs: 9 grams
Fiber: 2 grams
Protein: 9 grams
Fat: 15 grams
Calories: 200

Makes: 12 (1-scone) servings
Active Time: 10 minutes
Total Time: 20 minutes

WEEKDAY

To make this recipe suitable for Phase 2, increase the amount of baking mix to 1½ cups and omit the whole-wheat flour for a Net Carb count of 2 grams per scone. This recipe is extremely adaptable: instead of Cheddar, try Parmesan (use about half as much) with basil, mozzarella with oregano, or goat cheese with thyme. To make a sweet scone, increase the sugar substitute to 3 tablespoons and omit the cheese and dill.

- ¾ cup Atkins Cuisine All Purpose Baking Mix
- ¾ cup whole-wheat flour
- 1 tablespoon granular sugar substitute
- 1 tablespoon baking powder
- ½ teaspoon salt
- 5 tablespoons cold unsalted butter, cut into ½-inch pieces
- 2 large eggs, lightly beaten
- ¾ cup heavy cream
- 3 ounces sharp Cheddar cheese, shredded (¾ cup)
- 2 tablespoons chopped fresh dill or 1 teaspoon dried dill

1. Heat oven to 400°F. Pulse baking mix, flour, sugar substitute, baking powder, and salt in a food processor to combine. Add butter; pulse until mixture resembles coarse meal. Add eggs and heavy cream; pulse until just combined. Add cheese and dill; pulse until just combined.
2. Drop ¼-cup mounds onto an ungreased baking sheet or jelly roll pan. Bake until lightly golden, about 10 minutes. Serve warm or at room temperature.

TIP TIME

CRUMBLY, NOT DENSE

Don't overmix batters. Quick breads and scones get their structure from gluten, a protein in wheat flour. However, allow too much gluten to develop and the baked goods will be dense instead of light and crumbly.

Whole-Wheat Currant Scones

Phases 3, 4

Whole-wheat flour is higher in fiber and other micronutrients, fuller in flavor, and lower in carbs than white flour, but it can make for dense baked goods. Combining whole-wheat flour with low-carb baking mix keeps baked goods from resembling hockey pucks.

PER SERVING:
Net Carbs: 11 grams
Total Carbs: 14 grams
Fiber: 3 grams
Protein: 8 grams
Fat: 12 grams
Calories: 190

Makes: 12 (1-scone) servings
Active Time: 20 minutes
Total Time: 30 minutes

¼ cup currants
1 cup whole-wheat flour
1 cup Atkins Cuisine All Purpose Baking Mix
2 tablespoons granular sugar substitute
4 teaspoons baking powder
2 teaspoons ground ginger
⅛ teaspoon ground nutmeg
⅛ teaspoon salt
5 tablespoons cold unsalted butter, cut into small pieces
2 large eggs, lightly beaten
¾ cup heavy cream

1. Heat oven to 400°F. Soak currants in a cup of warm water.
2. Pulse flour, baking mix, sugar substitute, baking powder, ginger, nutmeg, and salt in a food processor to combine. Add butter; pulse until mixture resembles coarse meal. Add eggs and heavy cream; pulse until just combined. Drain currants and add; pulse until just combined.
3. Drop ¼-cup mounds on an ungreased baking sheet; press gently to flatten slightly. Bake until lightly golden, about 10 minutes. Serve warm or at room temperature.

TIP TIME

RAISINS TO THE RESCUE

If you have no currants on hand, raisins can step up to the job. Just sprinkle them with baking mix and chop roughly before substituting for an equal amount of currants. No need to soak them.

Peanut-Strawberry Breakfast Bars

Phases 3, 4

PER SERVING:
Net Carbs: 14 grams
Total Carbs: 17 grams
Fiber: 3 grams
Protein: 10 grams
Fat: 18 grams
Calories: 270

Makes: 12 (1-bar) servings
Active Time: 15 minutes
Total Time: 40 minutes

WEEKEND

Layered with peanut butter and fruit preserves, these protein-packed bars make a delicious on-the-go breakfast with a hard-boiled egg. Be sure to use old-fashioned oats, not the quick-cooking kind. Polaner and Smucker's sugar-free jellies and preserves are available in most supermarkets. We used Steel's low-carb preserves, available online and at selected specialty stores; the others add another gram of Net Carbs per serving.

- Olive oil cooking spray
- 1¼ cups old-fashioned rolled oats
- 1¼ cups granular sugar substitute
- ½ cup Atkins Cuisine All Purpose Baking Mix
- ¼ cup whole-wheat flour
- ¼ teaspoon salt
- ½ cup (1 stick) unsalted butter, melted
- 3 large eggs, lightly beaten
- ¾ cup unsweetened natural peanut butter
- ½ cup no-sugar-added strawberry jam

1. Heat oven to 350°F. Mist a 7-by-11-inch baking dish with cooking spray.
2. Combine oats, sugar substitute, baking mix, flour, and salt in a medium bowl; stir in butter and eggs until well combined. Press half the dough into the baking dish. Spread peanut butter evenly over dough; spread preserves evenly over peanut butter. Crumble remaining dough over preserves.
3. Bake until top and edges are golden brown, about 25 minutes. Cool completely before cutting into 12 pieces.

TIP TIME

CHILL FOR FRESHNESS

Because whole-wheat flour includes the valuable germ of the grain, which is a source of unsaturated fats, it can become rancid at room temperature. The best way to store whole-wheat flour is in a resealable plastic bag in the fridge or freezer.

Crunchy Tropical Berry and Almond Breakfast Parfait*

Phases 2, 3, 4

This sweet and tangy parfait layered with coconut, almonds, and fresh berries would also make a great dessert. If you can't find fresh raspberries, feel free to use thawed unsweetened frozen ones. To boost your protein intake, have this with a low-carb bar or a hard-boiled egg. Find unsweetened coconut in the baking section of a well-stocked supermarket or in a natural foods store.

PER SERVING:
Net Carbs: 9 grams
Total Carbs: 14 grams
Fiber: 5 grams
Protein: 6 grams
Fat: 21 grams
Calories: 260

Makes: 4 servings
Active Time: 10 minutes
Total Time: 20 minutes

WEEKDAY

- ½ cup heavy cream
- 1½ teaspoons granular sugar substitute, divided
- ¼ teaspoon coconut or pure vanilla extract
- ½ cup plain unsweetened whole-milk Greek yogurt
- 1 cup raspberries
- 1 cup blueberries or sliced strawberries
- 8 tablespoons Sweet and Salty Almonds (page 54)
- ½ cup unsweetened shredded coconut, toasted (see tip)

1. Combine cream, ½ teaspoon sugar substitute, and coconut extract in a medium bowl; whip with an electric mixer on medium speed until stiff peaks form. Fold in the yogurt.
2. Purée raspberries and remaining sugar substitute in a blender until smooth.
3. Using 4 parfait glasses, alternate layers of whipped cream, raspberry purée, blueberries, nuts, and coconut, making two layers of each. Serve right away.

TIP TIME

TOASTY TREAT

To toast coconut in the oven, spread it in a thin layer on a baking sheet and bake at 300°F for about 20 minutes, stirring every 5 minutes to ensure even browning.

*See photo on color page 3

Atkins Basic Muesli

Phases 3, 4

PER SERVING:
Net Carbs: 10 grams
Total Carbs: 14 grams
Fiber: 4 grams
Protein: 11 grams
Fat: 17 grams
Calories: 240

Muesli, which hails from Switzerland, is infinitely adaptable. Swap out the almonds for roughly chopped pecans or macadamias, or add dried berries without added sugar. Enjoy muesli with plain unsweetened soy milk or plain unsweetened whole-milk yogurt. Kamut is an ancient grain that's higher in protein and lower in carbs than wheat. Puffed kamut is sold in natural foods stores and well-stocked supermarkets under several brand names, including Arrowhead Mills.

Makes: 8 (½-cup) servings
Active Time: 10 minutes
Total Time: 10 minutes

1 cup old-fashioned rolled oats
1 cup puffed kamut cereal
1 cup slivered almonds, toasted
½ cup pepitas (green pumpkin seeds), toasted
½ cup unsalted sunflower seeds, toasted

Combine oats, kamut, almonds, pepitas, and sunflower seeds in a large bowl. Transfer to an airtight container and store in a cool, dry place for up to 2 weeks.

Cinnamon Granola

Phases 3, 4

Fiber-rich granola is a welcome breakfast treat with plain unsweetened soy milk or plain unsweetened whole-milk yogurt, or atop cottage cheese. You can also enjoy it on its own for a midday snack, or for dessert as a topping for low-carb ice cream or fruit salad. If the Brazil nuts are particularly large, chop them coarsely. Use a half-cup measure to scoop granola into small bags for easy portion control.

PER SERVING:
Net Carbs: 17 grams
Total Carbs: 22 grams
Fiber: 5 grams
Protein: 9 grams
Fat: 20 grams
Calories: 290

Makes: 8 (½-cup) servings
Active Time: 10 minutes
Total Time: 55 minutes

- 3 cups puffed kamut cereal (see page 26)
- 1 cup old-fashioned rolled oats
- 1 cup unsalted Brazil, macadamia, or other nuts
- ¾ cup salted hulled sunflower seeds
- ¾ cup sugar-free pancake syrup
- 1 tablespoon canola oil
- 1 teaspoon pure vanilla extract
- 1 teaspoon ground cinnamon
- ¼ teaspoon salt

1. Heat oven to 300°F. Line a baking sheet with parchment paper.
2. Combine kamut, oats, nuts, and sunflower seeds in a large bowl. Combine syrup, oil, vanilla, cinnamon, and salt in another bowl; pour over cereal mixture and toss well to coat.
3. Spread mixture onto baking sheet or jelly roll pan. Bake, stirring twice, until dry and lightly browned, about 30 minutes. Remove from oven; cool completely before serving or storing, about 15 minutes. Store granola in an airtight container in the refrigerator for up to 3 weeks.

Variation: Coconut-Orange Granola

Phases 3, 4

Prepare Cinnamon Granola as above, adding ¼ cup unsweetened shredded coconut and 2 tablespoons fresh orange zest before tossing with syrup.

Hot Wheat Cereal with Cherry-Walnut Butter

Phases 3, 4

PER SERVING:
Net Carbs: 16 grams
Total Carbs: 23 grams
Fiber: 7 grams
Protein: 4 grams
Fat: 11 grams
Calories: 200

Makes: 6 (½-cup) servings
Active Time: 15 minutes
Total Time: 45 minutes

WEEKEND

This hearty cereal offers a healthy boost of protein, fiber, and vitamins. Both the butter mix and the cereal can be made ahead. Reheat, adding a teaspoon or two of water if necessary.

Butter

¼ cup unsalted butter, at room temperature
¼ cup pitted chopped fresh or frozen unsweetened cherries
¼ cup chopped walnuts, toasted
¼ teaspoon sugar-free pancake syrup
¼ teaspoon salt

Cereal

3 cups water
1 cup medium bulgur
¾ teaspoon salt
¼ teaspoon ground cinnamon

1. For the butter, combine butter, cherries, walnuts, syrup, and salt in a small bowl until well blended. Transfer to a sheet of parchment or waxed paper; roll into a 4-inch log. Twist ends to close; freeze until firm, about 15 minutes (butter will keep, wrapped in plastic, in the refrigerator for up to 1 week and in the freezer for up to 2 months).
2. For the cereal, combine water, bulgur, salt, and cinnamon in a medium saucepan. Bring to a boil over high heat. Reduce heat to low, cover, and simmer until bulgur is soft and water is absorbed, about 15 minutes (cereal will keep in an airtight container in the refrigerator for up to 1 week). Divide cereal among serving bowls; top each with a ⅔-inch slice of the butter log.

Variation: Hot Wheat Cereal with Cherry-Almond Butter

Phases 3, 4

Prepare as above, substituting chopped toasted almonds for the walnuts and almond extract for the syrup. Add ½ teaspoon granular sugar substitute.

Western Omelet

Phases 1, 2, 3, 4

Omelets cook best in a small skillet with sloping sides. Keep individual portions warm in a 200°F oven while you prepare the others.

PER SERVING:
Net Carbs: 5 grams
Total Carbs: 6 grams
Fiber: 1 gram
Protein: 25 grams
Fat: 29 grams
Calories: 380

Makes: 4 servings
Active Time: 30 minutes
Total Time: 30 minutes

Filling
1 tablespoon virgin olive oil
¾ cup chopped red bell pepper
½ cup chopped yellow or white onion
¾ cup diced boiled deli ham (not honey-roasted)

Eggs
8 large eggs
¼ cup water
¼ teaspoon salt
⅛ teaspoon freshly ground black pepper
4 teaspoons butter
1 cup shredded Cheddar cheese (4 ounces)

1. Heat olive oil in a large skillet over medium-high heat. Add bell pepper and onion; cook until soft, about 5 minutes. Stir in ham and cook until all ingredients turn light golden, about 3 minutes. Remove from burner.
2. Whisk eggs, water, salt, and pepper in a medium bowl.
3. Melt 1 teaspoon butter in an 8-inch nonstick skillet over medium-high heat. Add scant ½ cup of the egg mixture and cook 1 minute, until slightly set. Lift edges of omelet with a heatproof spatula; tilt pan to let uncooked egg flow underneath. Cook just until eggs are set, about 2 minutes. Sprinkle ¼ cup cheese and ¼ of the filling over half of the omelet.
4. Fold the omelet to enclose the cheese and filling; transfer to serving plate. Repeat with remaining egg mixture, butter, cheese, and filling.

TIP TIME

SHRED ONCE

Packaged shredded cheese usually has a less favorable taste and texture than less costly block cheese. Shred it in a food processor, divide into half-cup portions, and freeze in resealable plastic bags.

Steak and Scrambled Eggs

Phases 1, 2, 3, 4

PER SERVING:
Net Carbs: 3 grams
Total Carbs: 3 grams
Fiber: 0 grams
Protein: 29 grams
Fat: 28 grams
Calories: 380

Makes: 6 servings
Active Time: 25 minutes
Total Time: 4 hours, 25 minutes

For a pretty brunch buffet, roll up the eggs in low-carb tortillas and serve with salsa and the sliced steak on the side.

1 small yellow or white onion, finely chopped
3 tablespoons red wine vinegar
3 tablespoons virgin olive oil
1 tablespoon chopped fresh thyme or 1½ teaspoons dried thyme
1½ teaspoons salt, divided
¾ teaspoon freshly ground black pepper, divided
1 pound flank steak
12 large eggs
¼ cup half-and-half
2 tablespoons chopped chives or scallions
2 tablespoons butter

1. Combine onion, vinegar, oil, thyme, 1 teaspoon salt, and ½ teaspoon pepper in a large resealable plastic bag or baking dish. Add steak. If using a bag, seal and turn to coat. If using baking dish, turn steak several times to coat; cover with plastic wrap. Marinate in refrigerator at least 4 hours, or preferably overnight.
2. Heat a large skillet over medium-high heat. Meanwhile, remove the steak and pat dry. Discard marinade. Add steak to skillet and sear to desired doneness, about 6 minutes per side for medium-rare. Transfer steak to a cutting board. Cover loosely to keep warm; let stand 10 minutes before slicing.
3. Meanwhile, whisk eggs, cream, chives, and remaining ½ teaspoon salt and ¼ teaspoon pepper in a large bowl.
4. Melt butter in a large nonstick skillet over medium heat. Add eggs and cook, stirring with a heatproof rubber spatula, until eggs are set but still moist, about 6 minutes. Remove from heat; cover to keep warm.
5. Thinly slice steak across the grain; serve with eggs on the side.

Sausage and Bell Pepper Frittata

Phases 1, 2, 3, 4

Frittatas are like open-face omelets. Fillings are mixed into the eggs rather than folded into partially cooked eggs like an omelet. Frittatas are started on the stovetop and finished in the oven, or sometimes under the broiler.

PER SERVING:
Net Carbs: 5 grams
Total Carbs: 7 grams
Fiber: 2 grams
Protein: 17 grams
Fat: 16 grams
Calories: 230

Makes: 6 servings
Active Time: 20 minutes
Total Time: 30 minutes

- 2 teaspoons virgin olive oil
- 4 ounces bulk hot or sweet Italian sausage
- 1 small yellow or white onion, chopped
- 1 medium red bell pepper, stemmed, seeds and ribs removed, and cut into ¼-inch strips
- 1 (5-ounce) bag baby spinach
- 8 large eggs
- ¼ cup water
- ¼ teaspoon salt
- ¼ teaspoon freshly ground black pepper
- 1 cup shredded Cheddar cheese (4 ounces)
- 1 teaspoon chopped fresh thyme or ½ teaspoon dried thyme

1. Heat oil in a 10-inch nonstick ovenproof skillet over medium-high heat. Add sausage and sauté until lightly browned, about 3 minutes. Add onion and bell pepper; sauté until vegetables are soft, about 5 minutes. Add spinach and sauté until wilted, about 2 minutes.
2. Heat broiler to high.
3. Meanwhile, whisk eggs, water, salt, and black pepper in a medium bowl. Add egg mixture, cheese, and thyme to skillet; cook until eggs are set on bottom but top remains slightly runny, about 5 minutes.
4. Transfer skillet to oven and broil until eggs are set and golden, about 2 minutes. Cut into wedges and serve.

Frittata Lorraine

Phases 1, 2, 3, 4

PER SERVING:
Net Carbs: 2 grams
Total Carbs: 2 grams
Fiber: 0 grams
Protein: 21 grams
Fat: 20 grams
Calories: 280

Makes: 6 servings
Active Time: 20 minutes
Total Time: 30 minutes

Lorraine refers to the classic mix of bacon and Gruyère cheese used in the Alsace-Lorraine region of France. Slab bacon is easy to cut into neat pieces; bacon strips may be too slippery to slice tidily. Simplify matters by cutting them with scissors and letting them fall directly into the skillet.

4 ounces bacon (3 or 4 strips), cut into small pieces
1 small yellow or white onion, chopped
8 large eggs
¼ cup water
¼ teaspoon salt
¼ teaspoon freshly ground black pepper
1 cup grated Gruyère (4 ounces)

1. Heat a 10-inch nonstick ovenproof skillet over medium-high heat. Add bacon and sauté until it begins to crisp, 3 to 5 minutes. Add onion and sauté until soft, about 5 minutes.
2. Whisk eggs, water, salt, and pepper in a medium bowl. Add egg mixture and cheese to skillet; cook until eggs are set on bottom but top remains slightly runny, about 5 minutes.
3. Heat broiler to high. Transfer skillet to oven and broil until eggs are set and golden, about 2 minutes. Cut into wedges and serve.

TIP TIME

TIME TO WRAP IT UP

An ovenproof skillet needs a handle that won't melt or warp when placed under the broiler or in the oven. Protect a handle made of wood or plastic by wrapping it heavy-duty foil or two layers of regular weight foil before finishing the frittata.

WEEKDAY

Turkey-Cauliflower Hash*

Phases 1, 2, 3, 4

Hash is usually made with corned beef, but this version is equally tasty and filling. Ask your deli to slice turkey breast (not turkey loaf) ¼-inch thick, and then cube it at home. Or use leftover roast turkey. Creamy, buttery cauliflower makes a perfect stand-in for potatoes. Top the hash with a poached egg, if desired.

PER SERVING:
Net Carbs: 4 grams
Total Carbs: 6 grams
Fiber: 2 grams
Protein: 29 grams
Fat: 12 grams
Calories: 250

Makes: 4 (1-cup) servings
Active Time: 25 minutes
Total Time: 30 minutes

½ small head cauliflower, trimmed and broken into florets (3 cups)
2 tablespoons butter
1 small yellow or white onion, chopped
1 teaspoon dried thyme
½ teaspoon salt
⅛ teaspoon freshly ground black pepper
1 pound roast turkey breast, cut into ¼-inch cubes
¼ cup heavy cream

1. Bring a medium pot of salted water to boil. Add cauliflower; cook until just tender, about 4 minutes. Drain, cool under cold water, drain again, and coarsely chop.
2. Meanwhile, melt butter in a large nonstick skillet over medium heat. Add onion, thyme, salt, and pepper; cook until soft and light brown, about 6 minutes. Add cauliflower and cook 2 minutes longer.
3. Increase heat to high. Add turkey and cook, stirring occasionally, until well browned, about 6 minutes. Add cream and cook until almost dry, about 2 minutes. Serve warm.

WEEKDAY

*See photo on color page 2

Ricotta with Melon and Pistachios

Phases 2, 3, 4

PER SERVING:
Net Carbs: 11 grams
Total Carbs: 12 grams
Fiber: 1 gram
Protein: 14 grams
Fat: 17 grams
Calories: 260

Makes: 4 servings
Active Time: 5 minutes
Total Time: 5 minutes

You might not think of ricotta as a breakfast cheese, but in fact its mild flavor is perfect topped with ripe melons and crunchy pistachios. Cantaloupe is an excellent source of vitamin C, beta-carotene, and potassium, while honeydew supplies plenty of vitamin C and zeaxanthin. To boost your protein intake, have this parfait with a muffin or scone.

1 (15-ounce) container whole-milk ricotta cheese (2 cups)
1 cup cantaloupe cubes or balls
1 cup honeydew cubes or balls
¼ cup shelled pistachio nuts, chopped
Sugar-free pancake syrup (optional)

Divide ricotta among 4 bowls. Top each with equal amounts of melon and nuts; drizzle with syrup if desired.

TIP TIME

HAVE A BALL

Dig out that melon baller from the back of your utensil drawer and use it to pretty up a fresh fruit dish. First cut a melon in half lengthwise. Using an ice cream scoop or a large spoon, scrape out the seeds and membranes. Holding the half melon with one hand, press the melon baller into the fruit, rotate it to form a ball, and remove.

Strawberry-Vanilla Protein Shake

Phases 2, 3, 4

This combination of almond butter and protein powder provides enough protein to replace a meal, making it a great on-the-go breakfast. Use peanut butter if you wish, but almond butter complements the strawberries better. You'll find many brands of unsweetened soy-based protein shake mix at natural foods stores and most well-stocked supermarkets.

PER SERVING:
Net Carbs: 11 grams
Total Carbs: 13 grams
Fiber: 2 grams
Protein: 25 grams
Fat: 22 grams
Calories: 350

Makes: 1 (1¾-cup) serving
Active Time: 10 minutes
Total Time: 10 minutes

¾ cup ice
¼ cup plain unsweetened soy milk (not low fat)
2 tablespoons heavy cream
½ cup sliced strawberries
1 tablespoon almond butter
1 scoop (24 grams) unsweetened soy-based protein shake mix
1 teaspoon pure vanilla extract
1 teaspoon granular sugar substitute

1. Purée ice, soy milk, cream, strawberries, almond butter, shake mix, vanilla, and sugar substitute in a blender.
2. Pour into a glass and serve.

TIP TIME

SUGAR SLEUTHING

A carton of soy milk may not list sugar or high-fructose corn syrup on the ingredient list, but if the carb count on the Nutrition Facts panel is more than 5 grams per serving, some form of sugar has been added, likely malted corn or malted barley (or barley malt), rice syrup, or cane juice. Even products marked "plain" or "original flavor" may be sweetened, so look for "unsweetened" or "no added sugar" on the package.

Mocha Smoothie

Phases 2, 3, 4

PER SERVING:
Net Carbs: 10 grams
Total Carbs: 11 grams
Fiber: 1 gram
Protein: 23 grams
Fat: 20 grams
Calories: 320

Makes: 2 (2-cup) servings
Active Time: 5 minutes
Total Time: 5 minutes

Protein from yogurt and tofu helps you start the day right. If you haven't frozen brewed coffee in an ice cube tray ahead of time, brew a pot that's double strength, pour ½ cup into a measure, and add ice to come to 1 cup. The texture won't be quite the same, but the flavor will be fine. Be sure to use unsweetened cocoa powder, not cocoa mix, which is full of sugar.

1 cup brewed coffee, frozen in an ice cube tray
2 (6-ounce) containers plain unsweetened whole-milk Greek or regular yogurt
1 (10-ounce) package firm silken tofu
2 tablespoons unsweetened cocoa powder
Granular sugar substitute

Purée coffee cubes, yogurt, tofu, and cocoa powder in a blender. Taste, add sugar substitute to taste, and blend again. Pour into glasses and serve immediately.

Chapter 4

SNACKS, APPETIZERS, AND HORS D'OEUVRES

Although snacks and their close kin, hors d'oeuvres and appetizers, can be the downfall of even a careful eater, snacking can actually help you lose (or maintain) your weight. Follow the old-school mantra of "no eating between meals" and you may find yourself going too long without eating, which can cause your blood sugar to plummet and make you overwhelmingly hungry. And *that* can leave you reaching for high-carb foods to stave off the pangs. That's why Atkins incorporates a midmorning and late afternoon snack into your eating program. On the other hand, not just any snack will do the trick. Not surprisingly, the ideal snack is low in carbs but has enough protein and fat to make you feel pleasantly full. The same goes for appetizers and hors d'oeuvres.

SMART SNACKS

This chapter is filled with great choices, whether you're looking for something as simple as Roasted Spiced Pecans, Roasted Garlic Hummus, or Spicy Black Bean Dip or for elegant appetizers such as Summer Rolls, Cheese-Stuffed Cherry Tomatoes, or Mild Mushroom-Lentil Pâté. Keep in mind as well that if you reduce the portion size, many of the main dish recipes in this book can also be eaten as a snack or served as an appetizer. Peel-and-Eat Shrimp (page 199) comes immediately to mind, as do Portobello Burgers with Blue Cheese Sauce (page 65)—minus the burger bun—and Sautéed Cocktail Meatballs (page 164). Also check out www.atkins.com for more delicious snacks and starters.

THE APPETIZING DEPARTMENT

First let's address the burning issue of whether appetizers and hors d'oeuvres are just different names in different languages for the same thing. They're not. An appetizer is served as a first course of a meal. The French term hors d'oeuvres roughly translates to "outside the meal," meaning the food is served separate from or prior to a meal. Typically, it's finger food that can be eaten standing up, perhaps with wine or cocktails. That said, feel free to use the recipes in this chapter in any way you wish.

Appetizers and hors d'oeuvres usually have great eye appeal. Their flavors are also zesty—horseradish, garlic, Worcestershire sauce, and ginger, for example, are used with a freer hand than they might be in an entrée. The result: a small amount of food is enough to satisfy. "Wait," you say; "if appetizers stimulate the palate, won't I end up eating more?" The opposite is more likely to be true. It can take 20 minutes or so after you begin eating to realize that you're sated. Eating a snack, a few hors d'oeuvres, an appetizer, or even a cup of soup will take the edge off your hunger. Have your serving and stop there. If you listen to your body, you're more likely to feel full after the meal that follows, rather than eyeing the leftovers.

Hors d'oeuvres can be as simple as a dish of roasted nuts or marinated olives or a platter of assorted cheeses, or as extravagant as an artfully arranged lavish buffet. If your guests will be standing, bite-size, drip-free morsels will be easier to manage, so save anything that requires cutlery for a seated course. Take care that party fare looks as good as it tastes. A variety of colors and shapes helps stimulate the palate. Prepare a selection, balancing flavor (garlicky, salty, tangy, and smoky) and texture (smooth pâtés, crisp crackers, creamy spreads, and succulent meats or seafood).

DO THE DIP

Crudités with dip are a terrific low-carb snack or appetizer, but you can only dunk so many broccoli florets into ranch dressing before you think, "Enough already!" To tickle your jaded taste buds, our colorful array of dips ranges from Speedy Spinach Dip to Olive Tapenade, Sun-Dried Tomato Dip, and Avocado Hummus. When it comes to dippers, conventional chips are out, but our recipes for Chili-Cheese Crisps and Italian Cheese Crisps can take up the slack. Also try low-carb tortillas and pitas along with crudités. The latter are usually raw, but some vegetables taste better when blanched (briefly cooked in boiling water). Follow these guidelines to achieve the best flavor and texture:

- *Asparagus:* Trim and blanch for 30 seconds.
- *Belgian endive:* Rinse and pat dry; separate leaves.
- *Bell peppers:* Set the pepper upright on a cutting board; holding the stem in one hand and a knife in the other, run the knife down the sides of the pepper, about an inch or so from the stem, and cut the pepper into 3 or 4 panels. Discard the core and seeds; cut the panels into strips or cracker-size pieces.
- *Broccoli:* Snap into florets and blanch for 1 minute.
- *Cauliflower:* Snap into florets and serve raw.
- *Celery:* Peel away the tough, stringy fibers, but don't remove the attractive leaves.
- *Cherry tomatoes:* Leave the stems attached to make dipping easier.
- *Cucumbers:* Halve lengthwise, and then cut each half into 3 spears. Or cut into ⅛-inch rounds.
- *Daikon:* Peel and cut into spears or ⅛-inch rounds.
- *Fennel:* Trim and cut into slices.
- *Green beans:* Trim ends and blanch for 15–30 seconds, and then plunge into ice water.
- *Jicama:* Peel and cut into ¼-inch rounds, and then into pie-wedge shapes.
- *Mushroom caps:* Choose bite-size cremini or button mushrooms; trim stems but leave attached. Wipe mushrooms clean.
- *Radishes:* Leave whole or slice large ones thinly and top with a spread.
- *Scallions:* Leave a few inches of green attached for an attractive presentation.
- *Snow peas/sugar snap peas:* Blanch snow peas for 15 seconds, sugar snap peas for 30 seconds; drain and rinse in ice water.

Now let's explore the world of guilt-free snacks and starters.

Sun-Dried Tomato Dip*

Phases 1, 2, 3, 4

Tangy sun-dried tomatoes play the starring role in this cheese-based dip. Serve it with celery, daikon, or cucumber spears or Chili-Cheese Crisps (page 46). Bring the dip to room temperature before serving.

PER SERVING:
Net Carbs: 0 grams
Total Carbs: 0 grams
Fiber: 0 grams
Protein: 4 grams
Fat: 7 grams
Calories: 80

Makes: 14 (2-tablespoon) servings
Active Time: 10 minutes
Total Time: 10 minutes

- 11 ounces fresh goat cheese, at room temperature
- 1 tablespoon heavy cream
- 3 tablespoons thinly sliced fresh basil
- 2 tablespoons minced oil-packed sun-dried tomatoes
- 2 tablespoons extra-virgin olive oil, divided
- ⅛ teaspoon freshly ground black pepper

1. Combine cheese and cream in a bowl; whip with a handheld mixer at medium speed until light and fluffy, about 3 minutes. Stir in basil, tomatoes, 1 tablespoon oil, and pepper.
2. Transfer to serving dish and drizzle top with remaining 1 tablespoon oil. Serve, or refrigerate in an airtight container for up to 1 week.

TIP TIME

THE TASTE OF SUMMER

Sun-dried tomatoes packed in oil are a convenient pantry item. Also try dry-pack tomatoes, which are less expensive and have a truer flavor.

Variation: Sun-Dried Tomato Dip with Walnuts

Phases 2, 3, 4

Prepare Sun-Dried Tomato Dip as above, adding ½ cup chopped toasted walnuts.

*See photo on color page 4

Speedy Spinach Dip*

Phases 1, 2, 3, 4

PER SERVING:
Net Carbs: 2 grams
Total Carbs: 3 grams
Fiber: 1 gram
Protein: 2 grams
Fat: 10 grams
Calories: 110

Makes: 12 (¼-cup) servings
Active Time: 20 minutes
Total Time: 20 minutes

Zingy and fresh-tasting, this dip is super-easy—it's made with frozen chopped spinach. Serve with crudités or Chili-Cheese Crisps (page 46).

- 1 (10-ounce) package frozen chopped spinach, thawed and well drained
- 1½ cups sour cream
- 1 cup regular (not low-fat) mayonnaise
- ½ small cucumber, peeled, seeded, and minced
- 2 celery ribs, trimmed and minced
- 3 scallions, thinly sliced
- 1 clove garlic, minced
- 1 teaspoon freshly squeezed lemon juice
- 1 teaspoon dried basil
- ½ teaspoon salt
- ⅛ teaspoon cayenne pepper

1. Combine spinach, sour cream, mayonnaise, cucumber, celery, scallions, garlic, lemon juice, basil, salt, and cayenne in a medium bowl, stirring well.
2. Transfer to a serving dish and serve, or refrigerate in an airtight container for up to 3 days.

TIP TIME

DEFROSTING FROZEN SPINACH

Thaw a box of frozen spinach overnight in the fridge in a pie plate. Then, snip off a corner of the box and holding it over a colander in the sink, press and twist it to squeeze out as much water as possible.

Variation: Curried Spinach Dip

Phases 1, 2, 3, 4

Prepare Spinach Dip as above, adding in 1½ teaspoons curry powder and 1 teaspoon ground cumin.

*See photo on color page 4

Olive Tapenade

Phases 1, 2, 3, 4

Tapenade comes from the Provençal word for caper, *tapeno*, though most of us think of it as an olive spread. Serve tapenade with crudités or Easy Low-Carb Chips (see tip). It also makes a great sandwich spread.

PER SERVING:
Net Carbs: 1 gram
Total Carbs: 1 gram
Fiber: 0 grams
Protein: 0 grams
Fat: 5 grams
Calories: 50

Makes: 16 (2-tablespoon) servings
Active Time: 15 minutes
Total Time: 15 minutes

1 cup Kalamata or other black olives, pitted
1 cup green olives, such as Provençal, Picholine, or Bella de Cerignola, pitted
1 clove garlic, minced
2 teaspoons freshly squeezed lemon juice
Pinch red pepper flakes
¼ cup extra-virgin olive oil

1. Pulse black olives, green olives, garlic, lemon juice, red pepper flakes, and oil in a food processor until finely chopped.
2. Transfer to a bowl and serve, or refrigerate in an airtight container for up to 1 week.

TIP TIME

EASY LOW-CARB CHIPS

Brush low-carb tortillas or pitas with oil. Then cut into 6 wedges, set on a baking sheet in a single layer, and bake in a preheated 300°F oven for 5 minutes. They're suitable for Phase 3 and Phase 4.

Variation: Classic Tapenade

Phases 1, 2, 3, 4

Prepare Olive Tapenade as above, adding 2 chopped anchovy fillets (from a jar or tin) and 1½ teaspoons rinsed and drained capers.

Baba Ghanoush

Phases 2, 3, 4

PER SERVING:
Net Carbs: 6 grams
Total Carbs: 6 grams
Fiber: 0 grams
Protein: 2 grams
Fat: 10 grams
Calories: 110

Makes: 12 (¼-cup) servings
Active Time: 10 minutes
Total Time: 1 hour 35 minutes

WEEKEND

You can use this lemony, nutty Middle Eastern eggplant spread on everything from low-carb pita sandwiches to crudités. Garnish it with pomegranate seeds, chopped fresh mint, a swirl of olive oil, or crushed pistachio nuts, if you wish. Tahini, made from ground sesame seeds, can be found in the ethnic foods section of the supermarket.

2 medium eggplants, cut in half
¼ cup plus 2 tablespoons extra-virgin olive oil, divided
¼ cup tahini
3 tablespoons freshly squeezed lemon juice
1 clove garlic, minced
½ teaspoon salt

1. Heat oven to 375°F. Line a baking sheet with parchment paper. Brush cut sides of eggplants with 2 tablespoons of the oil. Place eggplants, cut side down, on baking sheet and bake until very soft, about 45 minutes. Set aside until cool enough to handle, about 15 minutes.
2. Scoop eggplant flesh from skin; discard skin. Place flesh into a colander to drain for 30 minutes, pressing eggplant occasionally until all excess moisture is eliminated.
3. Transfer eggplant to a food processor. Add remaining ¼ cup oil, tahini, lemon juice, garlic, and salt; purée. Transfer to a bowl and serve, or refrigerate in an airtight container for up to 4 days.

TIP TIME

SELECT A PERFECT EGGPLANT

Whether you purchase baby eggplant, Japanese (long, thin, usually dark purple), Chinese (long, thin, usually white), American (the familiar rounded purple ones), or Italian (smaller version of American) eggplant, choose small yet heavy eggplants with no dents or blemishes.

Roasted Garlic Hummus*

Phases 2, 3, 4

Although hummus is widely available at supermarkets, it's quick and easy to make at home—at a fraction of the price. Chickpeas are a great source of fiber, protein, calcium, and iron. Roasting garlic makes it mellow, so this recipe has less bite than most hummus. Serve with crudités or low-carb pita.

PER SERVING:
Net Carbs: 7 grams
Total Carbs: 9 grams
Fiber: 2 grams
Protein: 3 grams
Fat: 7 grams
Calories: 110

Makes: 16 (scant ¼-cup) servings
Active Time: 10 minutes
Total Time: 70 minutes

- 1 large head garlic
- ¼ cup plus 2 teaspoons extra-virgin olive oil, divided
- 2 (15½-ounce) cans chickpeas, drained and rinsed
- 6 tablespoons freshly squeezed lemon juice
- ¼ cup extra-virgin olive oil
- ¼ cup tahini
- 2 teaspoons ground cumin
- 1 teaspoon salt
- ⅛ teaspoon freshly ground black pepper
- ½ cup water

1. Heat oven to 400°F. Cut the top ¼ inch off garlic head to expose the cloves. Set garlic cut side up on a piece of foil and drizzle with 2 teaspoons oil. Close tightly to form a packet. Bake until garlic is very soft, about 45 minutes. Remove from oven and let cool at room temperature.
2. Separate garlic into cloves. Squeeze roasted garlic out of skins.
3. Purée garlic, chickpeas, lemon juice, olive oil, tahini, cumin, salt, and pepper in food processor until smooth. With the motor running, pour water slowly through feed tube until hummus reaches desired consistency. Transfer to a bowl and serve right away or refrigerate in an airtight container for up to 2 days.

Variation: Avocado Hummus

Phases 2, 3, 4

Prepare as above, using 2 large cloves of raw garlic instead of the roasted garlic and adding 1 mashed Hass avocado.

*See photo on color page 4

WEEKEND

Spicy Black Bean Dip

Phases 2, 3, 4

PER SERVING:
Net Carbs: 7 grams
Total Carbs: 10 grams
Fiber: 3 grams
Protein: 2 grams
Fat: 3 grams
Calories: 50

Makes: 8 (¼-cup) servings
Active Time: 10 minutes
Total Time: 10 minutes

Black beans are a great source of protein and fiber. If you can find them, use canned black soybeans, which are significantly lower in carbs. Serve creamy black bean dip with crudités or Easy Low-Carb Chips (page 41).

1 tablespoon extra-virgin olive oil
½ medium red onion, chopped
1 jalapeño, seeded and chopped
1 clove garlic, chopped
1 teaspoon chili powder
½ teaspoon ground cumin
½ teaspoon salt
1 (15½-ounce) can black beans, drained (reserve 3 tablespoons liquid)

1. Heat oil in a small skillet over medium heat. Add onion, jalapeño, garlic, chili powder, cumin, and salt; sauté until onions are soft, about 3 minutes. Add beans; cook to heat through, about 3 minutes.
2. Transfer mixture to a food processor; purée with reserved bean liquid until smooth. Serve, or refrigerate in an airtight container for up to 3 days.

TIP TIME

FREEZE THOSE HOTTIES

Seeding and chopping jalapeños is no fun, but the flavor and heat are worth it. If you use chiles often, prepare a bunch at one time and freeze each one in a small resealable freezer bag. They defrost almost immediately, and freezing has no impact on taste.

Variation: Creamy Black Bean Dip

Phases 2, 3, 4

Prepare Spicy Black Bean Dip as above, stirring in ¼ cup sour cream after puréeing.

WEEKDAY

Garlicky White Bean Dip

Phases 2, 3, 4

At Italian restaurants, a version of this pungent dip is often brought to the table along with the breadbasket. Instead, serve it with Zucchini Crisps (see tip) or crudités.

PER SERVING:

Net Carbs: 6 grams

Total Carbs: 8 grams

Fiber: 2 grams

Protein: 2 grams

Fat: 2 grams

Calories: 60

Makes: 8 (¼-cup) servings

Active Time: 10 minutes

Total Time: 10 minutes

1 tablespoon extra-virgin olive oil
2 cloves garlic, sliced
Leaves from 1 sprig rosemary, chopped
1 (15½-ounce) can cannellini beans, drained, 3 tablespoons liquid reserved
½ teaspoon salt
⅛ teaspoon freshly ground black pepper

1. Heat oil in a small skillet over medium heat. Add garlic and rosemary; sauté until aromatic, about 1 minute. Add beans, salt, and pepper; cook to heat through, about 3 minutes.
2. Transfer mixture to a food processor; purée with reserved beans. Serve, or refrigerate in an airtight container for up to 3 days.

TIP TIME

ZUCCHINI CRISPS

Cut zucchini into ¼-inch slices (on a diagonal if they're small). Brush both sides with virgin olive oil and season with salt, pepper, and whatever strikes your fancy—garlic powder, grated Parmesan, Italian seasoning, rosemary, or dill. Set on a baking sheet in a single layer and bake in a preheated 400°F oven for 10 minutes, turning once. Cool on a wire rack. These are suitable for Phase 1 and beyond.

WEEKDAY

Chili-Cheese Crisps*

Phases 2, 3, 4

PER SERVING:
Net Carbs: 2 grams
Total Carbs: 3 grams
Fiber: 1 gram
Protein: 6 grams
Fat: 13 grams
Calories: 150

Makes 9 (5-cracker) servings
Active Time: 10 minutes
Total Time: 35 minutes

Almond meal provides a nutty quality to these crisps—and keeps the carb count down. Parchment paper makes it easy to transfer the unbaked crisps to the baking pan and also helps keep them from burning.

- 1 cup almond meal (see page 11)
- 4 ounces Cheddar cheese, shredded (1 cup)
- ¼ teaspoon baking soda
- ¼ teaspoon salt
- 1½ tablespoons canola oil
- 1 large egg, slightly beaten
- 1 teaspoon chili powder

1. Heat oven to 350°F.
2. Combine almond meal, cheese, baking soda, salt, oil, egg, and chili powder. Using your hands, form into a ball.
3. Place dough between two sheets of parchment paper. Flatten and roll into a rectangle about ⅛ inch thick. Remove the top piece of paper and score the dough with a knife into 45 (1½-inch) squares. Lift the dough, still on the parchment paper, onto a baking sheet.
4. Bake for 15 minutes. Remove from the oven and let rest for 5 minutes. Separate the crackers by cutting if necessary. Put back in the oven for 5 minutes just until crispy (do not overbake).
5. Cool crackers on the parchment paper. Store in an airtight container.

Variation: Italian Cheese Crisps

Phases 2, 3, 4

Prepare Chili-Cheese Crisps as above, but replace the Cheddar with 1 cup shredded Parmesan cheese (not the packaged grated version, which contains bitter anti-caking agents) and replace the chili powder with ½ teaspoon dried oregano, ½ teaspoon dried basil, and ¼ teaspoon red pepper flakes.

*See photo on color page 5

Cheese-Stuffed Cherry Tomatoes

Phases 1, 2, 3, 4

You can also stuff partially hollowed-out cucumber rounds or use the cheese filling as a spread for roll-ups. If you don't have a pastry tube, simply use a plastic bag with a cut-off corner to pipe the filling into the tomatoes.

PER SERVING:
Net Carbs: 2 grams
Total Carbs: 2 grams
Fiber: 0 grams
Protein: 3 grams
Fat: 7 grams
Calories: 80

Makes: 12 servings
Active Time: 25 minutes
Total Time: 25 minutes

24 cherry tomatoes
12 ounces cream cheese, softened
1½ ounces Italian cheese blend or mozzarella, shredded (6 tablespoons)
6 tablespoons grated Parmesan
8 tablespoons chopped fresh basil, divided
1½ tablespoons sour cream
1 clove garlic, minced
⅛ teaspoon freshly ground black pepper

1. Remove stems from tops of tomatoes. Turn over and scoop out tomatoes from the bottom with a melon baller; discard pulp. (See tip.) Invert tomatoes onto paper towels to drain.
2. Mix cream cheese, cheese blend, Parmesan, 6 tablespoons basil, sour cream, garlic, and pepper in a medium bowl until smooth. Transfer to a piping bag fitted with a round or star tip. Pipe mixture into tomatoes (see note above) and garnish with remaining 2 tablespoons basil.
3. Cover and refrigerate until ready to serve, but no more than 4 hours.

TIP TIME

NO-TIP TOMATOES

Most recipes for stuffed tomatoes instruct you to cut a thin slice off the bottom to keep them from rolling around. Instead, stuff tomatoes upside down, so the dimples on the top hold them steady.

WEEKDAY

Smoky Cheese Log*

Phases 1, 2, 3, 4

PER SERVING:
Net Carbs: 0 grams
Total Carbs: 0 grams
Fiber: 0 grams
Protein: 3 grams
Fat: 5 grams
Calories: 60

Makes: 32 servings
Active Time: 15 minutes
Total Time: 3 hours 15 minutes

Feel free to vary the ingredients in this recipe to suit your preferences—add your favorite herbs or condiments, or use any cheeses you happen to have on hand in place of our suggestions. Serve with Easy Low-Carb Chips (page 41) or low-carb flatbreads.

- 8 ounces extra-sharp Cheddar cheese, cut into ¾-inch cubes
- 6 ounces smoked Gouda, cut into ¾-inch cubes
- ¼ cup regular (not low-fat) mayonnaise
- 1 tablespoon grainy brown mustard
- 7 tablespoons minced fresh parsley, divided
- 1 tablespoon chopped scallion
- 1 teaspoon Worcestershire sauce
- 5 drops hot pepper sauce, or to taste

1. Combine Cheddar, Gouda, mayonnaise, mustard, 2 tablespoons parsley, scallion, Worcestershire sauce, and hot pepper sauce in a food processor; purée. Scrape onto a sheet of plastic wrap and shape into a 2-inch thick log. Refrigerate until firm, at least 3 hours.
2. Sprinkle remaining parsley in a circle on a sheet of plastic wrap. Unwrap cheese; set in center of parsley and roll until evenly coated. Transfer to a plate and serve.

Variation: Nut-Rolled Salmon-Cheese Ball

Phases 2, 3, 4

Prepare Smoky Cheese Log as above, omitting the Gouda and replacing with a 6-ounce can of salmon (drained). Also omit the mustard, replacing with 2 teaspoons prepared horseradish and 1 tablespoon lemon juice. Roll into a ball instead of a log and coat with ¼ cup chopped walnuts.

*See photo on color page 5

WEEKEND

Lime-Chili Grilled Wings

Phases 1, 2, 3, 4

Wings typically come in three segments. The parts closest to the body look something like miniature drumsticks and are sometimes sold as "drumettes." The middle part has two thin bones, and the tips are often discarded as they contain so little meat. Removing the wing tips has another benefit in this dish: it helps to ensure even cooking—the tips tend to burn on the grill.

PER SERVING:
Net Carbs: 1 gram
Total Carbs: 2 grams
Fiber: 1 gram
Protein: 20 grams
Fat: 7 grams
Calories: 150

Makes: 4 servings
Active Time: 30 minutes
Total Time: 2 hours 30 minutes

WEEKEND

- ¼ cup freshly squeezed lime juice
- 1 tablespoon virgin olive oil
- 2 teaspoons chili powder
- 2 teaspoons ground cumin
- 2 teaspoons salt
- 3 tablespoons chopped fresh cilantro
- 12 chicken wings, tips removed

1. Combine lime juice, oil, chili powder, cumin, salt, and cilantro in a large bowl. Add wings and toss to coat. Cover and refrigerate 2 hours, turning occasionally.
2. Prepare a charcoal or gas grill for medium-heat grilling or heat a grill pan. Grill wings until browned and cooked through, about 20 minutes. Serve hot.

Summer Rolls*

Phases 3, 4

PER SERVING:
Net Carbs: 4 grams
Total Carbs: 6 grams
Fiber: 2 grams
Protein: 15 grams
Fat: 7 grams
Calories: 150

Makes: 4 servings
Active Time: 25 minutes
Total Time: 50 minutes

These summer rolls replace the traditional rice paper wrapping with lettuce leaves. In Phase 2, replace the carrot with a second daikon.

- 1 teaspoon fresh lime juice
- 1 teaspoon dark (toasted) sesame oil
- 1 small red chile pepper, seeded and minced
- ½ teaspoon salt
- ½ pound medium shrimp, peeled and deveined
- 8 large green or red leaf lettuce leaves
- 1 medium carrot, julienned (see tip)
- 1 small daikon radish, julienned
- ½ cup mung bean sprouts
- ¼ cup peanuts, toasted and chopped

1. Combine lime juice, sesame oil, chile, and salt in a medium bowl; set aside.
2. Bring a medium pot of salted water to a boil. Add shrimp; simmer until pink, about 3 minutes. Drain; add to lime juice mixture and toss to coat. Refrigerate until cool, about 10 minutes.
3. Set lettuce leaves on a counter with stem ends toward you. Press against the "spines" until you hear a crunch to make it easier to roll.
4. Divide carrot, daikon, and sprouts among leaves, setting them in the centers toward the bottom. Divide shrimp among leaves; sprinkle with chopped peanuts. Roll lettuce from the bottom up.
5. Place each roll, seam side down, on a sheet of plastic wrap; wrap tightly and refrigerate for 15 minutes. Remove wrap; cut rolls in half and serve.

TIP TIME

SLICE TWICE

The French term "julienne" refers to thin, matchstick-like strips. You can simply cut the vegetable into ¼-inch-thick slices. Then lay each slice on its side and cut into ¼-inch thick strips.

*See photo on color page 6

Shrimp Satay with Nuoc Cham

Phases 2, 3, 4

Nuoc mam, or Vietnamese fish sauce, is integral to Vietnamese cooking. (You can also use Chinese fish sauce, known as nam pla.) In Phase 1, have 2 skewers and 2 tablespoons of sauce per serving.

PER SERVING:
Net Carbs: 4 grams
Total Carbs: 4 grams
Fiber: 0 grams
Protein: 26 grams
Fat: 2 grams
Calories: 140

Makes: 4 (3 skewers, 3 tablespoons sauce) servings
Active Time: 20 minutes
Total Time: 50 minutes

WEEKEND

Shrimp

2 tablespoons tamari (see page 11)
2 tablespoons fish sauce (nuoc mam or nam pla)
2 tablespoons water
2 teaspoons peeled and minced fresh ginger
2 teaspoons unseasoned, unsweetened rice vinegar
1 clove garlic, minced
1 teaspoon granular sugar substitute
1 pound shelled and deveined medium shrimp

Sauce

¼ cup fish sauce (nuoc mam or nam pla)
¼ cup unseasoned, unsweetened rice vinegar
2 tablespoons fresh lime juice
1 tablespoon granular sugar substitute
1 red chile, seeded and minced
2 cloves garlic, chopped

12 (10-inch) bamboo skewers

1. For the shrimp, soak skewers in water for 30 minutes. Meanwhile, combine tamari, fish sauce, water, ginger, vinegar, garlic, and sugar substitute in a large bowl. Add shrimp and toss to coat. Cover and refrigerate for 30 minutes. Discard marinade after removing shrimp.
2. Meanwhile, for the sauce, combine fish sauce, vinegar, lime juice, sugar substitute, chile, and garlic in a small bowl.
3. Heat gas or charcoal grill to high or grill-pan over very high heat. Thread shrimp on skewers, piercing them twice, once near the tail and once near the wider end so they won't spin when you turn them. Grill shrimp until pink, about 2 minutes per side. Serve hot with sauce.

Mild Mushroom-Lentil Pâté

Phases 3, 4

PER SERVING:
Net Carbs: 11 grams
Total Carbs: 18 grams
Fiber: 7 grams
Protein: 9 grams
Fat: 7 grams
Calories: 150

Makes: 8 (1¼-cup) servings
Active Time: 30 minutes
Total Time: 30 minutes

WEEKDAY

A mellow blend of mushrooms, lentils, and almonds, mildly seasoned with fresh basil and lemon, this vegetarian dish makes a great hors d'oeuvre or first course.

5 cups water
1 cup brown lentils
¼ cup extra-virgin olive oil
8 ounces mixed mushrooms, trimmed, wiped clean, and sliced
1 shallot, chopped
2 cloves garlic, chopped
½ cup fresh basil, chopped
2 tablespoons freshly squeezed lemon juice
1½ teaspoons salt
⅛ teaspoon cayenne
¾ cup slivered or sliced almonds, toasted

1. Bring water to a boil in a medium saucepan over high heat. Add lentils, reduce heat to low, cover, and simmer until tender, about 20 minutes. Strain, reserving any liquid.
2. Heat oil in a large skillet over high heat. Add mushrooms and shallot; sauté until golden, about 4 minutes. Add garlic and sauté until fragrant, about 30 seconds.
3. Transfer mushroom mixture to a blender and add lentils, basil, lemon juice, salt, and cayenne. Blend until a smooth paste forms, adding reserved cooking liquid as needed.
4. Transfer to a bowl, garnish with almonds, and serve, or refrigerate in an airtight container for up to 3 days and garnish with almonds just before serving.

Roasted Spiced Pecans

Phases 2, 3, 4

Although pecans are delicious with this mélange of spices and seasonings, feel free to substitute cashews, macadamia nuts, or almonds, singly or in combination.

PER SERVING:
Net Carbs: 2 grams
Total Carbs: 5 grams
Fiber: 3 grams
Protein: 3 grams
Fat: 22 grams
Calories: 220

Makes: 12 servings
Active Time: 10 minutes
Total Time: 25 minutes

2 tablespoons butter, melted
2 tablespoons Worcestershire sauce
1 teaspoon chili powder
¾ teaspoon garlic powder
¾ teaspoon onion powder
¾ teaspoon salt
½ teaspoon cayenne
1 (12-ounces) bag pecan halves (3 cups)

1. Heat oven 375°F. Line a baking sheet with foil.
2. Combine butter, Worcestershire sauce, chili powder, garlic powder, onion powder, salt, and cayenne in a medium bowl; add pecans and toss to coat thoroughly.
3. Spread evenly onto baking sheet in a single layer. Bake until lightly toasted, about 8 minutes, stirring once. Cool completely before serving. Store in an airtight container at room temperature for up to 3 days.

TIP TIME

NUTTY ADVICE

Because they're high in fat, nuts can go rancid quickly at room temperature and when exposed to light. Store them in a cool dry place or the fridge, where they'll stay fresh for up to six months, or in the freezer for up to a year. Toss out nuts that smell musty.

Variation: Tamari-Roasted Pecans

Phases 2, 3, 4

Prepare Roasted Spiced Pecans as above, substituting tamari for the Worcestershire, omitting the salt, and adding ¾ teaspoon ground ginger.

WEEKDAY

Sweet and Salty Almonds

Phases 2, 3, 4

PER SERVING:
Net Carbs: 1 gram
Total Carbs: 3 grams
Fiber: 2 grams
Protein: 3 grams
Fat: 7 grams
Calories: 80

Makes: 16 (2 tablespoon) servings
Active Time: 5 minutes
Total Time: 20 minutes

WEEKDAY

Keep some of these nuts in your desk drawer for a crunchy snack. Or add a couple of tablespoons to cottage cheese or yogurt and fruit for a quick breakfast or snack. Substitute nutmeg or other spices for the cinnamon if you prefer. Egg white acts as a binder for the sweetener and spice and also heightens the crispness of the nuts.

1 large egg white
⅓ cup granular sugar substitute
¾ teaspoon salt
2 teaspoons cinnamon
2 cups slivered blanched almonds

1. Heat oven to 350°F.
2. Combine the egg white, sugar substitute, salt, and cinnamon in a medium bowl. Beat with a fork until frothy. Add almonds and toss to coat. Spread out in a single layer on a nonstick baking sheet or a baking sheet lined with aluminum foil.
3. Bake for 12–15 minutes, turning once, until toasted and crisp. Remove from oven and place baking sheet on a baking rack. When the nuts are cool, remove from pan and store in an airtight container at room temperature up to one week.

TIP TIME

SAVE PRECIOUS MINUTES

You can certainly blanch and sliver almonds yourself, but why spend the time and risk a nasty cut when they're available in the baking section and the nut section of any supermarket? Slivered blanched almonds also make a great garnish for asparagus, broccoli, and other veggies.

Chapter 5

SANDWICHES, WRAPS, FILLINGS, AND PIZZA

Fast to make and convenient when you're at work or on the move, low-carb sandwiches—along with wraps, panini, and (yes!) even pizza—offer numerous ways to enjoy a hearty lunch or light dinner. In this chapter you'll also find plenty of fillings for sandwiches or to wrap in lettuce leaves or serve atop fresh greens. As always, these recipes are just the tip of the iceberg: you'll find many more at www.atkins.com, including a raft of burgers, pizza, calzones, and plenty more.

THE STAFF OF LIFE

But wait, isn't bread the last thing you want to eat on the Atkins Diet? Well, yes and no. It's true that a slice of conventional bread can run anywhere from 15–25 grams of Net Carbs or even more, plus it's also usually made with refined white flour and often sugar—the very ingredients you want to avoid. In Phases 3 and 4, 100 percent whole-grain bread is a fine option. But where does that leave you in the earlier phases of the program?

In Phase 1, we recommend you forgo any form of bread, but food scientists have made significant developments in modifying ingredients such as wheat flour to isolate and modify its carbohydrate component (thereby reducing the carb component) and retain the fiber (bran) and protein (wheat gluten). Atkins Cuisine All Purpose Baking Mix employs this technology, combining wheat gluten, modified wheat starch, and wheat bran with soy flour. More on the baking mix below.

Now things get a bit complicated. Online retailers that specialize in low-carb products offer a number of loaf breads, some of which are low enough in carbs to qualify as Phase 2 foods, assuming the grains in them have been modified. Some are remarkably low in carbs, but other products rely on some mixture of soy flour, flaxseeds, oat flour, whole-wheat flour, oat bran, and wheat bran. If they contain no unmodified wheat or other conventional flour made from grains, they may also be acceptable in Phase 2, but it's impossible to generalize. Again, you have to read the Nutrition Facts panel as well as the list of ingredients to ascertain whether or not bread contains regular wheat (including whole-wheat flour) or modified flour. The latter is acceptable in Phase 2; the former is not.

Creating a tasty low-carb bread is challenging. That's because alternatives to conventional wheat flour don't readily rise with yeast or other leavening agents. As a result, low-carb bread tends to be denser than conventional bread and each slice is thus smaller. (We've found that toasting it enhances the taste and texture.) The good news is that it's easier to produce a tasty unleavened low-carb pita, flatbread, or wrap. Ditto for low-carb tortillas. Neither seem to suffer in flavor or texture compared to high-carb products. Most supermarkets carry some low-carb flatbreads. You should be able to easily find flatbreads with 6–8 grams of Net Carbs per serving in most well-stocked supermarkets.

Again, read labels carefully, because one product may serve your needs well, but another from the same company may be too high in carbs for anyone following the Atkins Diet. For example, Flatout's Light line clocks in at 6–8 grams of Net Carbs per flatbread, making them acceptable in Phase 3 and 4 of Atkins. You should be able to easily find low-carb tortillas with 3–4 grams of Net Carbs. However, other so-called low-carb tortillas can be considerably higher.

FLOUR 101

When considering bread products, be aware of the following:

- *White flour.* Whether it says bleached or unbleached, enriched, bromated, or whatever, this is refined white flour made from wheat. It's high in carbs—and contains precious few nutrients.
- *Rye flour.* High in fiber, making it relatively low in Net Carbs compared to wheat flour, rye flour adds a chewy texture and distinctive flavor to breads. If it isn't combined with wheat flour, rye bread will be very dense and friable. Breads made from all rye flour are suitable in Phases 3 and 4 of the Atkins Diet.
- *Whole-wheat flour.* Made from hard wheat, it can be combined with soy flour, rye flour, or Atkins Cuisine All Purpose Baking Mix in most recipes. As the name implies, the flour includes both the wheat germ and the bran, where the nutrients lie. Again, bread made with 100 percent whole-wheat flour or combined with other whole-grain flours is acceptable only in the last two phases of the program.

BECOME A (LOW-CARB) BAKER

Another alternative is to make your own bread using Atkins Cuisine All Purpose Baking Mix. A slim slice of Atkins Cuisine Bread—the recipe is at www.atkins.com—logs in at less than 2 grams of Net Carbs, making it suitable for Phase 2 and beyond. (We've used this bread in calculating the nutritionals for each sandwich, unless otherwise stated. If you use store-bought low-carb bread, it may well be higher in carbs.) We've also provided a recipe for Atkins Hamburger Buns (page 60) that combines the baking mix with whole-wheat flour. At 13 grams of Net Carbs, they're suitable for Phases 3 and 4. If you're in Phase 1, you can always wrap your sandwich fillings in a lettuce leaf.

SANDWICH SAVVY

Classic sandwich combos exist for a reason—these tried-and-true flavors and textures work. Think of a sauerkraut-laden Reuben on rye or a lamb gyro stuffed into a pita and slathered with yogurt sauce. That doesn't mean you can't tinker with perfection, especially as your tastes change. If you've moved beyond American cheese, try our Grown-Up Grilled Cheese, featuring three kinds of cheese jazzed up with mustard. Then try the variations with tomatoes or ham, if you like. Instead of that old standby egg salad, kick it up a notch with our Indian-inspired Curried Egg Salad or Spicy Shrimp-Egg Salad. And rather than the usual comforting but bland chicken salad, how about Chicken-Pesto Salad? Note that our salad sandwich fillings can be served right away, although refrigerating them for half an hour or so blends the flavors more.

Also check out our dips and spreads in "Snacks, Appetizers, and Hors d'Oeuvres" (page 37). Several of these would make a great sandwich filling in a low-carb pita with a lettuce leaf and a slice of tomato.

So go ahead. Experiment, eat, and enjoy sandwiches and their kin, while remaining true to your low-carb convictions!

Grown-Up Grilled Cheese

Phases 2, 3, 4

PER SERVING:
Net Carbs: 5 grams
Total Carbs: 8 grams
Fiber: 3 grams
Protein: 32 grams
Calories: 410

Makes: 4 servings
Active Time: 10 minutes
Total Time: 10 minutes

Feel free to vary the cheeses in this recipe. Swap Emmentaler or Swiss for the Gruyère; try sharp provolone instead of Cheddar. Or, for a zestier sandwich, substitute pepper Jack for the mozzarella. Any of these would be delicious served with Tomato Bisque (page 132).

4 teaspoons Dijon mustard
8 slices Atkins Cuisine Bread or other low-carb bread (see page 56)
3 ounces whole-milk mozzarella, preferably fresh, cut into 8 slices
2 ounces sharp Cheddar cheese, cut into 4 slices
2 ounces Gruyère, cut into 4 slices
4 tablespoons (½ stick) butter, at room temperature

1. Spread 1 teaspoon mustard on each of 4 slices of bread. Top each with 2 slices mozzarella, 1 slice Cheddar, and 1 slice Gruyère. Cover with remaining bread. Spread butter on both sides of exposed bread slices.
2. Heat a large nonstick skillet over medium heat. Add sandwiches; cover and cook until bread is golden and cheese is melted, about 2 minutes per side. Cut in half on the diagonal and serve.

Variations: Grilled Cheese with Tomato

Phases 2, 3, 4

Prepare Grown-Up Grilled Cheese as above, dividing 1 large plum tomato, cut into 12 slices, among the sandwiches and placing it between the mozzarella and the Cheddar cheese.

Grilled Cheese with Ham

Phases 2, 3, 4

Prepare Grown-Up Grilled Cheese as above, dividing 4 ounces thinly sliced deli ham (not honey-roasted) among the sandwiches and placing it between the mozzarella and the Cheddar cheese.

Tuna Melt

Phases 2, 3, 4

Make the tuna salad a few hours ahead (or up to 4 days ahead if kept in an airtight container) and this tasty diner classic can be on the table in no time. To cut the carbs (especially if you're using low-carb bread with a relatively high carb count instead of Atkins Cuisine Bread), omit the second piece of bread for an open-face version.

PER SERVING:
Net Carbs: 4 grams
Total Carbs: 8 grams
Fiber: 4 grams
Protein: 38 grams
Fat: 30 grams
Calories: 450

Makes: 4 servings
Active Time: 15 minutes
Total Time: 20 minutes

- 4 (6-ounce) cans oil-packed solid white tuna, drained
- 1 large celery stalk, trimmed and finely chopped
- ⅓ cup plus 2 tablespoons regular (not low-fat) mayonnaise, divided
- ¼ cup finely chopped yellow or white onion
- 1 tablespoon Dijon mustard
- ½ teaspoon salt
- ¼ teaspoon freshly ground black pepper
- 8 slices Atkins Cuisine Bread (see page 56) or other low-carb bread, lightly toasted
- 4 slices Swiss or Cheddar cheese (2 ounces)

1. Combine tuna, celery, ⅓ cup mayonnaise, onion, mustard, salt, and pepper in a medium bowl.
2. Set oven rack to 6–8 inches from broiler element. Heat broiler.
3. Spread 2 tablespoons mayonnaise on toasted bread. Divide tuna salad on the bread; top each with a slice of cheese. Set on a baking sheet; broil until cheese is melted, about 2 minutes. Top with remaining bread. Serve hot.

TIP TIME

OPT FOR TASTE

Tuna packed in oil—preferably olive oil—tastes much richer than its watery counterpart. If you can't find it with other canned tuna, check the Italian foods section of the ethnic foods aisle.

WEEKDAY

Atkins Hamburger Buns*

Phases 3, 4

PER SERVING:
Net Carbs: 13 grams
Total Carbs: 19 grams
Fiber: 6 grams
Protein: 16 grams
Fat: 11 grams
Calories: 230

Makes: 6 servings
Active Time: 10 minutes
Total Time: 1 hour, 25 minutes

These hearty buns are denser than store-bought ones made from white flour (and full of air). Use them for beef burgers, chicken or turkey burgers, or Sloppy Joes (page 62). Have half a bun to drop the carb count.

¼ cup heavy cream
½ cup warm water
2 teaspoons active dry yeast
1 large egg
1½ tablespoons canola oil
1 tablespoon granular sugar substitute
½ teaspoon salt
¾ cup whole-wheat flour
1¼ cups Atkins Cuisine All Purpose Baking Mix

1. Heat cream and water in a small saucepan to 115°F. Add yeast and allow to proof for 5 minutes or until it foams.
2. Add yeast and milk mixture to the bowl of an electric mixer. Add egg, oil, sugar substitute, and salt. Mix thoroughly.
3. Add the whole-wheat flour and mix on slowest setting for 10 seconds. Add the baking mix and combine until the mixture comes together as a wet dough, about 10 seconds. Do not overbeat.
4. Form dough into a ball and place into a lightly oiled bowl. Cover with plastic wrap and allow to double in size, about 30–40 minutes.
5. Punch down dough and separate into 6 equal portions. Form each portion into a disk on a sheet pan, cover with plastic wrap, and allow to double in size, about 20–30 minutes.
6. Bake in a preheated 400°F oven for 13–15 minutes until golden brown. Serve immediately or keep in an airtight container for up to 3 days.

*See photo on color page 7

Open-Faced Fried Catfish Sandwiches with Spicy Mayonnaise

Phases 2, 3, 4

Although Spicy Mayonnaise is the perfect complement to the mild taste of catfish, if you're in a hurry or don't like spicy foods, simply use mayo right out of the jar.

PER SERVING:
Net Carbs: 5 grams
Total Carbs: 10 grams
Fiber: 5 grams
Protein: 34 grams
Fat: 37 grams
Calories: 510

Makes: 4 servings
Active Time: 20 minutes
Total Time: 20 minutes

WEEKDAY

Spicy Mayonnaise

¼ cup regular (not low-fat) mayonnaise
1½ teaspoons capers, drained and chopped
½ teaspoon paprika
¼ teaspoon chipotle powder (or medium-hot chili powder)
¼ teaspoon garlic powder
¼ teaspoon onion powder
⅛ teaspoon dried thyme
⅛ teaspoon ground allspice

Fish

2 teaspoons paprika
1 teaspoon dried oregano
1 teaspoon salt
¼ teaspoon freshly ground black pepper
4 (6-ounce) catfish fillets
3 tablespoons virgin olive oil
4 slices Atkins Cuisine Bread (see page 56), or other low-carb bread, toasted
4 small Boston or Bibb lettuce leaves
4 (¼-inch-thick) tomato slices

1. For the spicy mayonnaise, combine mayonnaise, capers, paprika, chipotle powder, garlic powder, onion powder, thyme, and allspice in a bowl, mixing well. Set aside.
2. Combine paprika, oregano, salt, and pepper in a small bowl; mix well. Sprinkle over the catfish.
3. Heat oil in a large nonstick skillet over medium-high heat. Add fillets and sear, turning once, until cooked through, 4 to 5 minutes per side.
4. To assemble, put one slice of toasted bread on each of 4 plates. Top each with 1 lettuce leaf, 1 slice of tomato, and 1 catfish fillet. Top with Spicy Mayonnaise and serve right away.

Sloppy Joes

Phases 3, 4

PER SERVING:
Net Carbs: 18 grams
Total Carbs: 26 grams
Fiber: 8 grams
Protein: 32 grams
Fat: 25 grams
Calories: 440

Makes: 6 servings
Active Time: 25 minutes
Total Time: 55 minutes

Bored with burgers? Robustly seasoned sloppy Joes are beloved by little and big kids alike. If you're not making 6 sandwiches, freeze the extra filling for up to a month. For Phase 2, serve over toasted Atkins Cuisine Bread for a Net Carb count of about 7 grams. (Find the recipe at www.atkins.com.)

2½ tablespoons virgin olive oil
1 small yellow or white onion, chopped
½ green bell pepper, stemmed, ribs and seeds removed, and chopped
2 celery stalks, trimmed and chopped
1 teaspoon dried oregano
1 pound ground sirloin
1 (14-ounce) can crushed tomatoes
1 cup cold water
4 teaspoons red wine vinegar
1 tablespoon granular sugar substitute
1 teaspoon tamari (see page 11)
1 teaspoon salt
6 Atkins Hamburger Buns (page 60)

1. Heat oil in a large skillet over medium-high heat. Add onion, pepper, celery, and oregano; sauté until onions are translucent and pepper and celery begin to soften, 5–7 minutes.
2. Add beef, breaking it apart with a wooden spoon, and sauté until browned, about 4 minutes. Drain off any fat.
3. Add tomatoes, water, vinegar, sugar substitute, tamari, and salt. Stir well and bring to a boil. Reduce heat to medium and simmer, stirring occasionally, until sauce is reduced and very thick, about 30 minutes.
4. Scoop ½ cup beef mixture onto each bun and serve hot.

Chicken Teriyaki Burgers

Phases 1, 2, 3, 4

Purchase ground chicken, not ground chicken breast. The latter is dry and bland compared to ground chicken. If you can't find Seal Sama Teriyaki Sauce, which is low carb, simply substitute 2 tablespoons tamari sauce mixed with 1 packet granular sugar substitute.

PER SERVING:
Net Carbs: 1 gram
Total Carbs: 1 gram
Fiber: 0 grams
Protein: 25 grams
Fat: 19 grams
Calories: 280

Makes: 4 servings
Active Time: 10 minutes
Total Time: 20 minutes

- 1 pound ground chicken
- 2 scallions, finely chopped
- 1 clove garlic, chopped
- 2 tablespoons Seal Sama low-carb teriyaki sauce (see page 8)
- 1 teaspoon peeled and grated fresh ginger
- 1 teaspoon dark (toasted) sesame oil
- ¼ teaspoon freshly ground black pepper
- 1 tablespoon canola oil

1. Combine chicken, scallions, garlic, teriyaki sauce, ginger, sesame oil, and pepper in a medium bowl; shape into four ¾-inch-thick patties.
2. Heat oil in a large skillet over medium heat. Add patties and sear until browned and no longer pink inside, about 5 minutes per side. Serve right away on Atkins Hamburger Buns (page 60) or wrapped in lettuce leaves.

Lamb Gyros

Phases 2, 3, 4

PER SERVING:
Net Carbs: 10 grams
Total Carbs: 19 grams
Fiber: 9 grams
Protein: 26 grams
Fat: 25 grams
Calories: 410

Makes: 6 servings
Active Time: 20 minutes
Total Time: 20 minutes

WEEKDAY

Whole-milk yogurt is an acceptable substitute for Greek yogurt, but pass on low-fat or non-fat types. They're higher in carbs and simply not rich enough to give the sauce body. To get this meal on the table even faster, make the sauce earlier in the day and refrigerate. You can also wrap each lamb patty in a lettuce leaf and enjoy this dish in Phase 1.

Sauce

¾ cup plain unsweetened whole-milk Greek yogurt
½ small yellow or white onion, chopped
¼ cup finely chopped peeled cucumber
1 tablespoon chopped fresh mint
½ teaspoon salt
⅛ teaspoon freshly ground black pepper

Gyros

1 pound ground lamb
½ small yellow or white onion, finely chopped
2 cloves garlic, chopped
1½ teaspoons dried oregano
1 teaspoon salt
½ teaspoon freshly ground black pepper
½ teaspoon dried thyme
1 tablespoon virgin olive oil

6 (6-inch) low-carb pita breads (see page 9), warmed

1. For the sauce, combine yogurt, onion, cucumber, mint, salt, and pepper in a small bowl. Set aside.
2. For the gyros, combine lamb, onion, garlic, oregano, salt, pepper, and thyme in a large bowl; shape into six ¾-inch-thick patties.
3. Heat oil in a large skillet over medium-high heat. Add patties and sear until browned and no longer pink inside, about 3 minutes per side.
4. Stuff each pita with a lamb patty and top with sauce.

Portobello Burgers with Blue Cheese Sauce*

Phases 3, 4

Large portobello mushrooms are easy to grill, but you can also cook them under the broiler or on a grill pan. To serve as an appetizer or side dish, omit the burger bun. Do likewise if you're in Phase 2.

PER SERVING (without bun):
Net Carbs: 5 grams
Total Carbs: 7 grams
Fiber: 2 grams
Protein: 7 grams
Fat: 31 grams
Calories: 320

PER SERVING (with bun):
Net Carbs: 17 grams
Total Carbs: 25 grams
Fiber: 8 grams
Protein: 23 grams
Fat: 42 grams
Calories: 550

Makes: 4 servings
Active Time: 25 minutes
Total Time: 45 minutes

- 2 cloves garlic, minced
- 1 tablespoon sherry or red wine vinegar
- 1 tablespoon tamari (see page 11)
- ½ teaspoon granular sugar substitute (optional)
- ½ teaspoon salt
- ¼ teaspoon freshly ground black pepper
- 3 tablespoons virgin olive oil
- 4 large portobello mushroom caps, wiped clean
- ¾ cup crumbled blue cheese (3 ounces)
- ¼ cup mayonnaise
- 2 tablespoons heavy cream
- 1 teaspoon Worcestershire sauce
- 4 Atkins Hamburger Buns (page 60)
- 1 cup loosely packed arugula or watercress
- 4 (¼-inch-thick) tomato slices
- 4 slices red onion (optional)

1. Heat a grill to medium-high.
2. Meanwhile, combine garlic, vinegar, tamari, sugar substitute (if using), salt, and pepper in a bowl. Slowly whisk in oil; brush over mushrooms and let stand 20 minutes. Remove mushrooms from bowl and discard marinade.
3. Set mushrooms on grill rack and grill until tender, 4 to 6 minutes per side.
4. Meanwhile, combine blue cheese, mayonnaise, cream, and Worcestershire sauce in a bowl; mix well, mashing chunks of cheese with the back of a spoon or fork.
5. To assemble, place half a bun on each of 4 plates; top with ¼ cup arugula, a mushroom cap, a tomato slice, and optional onion slice. Spoon 2 tablespoons of the blue cheese sauce over each and top with the other half of the bun. Serve warm or at room temperature. (If serving without the bun, place the mushroom on the arugula, and top with the tomato slice and sauce.)

*See photo on color page 7

Chicken Caesar Wraps

Phases 2, 3, 4

PER SERVING:
Net Carbs: 5 grams
Total Carbs: 13 grams
Fiber: 8 grams
Protein: 34 grams
Fat: 21 grams
Calories: 360

Makes: 4 servings
Active Time: 15 minutes
Total Time: 15 minutes

We used La Tortilla Factory Smart & Delicious Original Low Carb High Fiber Tortillas, which have 3 grams of Net Carbs each, as do Mama Lupe's Low Carb Tortillas. If you're in Phase 1, simply wrap the filling in lettuce leaves instead.

- ⅓ cup regular (not low-fat) mayonnaise
- 1 tablespoon freshly squeezed lemon juice
- 2 teaspoons Worcestershire sauce
- 2 teaspoons anchovy paste
- 3 tablespoons grated Parmesan
- ¼ teaspoon freshly ground black pepper
- 4 (6- or 7-inch) low-carb tortillas, warmed
- ½ head romaine lettuce, shredded (3 cups)
- ¾ pound deli-style chicken, thinly sliced
- 2 small plum tomatoes, diced

1. Combine mayonnaise, lemon juice, Worcestershire sauce, anchovy paste, Parmesan, and pepper in a bowl; spread each tortilla with 1 tablespoon of the dressing, leaving a 1-inch border around the edges. Add lettuce to remaining dressing and toss to coat.
2. Divide chicken among tortillas, mounding it in center; top with one-fourth of the lettuce and one-fourth of the tomatoes. Fold in sides of tortilla over filling; roll up tightly to enclose. Serve right away.

TIP TIME

IT'S A WRAP

Wrapping a tortilla or flatbread around a filling burrito-style makes the sandwich fairly leakproof. Spoon filling slightly below the center of the wrap; fold up the bottom, leaving an inch around the edges, and then fold in the sides before rolling it up.

Chicken-Pesto Salad

Phases 2, 3, 4

Chicken salad is a simple way to use leftover chicken. Use white or dark meat or a combination, but be sure to pick off any bits of fat or skin; their texture can be unpleasant in a cold salad. Scoop the salad onto a lettuce leaf or serve it on toasted low-carb bread.

PER SERVING:
Net Carbs: 2 grams
Total Carbs: 3 grams
Fiber: 1 gram
Protein: 23 grams
Fat: 21 grams
Calories: 300

Makes: 4 (½-cup) servings
Active Time: 25 minutes
Total Time: 25 minutes

- 2 cups (½ pound) chopped cooked chicken
- 1 celery stalk, trimmed and finely chopped
- ⅓ cup regular (not low-fat) mayonnaise
- ⅓ cup finely chopped onion
- 2 tablespoons chopped fresh parsley
- 2 tablespoons jarred pesto
- ¼ teaspoon salt
- ⅛ teaspoon freshly ground black pepper

Combine chicken, celery, mayonnaise, onion, parsley, pesto, salt, and pepper in a bowl. Serve right away or refrigerate in an airtight container for up to 3 days.

TIP TIME

POACH AND CHILL

Use chilled poached chicken breasts in your favorite chicken salad recipe, or atop a green salad, or to make a speedy curry. After poaching, transfer chicken to a plate and refrigerate, uncovered, until cool. If you like, strain and reserve the poaching stock for another recipe.

Deviled Ham Salad

Phases 1, 2, 3, 4

PER SERVING:
Net Carbs: 2 grams
Total Carbs: 2 grams
Fiber: 0 grams
Protein: 12 grams
Fat: 21 grams
Calories: 250 grams

Makes: 6 (½-cup) servings
Active Time: 10 minutes
Total Time: 10 minutes

Deviled refers to spicy or pungent flavors, usually from mustard or hot peppers. Use this retro recipe as a sandwich filler or a dip for fresh vegetables. Increase the amount of mustard if you like a spicier filling.

4 cups (1 pound) cubed boiled ham (not honey-roasted)
½ cup plus 2 tablespoons regular (not low-fat) mayonnaise
1 tablespoon Dijon mustard
¼ teaspoon freshly ground black pepper

Combine ham, mayonnaise, mustard, and pepper in a food processor and pulse until fairly smooth, about 2 minutes. Serve immediately or refrigerate in an airtight container for up to 3 days.

Variation: Cheddar–Deviled Ham Salad

Phases 1, 2, 3, 4

Prepare Deviled Ham Salad as above, stirring in 1 cup shredded Cheddar cheese after processing.

Curried Egg Salad

Phases 1, 2, 3, 4

You can hard-boil eggs in advance—simply refrigerate them, unpeeled, in the carton for up to 4 days. Just remember that if you do boil the eggs ahead of time, it will reduce the number of days you can store the salad.

PER SERVING:
Net Carbs: 3 grams
Total Carbs: 3 grams
Fiber: 0 grams
Protein: 17 grams
Fat: 36 grams
Calories: 410

Makes: 4 (¾-cup) servings
Active Time: 15 minutes
Total Time: 15 minutes

1 dozen large hard-boiled eggs
½ cup regular (not low-fat) mayonnaise
¼ cup finely chopped red onion
1 tablespoon chopped fresh parsley
2 tablespoons curry powder
1 teaspoon Worcestershire sauce
½ teaspoon salt
½ teaspoon freshly ground black pepper

1. Peel and halve the eggs. Separate the egg yolks from the whites. Using a fork or spatula, mash the yolks. Finely chop the whites.
2. Combine egg yolks, mayonnaise, onion, parsley, curry powder, Worcestershire sauce, salt, and pepper in a medium bowl. Gently fold in the whites.
3. Serve right away or refrigerate in an airtight container for up to 4 days.

TIP TIME

PEEL AWAY

Fresh eggs are the easiest to peel. Plunge newly boiled eggs into a bowl of ice water for 30 seconds, or run chilled eggs under hot water. The change in temperature makes them easier to peel. Roll the egg on a counter to crack the entire surface before removing the shell.

Variation: Spicy Shrimp-Egg Salad

Phases 1, 2, 3, 4

Prepare as above, omitting curry powder and adding 6 ounces chopped cooked peeled shrimp, 2 teaspoons Dijon mustard, ¼ teaspoon paprika, and hot sauce to taste.

Tofu "Egg" Salad

Phases 1, 2, 3, 4

PER SERVING:
Net Carbs: 2 grams
Total Carbs: 3 grams
Fiber: 1 gram
Protein: 10 grams
Fat: 28 grams
Calories: 290

Makes: 4 (¾-cup) servings
Active Time: 15 minutes
Total Time: 15 minutes

If you're a vegan, use tofu mayonnaise, which is made without eggs. You can find it at natural foods stores and in the organic section of many supermarkets. Turmeric gives the mixture the pleasing yellow hue of egg salad.

1 (12-ounce) package soft tofu, drained, patted dry, and chopped
½ cup regular (not low-fat) mayonnaise or tofu mayonnaise
1 medium celery stalk, trimmed and finely chopped
¼ cup finely chopped yellow or white onion
2 tablespoons chopped fresh parsley
½ teaspoon turmeric (optional)
½ teaspoon salt
¼ teaspoon freshly ground black pepper

1. Combine tofu, mayonnaise, celery, onion, parsley, turmeric if using, salt, and pepper in a medium bowl.
2. Serve right away or refrigerate in an airtight container for up to 5 days.

Variation: Spicy Tofu "Egg" Salad

Phases 1, 2, 3, 4

Prepare Tofu "Egg" Salad as above, substituting chopped scallions for the onion, chopped cilantro for the parsley, and 2 tablespoons tamari for the salt. Add Asian chili sauce to taste.

Mediterranean-Style Tuna Salad*

Phases 1, 2, 3, 4

This tuna salad has all the flavors of the Mediterranean. Make a batch for quick low-carb sandwiches or serve it rolled in lettuce leaves or over a bed of greens.

PER SERVING:
Net Carbs: 2 grams
Total Carbs: 3 grams
Fiber: 1 gram
Protein: 50 grams
Fat: 19 grams
Calories: 390

Makes: 4 (¾-cup) servings
Active Time: 15 minutes
Total Time: 15 minutes

- 4 (6-ounce) cans olive-oil-packed tuna, drained
- ¼ cup chopped red onion
- 3 tablespoons red wine vinegar
- 2 tablespoons extra-virgin olive oil
- 2 tablespoons capers, rinsed and drained
- 2 tablespoons chopped roasted red pepper
- 2 tablespoons chopped pitted Niçoise or Kalamata olives
- 2 tablespoons chopped fresh parsley
- 2 tablespoons chopped anchovies (optional)
- ⅛ teaspoon salt
- ⅛ teaspoon freshly ground black pepper

1. Combine tuna, onion, vinegar, oil, capers, red pepper, olives, parsley, anchovies if using, salt, and ground pepper in a bowl; toss gently to combine.
2. Serve right away or refrigerate in an airtight container for up to 3 days.

TIP TIME

LITTLE FISH, BIG FLAVOR

Look for anchovies in glass jars, which are easier to reseal than the tins. Anchovy fillets disintegrate when heated. Add some to garlic as you sauté vegetables, or toss a few into a dip before you purée. Their somewhat off-putting texture vanishes, and their pungent flavor is distributed throughout the dish.

*See photo on color page 8

Smoked Whitefish Salad

Phases 1, 2, 3, 4

PER SERVING:
Net Carbs: 1 gram
Total Carbs: 1 gram
Fiber: 0 grams
Protein: 18 grams
Fat: 15 grams
Calories: 220

Makes: 6 (½-cup) servings
Active Time: 15 minutes
Total Time: 15 minutes

This salad is a traditional Jewish favorite, but deli whitefish salad may have sugar in it. Try to find skinned and deboned smoked whitefish or ask the person at the fish counter or delicatessen to clean it for you—it's a real time-saver.

1 pound smoked whitefish meat
½ cup regular (not low-fat) mayonnaise
⅓ cup coarsely chopped white or yellow onion
2 tablespoons freshly squeezed lemon juice
¼ teaspoon salt
¼ teaspoon freshly ground black pepper

Combine fish, mayonnaise, onion, lemon juice, salt, and pepper in a food processor and pulse until fairly smooth, about 2 minutes. Serve right away, or refrigerate in an airtight container for up to 3 days.

WEEKDAY

Mozzarella, Kalamata, and Tomato Panini

Phases 2, 3, 4

Panini are Italian sandwiches that are often grilled in a special press that flattens them, but our method needs no special equipment.

PER SERVING:
Net Carbs: 9 grams
Total Carbs: 17 grams
Fiber: 8 grams
Protein: 24 grams
Fat: 31 grams
Calories: 430

Makes: 4 servings
Active Time: 20 minutes
Total Time: 20 minutes

WEEKDAY

- ⅔ cup coarsely chopped pitted Kalamata or other black olives
- ¼ cup extra-virgin olive oil
- 1 tablespoon capers, rinsed and drained
- 1 clove garlic, chopped
- 8 slices Atkins Cuisine Bread or other low-carb bread (see page 56).
- 1 medium tomato, cut into 4 slices
- 6 ounces whole-milk mozzarella, preferably fresh, cut into 4 slices
- 4 tablespoons chopped fresh basil
- Olive oil cooking spray

1. Combine olives, oil, capers, and garlic in a small bowl. Spread on 4 slices of the bread; top each with 1 slice tomato, 1 slice mozzarella, and 1 tablespoon basil. Top with remaining bread.
2. Heat a large nonstick skillet over medium heat until hot, then mist it generously with cooking spray. Add panini; set a large heavy skillet or pot on top to weight them down, pressing down if needed. Cook until sandwiches are golden and cheese has melted, about 3 minutes per side. Cut in half on the diagonal and serve.

Variation: Smoked Mozzarella, Kalamata, and Prosciutto Panini

Phases 2, 3, 4

Prepare Mozzarella, Kalamata, and Tomato Panini as above, substituting smoked mozzarella for fresh mozzarella and 8 ounces thinly sliced prosciutto for the tomato. Omit the basil.

Sautéed Onion, Black Olive, and Goat Cheese Pizza*

Phases 3, 4

PER SERVING:
Net Carbs: 15 grams
Total Carbs: 20 grams
Fiber: 5 grams
Protein: 17 grams
Fat: 18 grams
Calories: 300

Makes: 4 (2-slice) servings
Active Time: 15 minutes
Total Time: 1 hour

WEEKEND

Vegetables and other high-moisture ingredients can soak into pizza crust and make it soggy. Partially baking the dough and flipping it over before adding the topping creates another step but ensures a well-browned and crispy crust. To make this recipe suitable for Phase 2, substitute the non-yeasted crust used in Atkins Cuisine Pizza at www.atkins.com.

Dough

1 teaspoon active dry yeast
½ cup warm (110°F) water
1 teaspoon granular sugar substitute
½ teaspoon salt
½ cup whole-wheat flour
½ cup Atkins Cuisine All Purpose Baking Mix
2 teaspoons virgin olive oil

Topping

1 tablespoon virgin olive oil
1 medium yellow or white onion, sliced
¼ teaspoon salt
⅛ teaspoon freshly ground black pepper
4 ounces fresh goat cheese, crumbled
¼ cup sliced black olives
3 tablespoons thinly sliced basil (garnish)

1. To make the dough, add the yeast to the water, gently stir, and allow to sit for about 5 minutes until it becomes foamy. (This indicates the yeast is still active.) In the bowl of an electric mixer, combine the sugar substitute, salt, whole-wheat flour, baking mix, and olive oil. Add yeast mixture and mix until thoroughly combined to form a wet dough, about 1 minute. Shape into a ball and place into a lightly oiled bowl. Cover with plastic wrap and allow to double in size, about 30–40 minutes.
2. Meanwhile, heat olive oil in a large skillet over medium heat. When fragrant, add onion, salt, and pepper; cook until golden brown, about 8 minutes. Set aside.

*See photo on color page 9

3. Heat oven to 450°F. Set one rack at the lowest position and a second rack at the highest position near the broiler.
4. When dough has risen, punch it down and form into a disk. Place onto a greased sheet pan or pizza stone and continue to press it outward until it forms a disk about 12 inches in diameter. Bake on the bottom oven rack for 8 minutes, until the top outer edges are beginning to turn golden brown. Remove from the oven and turn over the crust.
5. Top with sautéed onions, goat cheese, and olives. Return to the oven and place on the top rack. Broil for 3–4 minutes until the cheese has melted. Garnish with basil if desired, and serve immediately.

TIP TIME

SMALL IS GOOD

To make mini pizzas as single servings, simply divide the dough into four equal pieces. Chill or freeze any you don't need, and top the remaining ones as you like. Check to see if they're done a few minutes before the recipe instructs you to.

Variation: Zucchini and Roasted Red Pepper Pizza

Phases 3, 4

Prepare dough for Sautéed Onion, Black Olive, and Goat Cheese Pizza as above, but instead of the onion topping, heat 1 tablespoon olive oil in a large skillet over high heat. Add 1 thinly sliced small zucchini, ¼ teaspoon dried oregano, ¼ teaspoon salt, and ⅛ teaspoon pepper; cook until soft and brown, about 5 minutes. Stir in ⅓ cup drained roasted red peppers (from a jar) before topping the crust with the mixture.

Chapter 6

SALADS AND DRESSINGS

Salads are a particularly important part of your meals when you're watching your carbs, making them a key component of the Atkins lifestyle. They fill you up and provide lots of fiber and other nutrients, usually with minimal carb impact. Our salad bar of choices goes far beyond iceberg lettuce topped with a tomato wedge and some bottled orange dressing. Many of the salads that follow are inspired by various and varied cuisines. Only three of them—Caprese Salad, New York Strip Steak Salad, and Mushrooms and Greens with Bacon and Eggs—are main course salads. But it's easy to turn others, such as Athenian Salad, Shaved Fennel Salad with Lemon Dressing, and Tomato and Red Onion Salad into main dishes with the addition of cheese, eggs, tuna, shrimp, leftover chicken, or other protein sources.

Look for other main dish salads in "Sandwiches, Wraps, Fillings, and Pizza" (page 55), as well as many more salads, including such classics as Chef Salad, Cobb Salad, and Caesar Salad, at www.atkins.com.

GREENS AND MORE

From arugula to watercress, supermarkets stock a wonderful variety of salad greens, which can be combined with mung bean sprouts, olives, capers, bell peppers, artichoke hearts, jicama, scallions, and any number of other veggies to make an endless array of salads. We at Atkins call leafy greens and other non-starchy vegetables "foundation vegetables" because they're the primary source of carbs consumed in the first phase of Atkins and those upon which you build as you increase and diversify your carb intake.

In addition to being extremely low in carbs and high in vitamins, minerals, and fiber, salad greens add flavor and variety to your meals. Greens should always be part of your eating plan, and not just if you're slimming down. As you move through the phases of the Atkins Diet, your salad options broaden dramatically. Greens continue to be important, but your salad buffet can now include salads based on such grains as quinoa, brown rice, and wheat berries.

MASTERING HOMEMADE DRESSINGS

It takes no time at all to make salad dressings, and each of our salads includes a dressing that is designed to complement it. Not only are homemade dressings easy to make, but their flavor is vastly superior to bottled stuff. Just as greens and garnishes should be chosen for flavor, texture, and color, so should their companion dressings. Thick, creamy dressings stand up to sturdy greens and grains; oil-based dressings are ideal with delicate greens such as baby spinach. Arugula and other strongly flavored greens such as watercress compete with complex dressings; they're often best served with simple oil-and-vinegar dressings.

Most of the dressings that follow combine three to four parts oil with one part acid, and are enhanced with seasonings that can range from mustard to garlic and fresh herbs. Our oil of choice is usually olive oil—preferably high-quality extra-virgin olive oil—but some dressings benefit from neutral oil, such as canola. The pronounced flavor of dark sesame oil is appropriate for some salads. Walnut oil also lends a distinct flavor. The acid you choose should depend on the oil and other ingredients in the salad. Feel free to improvise. If you prefer a sweet dressing, use vinegars that are less acidic, such as rice or balsamic.

Vinaigrettes are the easiest dressings to make. If you're making a small batch—just enough for one recipe—mix the dressing directly in the salad bowl before you add the greens. Otherwise, combining the ingredients in a glass jar makes mixing the dressing a snap. Simply screw the cap on tightly and shake the jar vigorously. (Add the oil in three or four batches to aid in emulsifying it.)

CARBS AND PHASES

Any salad with more than 3 grams of Net Carbs per serving is coded for Phase 2 and beyond. But if the recipe contains only Phase 1 ingredients, feel free to simply have a smaller portion. Or if you turn the salad into a main dish by adding a protein source, you can go up to 7 grams of Net Carbs per serving.

Time to get out your salad bowl and tongs and explore the world of salads!

Athenian Salad

Phases 2, 3, 4

PER SERVING:
Net Carbs: 7 grams
Total Carbs: 9 grams
Fiber: 2 grams
Protein: 4 grams
Fat: 27 grams
Calories: 280

Makes: 4 (2-cup) servings
Active Time: 15 minutes
Total Time: 15 minutes

WEEKDAY

Unlike a classic Greek salad, this recipe has no iceberg lettuce or spinach. Instead, mild cucumbers are a perfect foil for the big Greek flavors of Kalamata olives, feta cheese, and lemon-garlic dressing. In Phase 1, simply have a smaller portion or add grilled shrimp to turn it into a main dish.

6 tablespoons extra-virgin olive oil
1 clove garlic, finely minced
1½ teaspoons dried oregano, crumbled, or 1 tablespoon fresh oregano, chopped
½ teaspoon salt
¼ teaspoon freshly ground black pepper
2 tablespoons plus 1 teaspoon freshly squeezed lemon juice
½ small red onion, thinly sliced
1½ medium cucumbers, peeled, halved lengthwise, seeded, and thinly sliced
1 medium green bell pepper, stemmed, ribs removed, and thinly sliced
½ cup quartered pitted Kalamata or other black olives
12 cherry tomatoes, quartered
½ cup crumbled feta cheese

1. Whisk together oil, garlic, oregano, and salt and pepper in a small bowl; whisk in lemon juice.
2. Put onion, cucumbers, bell pepper, and olives in a bowl and toss with the dressing. Arrange on a large platter or four individual plates, top with tomatoes and cheese, and serve.

TIP TIME

KEEP FETA FRESH

When exposed to air, feta dries out and gets a sour taste. Instead, refrigerate it in brine for up to two weeks. Or leave it in the wrapping paper (even if it's soggy) and wrap it in plastic wrap or put it in a plastic bag. Or cover it completely with extra-virgin olive oil in a tightly sealed glass jar and store out of the light at room temperature.

Caprese Salad

Phases 1, 2, 3, 4

Named for Capri, the island off the coast of Italy where it originated, this salad evokes the colors of the Italian flag. Make it in summer, when garden-fresh tomatoes are at their best.

PER SERVING:

Net Carbs: 5 grams

Total Carbs: 6 grams

Fiber: 1 gram

Protein: 24 grams

Fat: 42 grams

Calories: 500

Makes: 4 servings

Active Time: 10 minutes

Total Time: 10 minutes

- 1 pound fresh mozzarella, cut into ¼-inch slices
- 4 medium tomatoes, cored and cut into ¼-inch slices
- ¼ cup extra-virgin olive oil
- 4 teaspoons red wine vinegar
- 1 teaspoon granular sugar substitute
- ½ teaspoon salt
- ¼ teaspoon freshly ground black pepper
- 6 basil leaves, cut into thin strips

Arrange mozzarella and tomatoes on a platter, alternating and overlapping the slices decoratively. Whisk together oil, vinegar, sugar substitute, salt, and pepper in a small bowl. Drizzle over cheese and tomatoes, and then scatter basil on top.

TIP TIME

FRESH FROM THE DAIRY

Unlike regular mozzarella, which is semisoft, chewy, and elastic (think of most pizza toppings), fresh mozzarella has a softer texture and a more delicate flavor. Fresh mozzarella was originally made from the milk of water buffaloes, but it's now more commonly made from cow's milk or a combination of the two.

Mexican Avocado Salad*

Phases 1, 2, 3, 4

PER SERVING:
Net Carbs: 3 grams
Total Carbs: 7 grams
Fiber: 4 grams
Protein: 2 grams
Fat: 9 grams
Calories: 100

Makes: 8 (1-cup) servings
Active Time: 15 minutes
Total Time: 1 hour 15 minutes

This salad of Mexican flavors is a takeoff on guacamole. Serve it as is, or omit the lettuce, mix the avocado into the tomato mixture, and serve as a salsa over grilled chicken breast or fish. Marinating the tomatoes enhances their flavor, but it you want to get this tasty side dish on the table ASAP, omit Step 1.

24 cherry tomatoes, quartered
1 tablespoon extra-virgin olive oil
2 teaspoons red wine vinegar
1 teaspoon salt
¼ teaspoon freshly ground black pepper
½ medium yellow or white onion, finely chopped
1 jalapeño, seeded and finely chopped
2 tablespoons chopped fresh cilantro
¼ medium head iceberg lettuce, cut into ½-inch ribbons
2 ripe Hass avocados, seeded, peeled, and chopped

1. Combine tomatoes, oil, vinegar, salt, and pepper in a medium bowl; let stand at room temperature for 1 hour. Add onion, jalapeño and cilantro; toss well.
2. Arrange lettuce on a platter and top with avocado. Spoon tomato mixture on top and serve.

TIP TIME

ICEBERG REVISITED

Don't dismiss iceberg lettuce. Its crisp texture makes it the perfect foil to the creamy smoothness of avocado, and its mild flavor plays well with more assertive greens. To core iceberg lettuce, hit it firmly against the counter, core side down. The cone-shaped core should come right out.

*See photo on color page 25

Endive and Almond Salad

Phases 2, 3, 4

Choose heads of endive that are white or palest yellow, never green, which is a sign they'll be too bitter. Endive discolors after being cut, so don't prepare it more than half an hour or so in advance.

PER SERVING:
Net Carbs: 3 grams
Total Carbs: 8 grams
Fiber: 5 grams
Protein: 6 grams
Fat: 27 grams
Calories: 280

Makes: 4 (1¼-cup) servings
Active Time: 10 minutes
Total Time: 15 minutes

- 3 tablespoons cider vinegar
- 1 teaspoon Dijon mustard
- ½ teaspoon salt
- ¼ teaspoon freshly ground black pepper
- ⅓ cup walnut oil or extra-virgin olive oil
- 4 medium heads Belgian endive, cored and cut lengthwise into ¼-inch slices
- ⅓ cup slivered almonds, toasted and coarsely chopped
- ½ cup crumbled Gorgonzola or other blue cheese

1. Combine vinegar, mustard, salt and pepper in salad bowl. Add oil in a slow, steady stream, whisking until dressing thickens (this can also be done in a blender or by combining all ingredients in a jar with a tight-fitting lid and shaking vigorously). Add endive and toss gently to coat.
2. Divide among four plates and top with almonds and Gorgonzola.

TIP TIME

AVOID SEPARATION ANXIETY

Oil and vinegar separate quickly, so dressings frequently contain ingredients that help to keep the two emulsified, such as prepared mustard, sugar-free pancake syrup, tomato paste, cream, or mayonnaise.

Variation: Endive and Avocado Salad

Phases 2, 3, 4

Prepare Endive and Almond Salad as above, substituting 1 diced Hass avocado for the cheese and adding 2 tablespoons chopped fresh cilantro.

WEEKDAY

Shaved Fennel Salad with Lemon Dressing*

Phases 2, 3, 4

PER SERVING:
Net Carbs: 5 grams
Total Carbs: 8 grams
Fiber: 3 grams
Protein: 1 gram
Fat: 10 grams
Calories: 120

Makes: 6 (1-cup) servings
Active Time: 15 minutes
Total Time: 50 minutes

WEEKEND

Don't confuse fennel with anise, which looks similar but has a definite licorice flavor. Fennel is much milder, with a faintly sweet taste. A mandoline is the quickest way to slice fennel thinly, but a heavy sharp knife will work as well. Fennel's feathery, dill-like fronds make a pretty garnish.

¼ pound green beans, cut into 1½-inch pieces
¼ cup extra-virgin olive oil
3 tablespoons freshly squeezed lemon juice
1 teaspoon freshly grated lemon zest
1 teaspoon red wine vinegar
½ teaspoon salt
½ teaspoon freshly ground black pepper
¼ teaspoon granular sugar substitute
2 medium fennel bulbs, cored, quartered lengthwise, and thinly sliced crosswise
2 tablespoons chopped fresh basil

1. Bring a medium pot of well-salted water to a boil over high heat. Add green beans and cook until crisp-tender, about 4 minutes. Drain and rinse under cold running water to cool; set aside.
2. Combine oil, lemon juice, lemon zest, vinegar, salt, pepper, and sugar substitute in a salad bowl. Add green beans, fennel, and basil; cover and refrigerate at least 30 minutes but no more than 3 hours to let flavors blend. Stir gently before serving.

Variation: Fennel-Mushroom Salad with Parmesan

Phases 2, 3, 4

Prepare Shaved Fennel Salad with Lemon Dressing as above, substituting 1 cup sliced button mushrooms for the green beans and garnishing the salad with ½ cup Parmesan shavings.

*See photo on color page 22

Cucumber-Dill Salad

Phases 2, 3, 4

This salad is an ideal accompaniment to chicken or fish—it has a particular affinity for salmon. Leave the skin on unless the cucumber has been waxed. Serve smaller portions as a relish if you prefer, which also makes it suitable for Phase 1.

PER SERVING:
Net Carbs: 4 grams
Total Carbs: 5 grams
Fiber: 1 gram
Protein: 1 gram
Fat: 0 grams
Calories: 25

Makes: 4 (1-cup) servings
Active Time: 10 minutes
Total Time: 40 minutes

½ cup white wine vinegar
¼ cup chopped fresh dill
2 teaspoons granular sugar substitute
1 teaspoon salt
4 medium cucumbers, halved lengthwise, seeded, and thinly sliced

1. Combine vinegar, dill, sugar substitute, and salt in a medium bowl. Add cucumbers and toss gently to coat. Refrigerate 30 minutes to let flavors blend.
2. Drain excess liquid before serving.

TIP TIME

SEEDING A CUKE

Cucumber seeds and pulp can make a salad watery. To remove them, simply slice the cucumber in half lengthwise. Then, holding it with one hand and a teaspoon in the other hand, use the bowl of the spoon to gently remove the seeds and pulp.

Variation: Creamy Cucumber Salad

Phases 2, 3, 4

Prepare Cucumber-Dill Salad as above, substituting chopped fresh mint for the dill. Stir in ⅔ cup sour cream and 2 cloves garlic, chopped, after draining.

Tomato and Red Onion Salad*

Phases 1, 2, 3, 4

PER SERVING:
Net Carbs: 3 grams
Total Carbs: 4 grams
Fiber: 1 gram
Protein: 1 gram
Fat: 9 grams
Calories: 100

Makes: 8 (¾-cup) servings
Prep time: 15 minutes
Total Time: 15 minutes

WEEKDAY

Choose fully ripe tomatoes for this salad. If vine-ripened tomatoes are unavailable, substitute halved cherry or grape tomatoes.

- 3 tablespoons red wine vinegar
- 2 teaspoons Dijon mustard
- ¾ teaspoon salt
- ½ teaspoon freshly ground black pepper
- 5 tablespoons extra-virgin olive oil
- 3 large tomatoes, cut into 1-inch pieces
- ½ small red onion, thinly sliced
- ¼ cup chopped fresh basil or dill
- 2 tablespoons capers, rinsed and drained

1. Combine vinegar, mustard, salt, and pepper in a salad bowl. Add oil in a slow, steady stream, whisking until dressing thickens (this can also be done in a blender or by combining all ingredients in a jar with a tight-fitting lid and shaking vigorously).
2. Add tomatoes, onion, basil, and capers; toss gently and serve right away.

TIP TIME

PUNGENT PICKLES

Capers are the pickled or salted flower buds of a bush found in parts of Asia and the Mediterranean. They make an excellent garnish in many meat and vegetable dishes. Rinse salted capers before using.

Variation: Tomato Salad with Cucumbers and Olives

Phases 1, 2, 3, 4

Prepare Tomato and Red Onion Salad as above, substituting 1 cup sliced cucumbers for the onions and ½ cup pitted black olives for the capers.

*See photo on the front cover

Mushrooms and Greens with Sherry Vinaigrette

Phases 2, 3, 4

Use a large skillet so the mushrooms don't steam in their juices, inhibiting browning. In Phase 1, have a half portion.

PER SERVING:
Net Carbs: 6 grams
Total Carbs: 9 grams
Fiber: 3 grams
Protein: 6 grams
Fat: 23 grams
Calories: 260

Makes: 6 (2-cup) servings
Active Time: 30 minutes
Total Time: 30 minutes

Mushrooms

3 tablespoons virgin olive oil
1 pound mixed mushrooms, trimmed, wiped, and sliced
½ teaspoon salt
⅛ teaspoon freshly ground black pepper
2 cloves garlic, chopped
2 tablespoons sherry vinegar
2 tablespoons chopped fresh parsley

Salad

2 tablespoons sherry vinegar
1 small shallot, minced
1 teaspoon Dijon mustard
½ teaspoon salt
¼ teaspoon freshly ground black pepper
6 tablespoons extra-virgin olive oil
8 cups baby spinach or arugula
½ cup Parmesan shavings

1. Heat oil in a large nonstick skillet over high heat. Add mushrooms, salt, and pepper; cook until soft and golden, about 12 minutes. Add garlic and cook until fragrant, about 30 seconds. Add vinegar and cook until evaporated, about 1 minute. Remove from heat; stir in parsley.
2. For the salad, combine vinegar, shallot, mustard, salt, and pepper in a salad bowl. Add oil in a slow, steady stream, whisking until dressing thickens. Add spinach and mushrooms; toss gently to coat.
3. Divide among 6 plates; top with Parmesan shavings and serve.

Variation: Mushrooms and Greens with Bacon and Eggs

Phases 1, 2, 3, 4

Cut 2 slices of bacon crosswise into strips; cook until crisp. Drain bacon on paper towels; reserve bacon fat. Prepare recipe as above, sautéing the mushrooms in bacon fat instead of olive oil and substituting 2 sliced hard-boiled eggs for the cheese. Top with bacon before serving.

Orange and Goat Cheese Salad

Phases 3, 4

PER SERVING:
Net Carbs: 12 grams
Total Carbs: 17 grams
Fiber: 5 grams
Protein: 11 grams
Fat: 35 grams
Calories: 410

Makes: 6 (1-cup) servings
Active Time: 20 minutes
Total Time: 20 minutes

WEEKDAY

To save time, omit Step 1 by using a 20-ounce package of fresh-cut orange segments in their juice. Kalamata olives hail from Greece and can be found in most well-stocked supermarkets. Large, almond-shaped, black or dark purple, and salty, they bear little resemblance to the tasteless canned Mission olives that often turn up on pizza.

- 6 small oranges
- 2 tablespoons white wine vinegar
- 2 teaspoons Dijon mustard
- 1 teaspoon salt
- 1 teaspoon freshly ground black pepper
- ½ cup extra-virgin olive oil
- 1 small red onion, thinly sliced
- 1 cup pitted Kalamata olives
- ¼ cup chopped fresh tarragon
- ½ pound fresh goat cheese, crumbled
- ½ cup sliced almonds, toasted

1. Using a small, very sharp knife, cut peels and outer membrane from oranges. Holding oranges above a bowl to catch juice, cut between membranes to separate segments. Reserve segments and discard membranes.
2. Combine 6 tablespoons juice from the oranges, vinegar, mustard, salt, and pepper in a salad bowl. Add oil in a slow, steady stream, whisking until dressing thickens.
3. Add orange segments, onion, olives, and tarragon; toss gently to coat. Divide salad among 6 plates; top with goat cheese and almonds and serve.

Variation: Orange and Avocado Salad with Mint

Phases 3, 4

Prepare Orange and Goat Cheese Salad as above, substituting chopped fresh mint for the tarragon and 1 diced Hass avocado for the cheese.

Slaw with Vinegar Dressing

Phases 1, 2, 3, 4

Never had coleslaw with a vinaigrette-style dressing? This refreshing take on the classic cabbage salad, typically made with mayonnaise, is terrific for picnics and potlucks because there's no risk of spoilage.

PER SERVING:
Net Carbs: 3 grams
Total Carbs: 5 grams
Fiber: 2 grams
Protein: 1 gram
Fat: 19 grams
Calories: 190

Makes: 8 (¾-cup) servings
Active Time: 15 minutes
Total Time: 45 minutes

⅓ cup white or red wine vinegar
1 tablespoon Dijon mustard
1 clove garlic, minced
⅔ cup extra-virgin olive oil
¼ cup chopped fresh parsley
4 small scallions, thinly sliced
½ teaspoon salt
½ teaspoon freshly ground black pepper
½ large head red and/or green cabbage, shredded (8 cups)

1. Combine vinegar, mustard, and garlic in a salad bowl. Add oil in a slow, steady stream, whisking until dressing thickens (this can also be done in a blender or by combining all ingredients in a jar with a tight-fitting lid and shaking vigorously). Stir in parsley, scallions, salt, and pepper.
2. Add cabbage; toss to coat. Cover and refrigerate for at least 30 minutes before serving.

TIP TIME

BEYOND COLESLAW

Cabbage, including Chinese cabbage, adds a sweet crunch to any salad. Cut cabbage into very thin shreds before tossing them with other greens. Cabbage salads pair well with ham, bacon, or sausage.

Variation: Lemony Slaw with Capers

Phases 1, 2, 3, 4

Prepare Slaw with Vinegar Dressing as above, substituting lemon juice for vinegar and adding 3 tablespoons drained capers and 1 teaspoon freshly grated lemon zest with the parsley and scallions.

Broccoli and Jicama Slaw

Phases 3, 4

PER SERVING:
Net Carbs: 10 grams
Total Carbs: 11 grams
Fiber: 1 gram
Protein: 1 gram
Fat: 19 grams
Calories: 158

Makes: 6 (⅔-cup) servings
Active Time: 15 minutes
Total Time: 45 minutes

Underneath broccoli's tough skin lurks a tender stalk. Too often discarded, the flavorful stalks combine with jicama to make a delicious alternative to cabbage in a slaw. The skin of jicama can be quite thick, so a paring knife might be more effective than a vegetable peeler.

- 3 heads broccoli
- ⅓ cup freshly squeezed lime juice
- 1 teaspoon peeled and minced fresh ginger
- 1 clove garlic, minced
- 1 teaspoon sugar substitute
- ½ teaspoon salt
- ½ teaspoon red pepper flakes
- ⅓ cup extra-virgin olive oil
- 1 medium (1-pound) jicama, peeled and shredded
- ½ small red onion, sliced
- ¼ cup chopped fresh cilantro

1. Trim woody bottoms off broccoli and discard; remove florets and reserve for another use. Peel stalks carefully, discarding any that have a white core, which will be woody. Then shred with a box grater or a food processor fitted with the shredding attachment.
2. Combine lime juice, ginger, garlic, sugar substitute, salt, and red pepper flakes in a medium bowl. Add oil in a slow, steady stream, whisking until dressing thickens (this can also be done in a blender or by combining all ingredients in a jar with a tight-fitting lid and shaking vigorously).
3. Add broccoli, jicama, onion, and cilantro; toss to coat. Cover and refrigerate at least 30 minutes to let flavors blend. Serve chilled or at room temperature.

TIP TIME

LOOKS AREN'T EVERYTHING

A Mexican import, the homely jicama is delicious both raw and cooked. Its crisp white flesh is juicy and somewhat sweet. Smaller jicama roots are less woody than larger ones—choose those that weigh about a pound.

Tabbouleh Salad*

Phases 3, 4

Our version of tabbouleh minimizes carbs by changing the usual proportions of bulgur to herbs. The variation below is still lower in carbs. To eat tabbouleh in authentic Lebanese style, scoop it up with romaine lettuce leaves.

PER SERVING:
Net Carbs: 10 grams
Total Carbs: 13 grams
Fiber: 3 grams
Protein: 2 grams
Fat: 10 grams
Calories: 140

Makes: 6 (1-cup) servings
Active Time: 10 minutes
Total Time: 25 minutes

- ½ cup fine or medium bulgur
- 1 cup boiling water
- 2 plum tomatoes, seeded and cut into ¼-inch pieces
- 1 small cucumber, peeled, seeded, and thinly sliced
- ¾ cup chopped fresh parsley
- ½ cup chopped fresh mint
- ¼ cup freshly squeezed lemon juice
- ¼ cup extra-virgin olive oil
- 3 scallions, thinly sliced
- 1 teaspoon salt
- ½ teaspoon freshly ground black pepper

1. Combine bulgur and water in a large heatproof bowl; cover tightly with plastic wrap and let stand until water is absorbed, about 15 minutes.
2. Line a sieve with cheesecloth or a dishtowel, place bulgur in it, and press firmly with your hands to remove any excess water.
3. Add tomatoes, cucumber, parsley, mint, lemon juice, oil, scallions, salt, and pepper; toss gently to combine. Serve cold or at room temperature.

Variation: Green Tabbouleh Salad

Phases 3, 4

Prepare Tabbouleh Salad as above, reducing the bulgur to ¼ cup and water to ½ cup. Substitute 2 cups finely chopped romaine lettuce or watercress for the tomatoes and increase the parsley to 1¼ cups and mint to ½ cup.

WEEKDAY

*See photo on color page 19

Curried Quinoa with Snow Peas

Phases 3, 4

PER SERVING:
Net Carbs: 16 grams
Total Carbs: 18 grams
Fiber: 2 grams
Protein: 5 grams
Fat: 9 grams
Calories: 170

Makes: 8 (½-cup) servings
Active Time: 10 minutes
Total Time: 20 minutes

WEEKDAY

A staple of the ancient Incan diet, quinoa is higher in protein than any other grain and lower in carbohydrates than most. The tiny grains are bead-shaped and cook quickly, expanding to four times their original volume.

- 3 tablespoons unseasoned, unsweetened rice vinegar
- 1 clove garlic, chopped
- 1 teaspoon peeled and minced fresh ginger
- ½ teaspoon curry powder
- 1 teaspoon salt, divided
- ¼ teaspoon freshly ground black pepper
- ¼ teaspoon granular sugar substitute
- ¼ cup extra-virgin olive oil
- 2½ cups chicken or vegetable broth
- 1 cup quinoa, rinsed until water is almost clear
- ¼ pound snow peas
- 2 scallions, sliced
- ¼ cup fresh cilantro, chopped
- 1 jalapeño, seeded and minced

1. Combine vinegar, garlic, ginger, curry powder, ½ teaspoon salt, pepper, and sugar substitute in a salad bowl. Add oil in a slow, steady stream, whisking until dressing thickens (this can also be done in a blender or by combining all ingredients in a jar with a tight-fitting lid and shaking vigorously).
2. Bring broth and remaining ½ teaspoon salt to a boil in a medium saucepan over high heat. Add quinoa and reduce heat to low; cover and simmer for 10 minutes. Turn off heat and let quinoa stand, covered, until it absorbs the rest of the broth, about 10 minutes. Transfer to bowl with dressing.
3. Meanwhile, bring a medium pot of lightly salted water to a boil over high heat. Add snow peas and cook until crisp-tender, about 2 minutes. Drain and rinse under cold running water to cool. Cut snow peas lengthwise into thin strips; add to quinoa.
4. Add scallions, cilantro, and jalapeño to salad; toss to combine. Serve warm or at room temperature, or refrigerate in an airtight container for up to 2 days.

Wheat Berries with Sun-Dried Tomatoes and Feta

Phases 3, 4

There are two kinds of wheat berries, which are the hulled grain of whole wheat: the reddish-brown ones (hard wheat) are high in protein, and the blond ones (soft wheat) are lower in protein. We prefer the chewy texture of hard wheat berries for this recipe.

PER SERVING:
Net Carbs: 15 grams
Total Carbs: 18 grams
Fiber: 3 grams
Protein: 4 grams
Fat: 17 grams
Calories: 230

Makes: 6 (⅔-cup) servings
Active Time: 10 minutes
Total Time: 1 hour, 10 minutes

- 1 cup wheat berries
- 2 tablespoons red wine vinegar
- 1 clove garlic, minced
- ¾ teaspoon salt
- ½ teaspoon freshly ground black pepper
- ⅓ cup extra-virgin olive oil
- 1 small red onion, finely chopped
- ½ cup chopped fresh basil
- ½ cup chopped sun-dried tomatoes (oil-packed)
- ½ cup crumbled feta cheese

1. Bring a large pot of water to a boil over high heat. Add wheat berries, cover, and simmer until tender, about 1 hour. Drain.
2. Combine vinegar, garlic, salt, and pepper in a salad bowl. Add oil in a slow, steady stream, whisking until dressing thickens (this can also be done in a blender or by combining all ingredients in a jar with a tight-fitting lid and shaking vigorously).
3. Add wheat berries, onion, basil, tomatoes, and feta; toss gently to coat. Serve chilled or at room temperature.

Variation: Wheat Berries with Olives and Feta

Phases 3, 4

Prepare Wheat Berries with Sun-Dried Tomatoes and Feta as above, substituting ¼ cup chopped fresh dill for the basil and ½ cup chopped pitted Kalamata or other cured black olives for the tomatoes.

Creamy Potato and Cauliflower Salad

Phases 3, 4

PER SERVING:
Net Carbs: 7 grams
Total Carbs: 10 grams
Fiber: 3 grams
Protein: 6 grams
Fat: 15 grams
Calories: 190

Makes: 6 (⅔-cup) servings
Active Time: 15 minutes
Total Time: 1 hour 15 minutes

Red-skinned potatoes add color, but any waxy variety (such as Yukon golds or fingerlings) or an all-purpose potato can be substituted. Avoid the higher-carb starchy spuds such as russets (sometimes called Idaho or baking potatoes). If you enjoy a crunch in your salad, add some chopped celery.

¼ pound red new potatoes, cut into ½-inch slices
1 head cauliflower florets, cut into ½-inch slices
⅓ cup regular (not low-fat) mayonnaise
⅓ cup sour cream
3 large eggs, hard-boiled and chopped
½ small yellow or white onion, finely chopped
2 tablespoons chopped fresh parsley
¾ teaspoon salt
½ teaspoon freshly ground black pepper

1. Bring a large pot of well-salted water to a boil over high heat. Add potatoes; reduce heat to medium-low and simmer 5 minutes. Add cauliflower and simmer until vegetables are soft, about 7 minutes.
2. Drain vegetables and transfer to a medium bowl. Add mayonnaise, sour cream, eggs, onion, parsley, salt, and pepper; stir to combine. Cover and refrigerate to let flavors blend, about 1 hour and up to 2 days.

Variation: Curried Potato and Cauliflower Salad

Phases 3, 4

Prepare Creamy Potato and Cauliflower Salad as above, substituting chopped fresh cilantro for the parsley and adding ½ cup almonds, 1 tablespoon curry powder, and ½ teaspoon ground cumin.

Brown Rice Salad with Toasted Almonds

Phases 3, 4

Sautéing the rice prior to simmering adds flavor, especially when cooked with an onion. Using chicken or vegetable broth instead of salted water to cook the rice is another flavor booster.

PER SERVING:
Net Carbs: 11 grams
Total Carbs: 13 grams
Fiber: 2 grams
Protein: 3 grams
Fat: 12 grams
Calories: 170

Makes: 8 (½-cup) servings
Active Time: 20 minutes
Total Time: 1 hour 20 minutes

- 4 tablespoons extra-virgin olive oil, divided
- 1 small yellow or white onion, chopped
- ½ cup brown rice
- 1½ cups water
- 1 teaspoon salt
- ½ teaspoon freshly ground black pepper
- 2 medium cucumbers, peeled, seeded, and cut in ¼-inch dice
- ½ cup sliced almonds, toasted
- ½ cup chopped fresh parsley
- 1 tablespoon freshly grated lemon zest

1. Heat 1 tablespoon oil in a medium saucepan over high heat. Add onion and sauté until soft, about 3 minutes. Add rice and stir to coat with oil. Add water, salt, and pepper; bring to a boil. Reduce heat to medium, cover, and simmer until rice is tender and water is absorbed, about 45 minutes.
2. Transfer rice to bowl. Add remaining 3 tablespoons oil, cucumbers, almonds, parsley, and lemon zest; mix well. Let stand at least 15 minutes before serving to blend flavors. Serve at room temperature.

TIP TIME

A GREAT GRATER

When zesting a citrus fruit, the trick is to remove the colorful skin but avoid the unpleasantly bitter white pith below—and not scrape your knuckles in the process. A stainless-steel Microplane grater (similar to a woodworking tool) has tiny razor-sharp teeth that quickly and effortlessly produce finely grated zest. It's also super for grating hard cheese.

Garlicky Spinach and Feta Salad in Tomato Halves

Phases 2, 3, 4

PER SERVING:
Net Carbs: 4 grams
Total Carbs: 5 grams
Fiber: 1 gram
Protein: 7 grams
Fat: 15 grams
Calories: 180

Makes: 6 servings
Active Time: 30 minutes
Total Time: 30 minutes

WEEKDAY

This salad can be made two ways: either roll up your sleeves and mash the feta cheese into the julienned spinach or use a food processor and get the job done in half the time. The salad will have a smoother texture but retains the assertive taste. Note that baby spinach is too tender for this treatment. For Phase 1, use hollowed-out cucumber "boats" instead of tomato halves.

2 (5-ounce) bunches or bags spinach, well rinsed, spun, and patted dry
6 medium cloves garlic (or to taste), minced
3 tablespoons extra-virgin olive oil
8 ounces feta cheese, drained and roughly chopped
Freshly ground black pepper
3 medium ripe tomatoes, halved, seeded, drained, and hollowed out

1. Remove tough spinach stems. Stack several spinach leaves on top of each other and, using a sharp knife, cut into fine strips. Place in a large bowl.
2. Pour 3 tablespoons oil over the spinach and add the garlic. Add the feta to the bowl. Using your hands, mash or press the feta into the spinach until the feta is evenly distributed but the mixture is not too smooth. If necessary, add another tablespoon of oil. (Alternatively, place the garlic and spinach in a food processor, pulsing to chop roughly; work in batches as needed. Do not overprocess. When all the spinach is chopped, add 3 tablespoons oil and the feta. Pulse only until the feta and spinach are combined, but still distinct, not puréed. Add more oil only if necessary.) Add pepper to taste.
3. Spoon spinach-feta mixture into tomato halves and serve.

TIP TIME

BABY THAT SPINACH

Flat-leafed varieties of spinach are easier to clean than those with curly leaves, and they have a more delicate flavor and texture; the crinkly-leaved varieties can be leathery. Baby spinach is best for tossed salads.

Mung Bean Sprout, Mint, and Basil Salad

Phases 2, 3, 4

Mung beans, fresh herbs, and a sweet and salty Asian-inspired dressing are natural partners. If you don't have fish sauce, use tamari. In Phase 1, simply have a smaller portion of salad and omit the peanuts in the first two weeks. Or make it a Phase 1 and beyond main dish by adding a small can of drained salmon or tuna, or at least 4 ounces of sliced leftover grilled steak.

PER SERVING:
Net Carbs: 5 grams
Total Carbs: 7 grams
Fiber: 2 grams
Protein: 3 grams
Fat: 9 grams
Calories: 110

Makes: 4 (1¼-cup) servings
Active Time: 15 minutes
Total Time: 15 minutes

WEEKDAY

Dressing

- 1 tablespoon fish sauce (nam pla or nuoc mam)
- 1½ teaspoons granular sugar substitute
- 1 tablespoon freshly squeezed lime juice
- 1½ tablespoons dark (toasted) sesame oil
- 1 small clove garlic, crushed
- ½ jalapeño, seeded and minced (see tip on page 128)

Salad

- 1 cup chopped romaine lettuce or mixed baby greens
- 4 ounces fresh mung bean sprouts (2 cups), drained, rinsed, and patted dry
- 1 medium cucumber, seeded and coarsely chopped
- 1 cup fresh mint leaves, coarsely chopped
- ½ cup basil (preferably Thai basil), coarsely chopped
- 1 tablespoon chopped roasted peanuts
- ½ cup fresh cilantro, coarsely chopped

1. For the dressing, put fish sauce, sugar substitute, lime juice, sesame oil, garlic, and jalapeño in a small jar with a tight-fitting lid; shake vigorously. Set aside.
2. For the salad, combine lettuce, bean sprouts, cucumber, mint, and basil in a bowl; divide among 4 plates.
3. Remove garlic from dressing and drizzle over salads. Garnish with peanuts and cilantro.

New York Strip Steak Salad

Phases 1, 2, 3, 4

•

PER SERVING:
Net Carbs: 6 grams
Total Carbs: 8 grams
Fiber: 2 grams
Protein: 25 grams
Fat: 54 grams
Calories: 620

Makes: 4 servings
Active Time: 20 minutes
Total Time: 30 minutes

WEEKDAY

This salad is synonymous with satisfaction: crisp greens, tomatoes, red onion, and blue cheese are topped with steak hot off the grill!

Steak
1 (16-ounce) New York strip steak, ¾ inch thick
1 clove garlic, halved lengthwise
½ teaspoon salt
½ teaspoon freshly ground black pepper

Salad
⅓ cup extra-virgin olive oil
2 tablespoons red wine vinegar
½ teaspoon granular sugar substitute
1 clove garlic, minced
2 teaspoons Dijon mustard
¼ teaspoon salt
¼ teaspoon freshly ground black pepper
1 (6-ounce) bag baby greens
2 medium tomatoes, cut into wedges
1 small red onion, thinly sliced
½ cup blue cheese, crumbled (2 ounces)

1. Prepare a medium-hot charcoal or gas grill. Rub steak on both sides with cut sides of garlic and season with salt and pepper. Grill steak, turning once, about 10 minutes for medium-rare. Transfer to a cutting board and let stand for 5 minutes. Thinly slice steak across the grain.
2. Meanwhile, put oil, vinegar, sugar substitute, garlic, mustard, salt, and pepper in a small jar with a tight-fitting lid; shake vigorously to blend.
3. Line 4 plates with greens. Arrange tomatoes, onion, and blue cheese over lettuce. Drizzle dressing over salads and top with sliced steak.

TIP TIME

TREAT TOMATOES RIGHT

Never refrigerate a tomato—55°F or above is the optimum temperature. Chilling them changes their texture and mutes the taste.

Chopped Salad with Bacon and Blue Cheese

Phases 2, 3, 4

Six different veggies, bacon, and blue cheese team up for a salad that's as pretty as it is tasty. Serve this steakhouse favorite alongside a grilled steak, grilled chicken, or broiled fish. Or add a few chopped hard-boiled eggs or tuna to make it a main course salad suitable for Phase 1.

PER SERVING:
Net Carbs: 8 grams
Total Carbs: 12 grams
Fiber: 4 grams
Protein: 12 grams
Fat: 24 grams
Calories: 307

Makes: 8 (1½-cup) servings
Active Time: 30 minutes
Total Time: 30 minutes

Dressing

3 tablespoons red wine vinegar
1 teaspoon Dijon mustard
¾ teaspoon salt
½ teaspoon freshly ground black pepper
6 tablespoons extra-virgin olive oil

Salad

1 medium head romaine lettuce, chopped
2 large tomatoes, chopped
2 medium cucumbers, chopped
4 ounces blue cheese, crumbled (1 cup)
8 canned artichoke hearts, drained and coarsely chopped
4 ounces bacon, cooked and crumbled
1 large Hass avocado, chopped
6 scallions, chopped

1. For the dressing, combine vinegar, mustard, salt, and pepper in a small bowl. Add oil in a slow, steady stream, whisking until dressing thickens (this can also be done in a blender or by combining all ingredients in a jar with a tight-fitting lid and shaking vigorously).
2. For the salad, combine lettuce, tomatoes, cucumbers, cheese, artichoke hearts, bacon, avocado, and scallions in a salad bowl; toss to combine.
3. Add dressing and toss gently to coat. Serve right away.

TIP TIME

AVOCADO ADVISORY

Atkins recipes call for Hass avocados, which have a blackish pebbly surface and are smaller than the shiny medium-green Florida avocados. The Hass have fewer carbs and are less watery and richer in flavor.

WEEKDAY

Chapter 7

VEGETABLES AND OTHER SIDES

Along with salads, cooked vegetables are a key component of the Atkins Diet. In fact, with a few exceptions, nutrient-rich veggies are the core carbohydrates in the Atkins lifestyle. The parts of the plant that grow above ground—leaves, flowers, and "fruit" (anything that contains seeds)—are lower in carbs than those that grow below ground. Roots and tubers (such as carrots and potatoes) are carbohydrate rich because they provide the nutrients and energy for plants to grow. (A few low-carb roots, such as radishes and jicama, are acceptable in Phase 1.)

You'll focus mostly on the above-ground components—we call them "foundation vegetables" initially. However, once you get close to your goal weight and increase your carb intake, feel free to add higher-carb veggies, as well as modest portions of grains, to your menus.

To help you choose the most nutrient-rich produce, reach for foods with deeper, darker colors. Plant pigments contain potent compounds called phytochemicals (*phyto* means "plant") that can promote health and protect against diseases. By selecting produce in a variety of colors and by leaving the skins on vegetables with pale flesh you'll boost your intake of these compounds, as well as of vitamins and minerals—along with flavor.

COOKING VEGETABLES 101

Vegetables are nothing if not versatile. They can be prepared in a variety of ways to yield an array of textures, flavors, and colors. Each method has its advantages. Blanching and steaming yield the brightest colors and purest flavors; roasting, broiling, and grilling caramelize sugars in the vegetables to result in sweet, rich flavors. Sautéing and stir-frying in fat can help to boost the body's ability to absorb certain nutrients.

The recipes that follow make use of these techniques:

- *Baking* is the generic term for cooking foods in an oven, usually at moderate temperatures (around 350°F). It's best for whole or halved veggies such as winter squash, eggplant, carrots, fennel, onion, beets, and stuffed peppers.
- *Blanching* means plunging vegetables into boiling water briefly (sometimes only a few seconds) to set the color, soften the texture, or loosen skins.
- *Simmering*. Although few vegetables should be boiled in water that is vigorously bubbling, most, such as asparagus, snap beans, and artichokes, do well when simmered in liquids

where bubbles break the surface slowly and gently.

- *Stewing* refers to cooking several foods together in a small amount of liquid in a covered pot, which allows the juices to condense on the lid and fall back on the food, helping to keep it moist and flavorful.
- *Braising* is similar to stewing but generally refers to one food and uses even less liquid. Some veggies that take well to braising are leeks, celery, cabbage, collards, fennel, tomatoes, and summer squash.
- *Broiling and grilling* are both quick cooking methods under or over direct and intense heat. The food should be fairly flat and tender, so slices of zucchini or eggplant rather than the whole vegetable are better suited to broiling and grilling.
- *Deep-frying* is only suitable for foods with a low moisture content; foods with more moisture spatter violently when they hit the hot fat. Batters can help to reduce spattering, and it's important to use a deep pot.
- *Roasting* requires higher heat than baking (usually around 400° to 450°F) and is almost always done an uncovered shallow pan. Dense vegetables need to be cut into smaller pieces so the insides will be tender before the outsides char.
- *Sautéing* calls for a hot pan, hot fat, food cut to uniform size, and frequent stirring. Done properly, the surface of the food sears upon contact so it doesn't stick to the pan.
- *Stir-frying* involves bite-size pieces of food and constant stirring; the pan and oil are typically much hotter than in sautéing.
- *Steaming* cooks food above, not in, simmering liquid. The vapor actually cooks the food. Steaming requires a covered pan and a device to keep the food above the liquid. Almost any vegetable can be steamed.

For more on these techniques, see the Glossary (page 253).

VEGGIE VARIETY

Our side dishes include such familiar vegetables as asparagus and sweet potatoes, but you'll also find some others worth sampling. Give Sautéed Baby Bok Choy with Garlic and Lemon Zest a try. Or consider a new cooking method: roasting Brussels sprouts, for example, instead of steaming them. Have you ever thought about cooking lettuce? It's deliciously mild, as you'll find when you try Braised Lettuce. Or how about Edamame Succotash, that old Native American recipe updated with green soybeans in lieu of carb-heavy lima beans? We guarantee you'll come away with some new favorite vegetables or a new appreciation for vegetables in general. As always, check out www.atkins.com for a host of other delicious side dishes.

PHASE CODING

As with salads, if a dish is coded for Phase 2 because the count is more than 3 grams of Net Carbs per serving but all ingredients are acceptable in Phase 1, simply serve yourself a smaller portion. And, again, dishes with nuts or seeds, coded for Phase 2 and beyond are acceptable after two weeks in Phase 1 if they don't exceed 3 grams of Net Carbs and have no other ingredients unsuitable for Phase 1.

Roasted Asparagus and Red Peppers with Dijon and Thyme*

Phases 2, 3, 4

PER SERVING:
Net Carbs: 6 grams
Total Carbs: 8 grams
Fiber: 2 grams
Protein: 2 grams
Fat: 13 grams
Calories: 150

Makes: 4 (1-cup) servings
Active Time: 5 minutes
Total Time: 15 minutes

This dish is equally good on the grill (place the veggies in a grill basket). Use a white or yellow onion instead of the shallot, if necessary.

- 16 asparagus spears
- 1 large red bell pepper, cored, seeded, and cut into 8 strips
- 2 tablespoons chopped shallot
- 2 tablespoons butter
- 2 tablespoons grainy Dijon mustard
- 2 tablespoons freshly squeezed lemon juice
- 2 tablespoons virgin olive oil
- 1 tablespoon fresh thyme
- 2 teaspoons freshly grated lemon zest
- Salt
- Freshly ground black pepper

1. Heat oven to 425°F. Place the asparagus and bell pepper on a rimmed sheet pan covered with aluminum foil; set aside.
2. Sauté shallot in butter in a small saucepan over medium heat until translucent, about 3 minutes. Transfer to a small bowl; add mustard, lemon juice, oil, thyme, and lemon zest; whisk the dressing together.
3. Brush asparagus and red peppers with the dressing; set remainder aside. Roast vegetables in oven for 10–15 minutes, until asparagus is tender.
4. Drizzle with remaining sauce, season with salt and black pepper to taste, and serve right away.

TIP TIME

SNAP, DON'T CUT ASPARAGUS

Snap off the woody portion at the bottom of each spear. It will break at the naturally weak juncture of the tender and fibrous parts.

*See photo on color page 13

WEEKDAY

Sautéed Greens with Pecans

Phases 2, 3, 4

Darker outer leaves of greens are higher in nutrients, but the inner leaves are more tender. Blanching greens before sautéing reduces bitterness.

PER SERVING:
Net Carbs: 3 grams
Total Carbs: 6 grams
Fiber: 3 grams
Protein: 3 grams
Fat: 10 grams
Calories: 120

Makes: 4 (½-cup) servings
Active Time: 20 minutes
Total Time: 20 minutes

- 1 (1-pound) bunch Swiss chard or mustard, beet, or turnip greens
- 1 tablespoon extra-virgin olive oil
- 2 cloves garlic, chopped
- ⅓ cup pecans, toasted and coarsely chopped
- ½ teaspoon salt
- ⅛ teaspoon freshly ground black pepper

1. Chop the leaves of the greens crosswise into 1-inch slices; cut stems into ½-inch pieces. Rinse thoroughly.
2. Bring a large pot of salted water to a boil over high heat. Add stems, reduce heat to medium-low, and simmer 2 minutes; add leaves and cook until stems are tender, about 3 minutes longer. Drain, squeezing out as much water as possible.
3. Heat oil in a large skillet over high heat. Add garlic and sauté until fragrant, about 30 seconds. Add greens, pecans, salt, and pepper; sauté to heat through, about 2 minutes. Serve hot.

TIP TIME

SNIP THOSE TOPS

If you purchase beets or turnips with the greens attached, remove the tops and store them separately, as they lose nutrients if left intact.

Variation: Sautéed Greens with Balsamic Vinaigrette

Phases 1, 2, 3, 4

Prepare Sautéed Greens as above, omitting pecans and adding 1 tablespoon balsamic vinegar and ½ teaspoon Dijon mustard along with the greens.

WEEKDAY

Stir-Fried Broccolini with Cashews

Phases 2, 3, 4

PER SERVING:
Net Carbs: 7 grams
Total Carbs: 10 grams
Fiber: 3 grams
Protein: 5 grams
Fat: 11 grams
Calories: 150

Makes: 4 (1-cup) servings
Active Time: 20 minutes
Total Time: 20 minutes

Broccolini, sometimes called baby broccoli, is actually a cross between broccoli and Chinese broccoli (kai-lan). It's crunchier and more delicately flavored than broccoli. Select the smallest broccolini you can find—larger ones are tougher and more pungent—with firm stalks, deep green leaves, and compact heads. You can also use broccoli or broccoli rabe in this recipe.

2 tablespoons canola oil
1 scallion, thinly sliced
2 teaspoons peeled and minced fresh ginger
2 cloves garlic, minced
1 pound broccolini, trimmed and cut into ½-inch slices
¾ cup water
¼ cup cashews, toasted and chopped
3 tablespoons tamari (see page 11)
¼ teaspoon red pepper flakes
⅛ teaspoon dark (toasted) sesame oil

1. Heat the canola oil in a large skillet or wok over high heat. Add scallion, ginger, and garlic; sauté until fragrant, stirring constantly, about 45 seconds.
2. Add broccolini and water; simmer until water has evaporated and broccolini is crisp-tender, about 2–3 minutes.
3. Add cashews, tamari, and red pepper flakes; cook to heat through, about 1 minute. Stir in sesame oil and serve.

WEEKDAY

Roasted Lemon-Garlic Brussels Sprouts

Phases 2, 3, 4

These are not your grandmother's Brussels sprouts! Roasting this fiber-rich vegetable is easy and brings out its natural sweetness, making it a natural accompaniment to roast pork, beef, and poultry.

PER SERVING:
Net Carbs: 5 grams
Total Carbs: 9 grams
Fiber: 4 grams
Protein: 3 grams
Fat: 12 grams
Calories: 150

Makes: 6 (¾-cup) servings
Active Time: 10 minutes
Total Time: 30 minutes

- 2 (10-ounce) containers Brussels sprouts, trimmed and halved
- 5 tablespoons virgin olive oil
- 1 tablespoon freshly grated lemon zest
- 2 cloves garlic, chopped
- 1 teaspoon chopped fresh thyme
- 1 teaspoon salt
- ¼ teaspoon freshly ground black pepper

1. Heat oven to 375°F.
2. Combine sprouts, oil, lemon zest, garlic, thyme, salt, and pepper in a large jelly roll pan or shallow baking dish; toss well. Arrange sprouts in a single layer; roast, stirring occasionally, until tender and light brown, about 20 minutes. Serve hot.

TIP TIME

GO FOR THE GREEN

Avoid large or yellowish sprouts; instead, select very small bright or deep green ones—they'll be most tender. Look for them from mid-fall to early winter. Don't wash Brussels sprouts before refrigerating them, but do trim any yellow or wilted outer leaves.

WEEKDAY

Sautéed Baby Bok Choy with Garlic and Lemon Zest

Phases 1, 2, 3, 4

PER SERVING:
Net Carbs: 1 gram
Total Carbs: 1 gram
Fiber: 0 grams
Protein: 1 gram
Fat: 5 grams
Calories: 45

Makes: 6 servings
Active Time: 10 minutes
Total Time: 10 minutes

Bok choy is a form of Chinese cabbage. Baby bok choy has green stems, rather than the white of its full-grown counterpart. This quick, aromatic preparation also works beautifully with tender young spinach. Or try it with chard, escarole, collards, or mature bok choy—just increase the cooking times as needed. If you are using a small skillet, you may need to add the bok choy in batches, letting it cook down before adding more.

2 tablespoons virgin olive oil
2 cloves garlic, chopped
2 teaspoons freshly grated lemon zest
18 baby bok choy, trimmed
¼ teaspoon salt
⅛ teaspoon freshly ground black pepper

1. Heat oil in a large skillet over medium-high heat. Add garlic and lemon zest and sauté until fragrant, about 30 seconds.
2. Add bok choy, salt, and pepper; sauté until just wilted, about 2 minutes. Serve hot.

TIP TIME

PICTURE PERFECT—OR NOT?

When selecting vegetables, don't confuse perfection with quality. Minor imperfections such as healed peel damage have far less impact on quality than recently inflicted damage from neighboring veggies, soft sunken areas, or torn leaves.

WEEKDAY

Kale with Sweet-and-Sour Vinaigrette

Phases 2, 3, 4

Drizzling cooked kale with warm vinaigrette is a perfect way to dress up greens. Swiss chard or a mix of bitter greens can be used in place of kale. This dish is wonderful with pork, from Italian sausage to an elegant roast.

PER SERVING:
Net Carbs: 5 grams
Total Carbs: 7 grams
Fiber: 2 grams
Protein: 2 grams
Fat: 8 grams
Calories: 100

Makes: 6 servings
Active Time: 30 minutes
Total Time: 30 minutes

- 1 (1½-pound) bunch Tuscan kale or another tender variety
- 3 tablespoons virgin olive oil, divided
- 2 cloves garlic, chopped
- ½ teaspoon salt
- ¼ teaspoon freshly ground black pepper
- 3 tablespoons red wine vinegar
- 1 tablespoon granular sugar substitute
- 1 teaspoon Dijon mustard
- ¼ teaspoon red pepper flakes

1. Remove and discard kale stems (or save for another use); chop leaves coarsely and rinse thoroughly.
2. Bring a large pot of salted water to a boil over high heat. Add kale and simmer until almost tender, about 3 minutes. Drain, squeezing out as much water as possible.
3. Heat 1 tablespoon oil in a large skillet over high heat. Add garlic and sauté until fragrant, about 30 seconds. Add kale, salt, and pepper; sauté until tender, about 3 minutes. Transfer to a bowl.
4. Reduce heat to medium; add remaining 2 tablespoons oil, vinegar, sugar substitute, mustard, and red pepper flakes. Sauté just long enough to heat through, about 1 minute.
5. Pour vinaigrette over kale; toss to coat. Serve hot.

TIP TIME

WAIT FOR JACK FROST

Kale tastes best after it has been hit with frost, meaning it's at its peak from October through March. Kale keeps for up to a week, though its flavor becomes more pronounced over time.

Creamy Red Cabbage with Dill*

Phases 3, 4

PER SERVING:
Net Carbs: 10 grams
Total Carbs: 14 grams
Fiber: 4 grams
Protein: 3 grams
Fat: 11 grams
Calories: 160

Makes: 6 (1-cup) servings
Active Time: 10 minutes
Total Time: 20 minutes

A natural with roast pork loin or tenderloin, this colorful dish is also delicious with chicken sausages or kielbasa.

3 tablespoons canola oil
1 medium yellow or white onion, thinly sliced
1 teaspoon caraway seeds
1 medium (1- to 1½-pound) head red cabbage, cored and thinly sliced
⅓ cup red wine vinegar
2 teaspoons granular sugar substitute
½ teaspoon salt
¼ teaspoon freshly ground black pepper
1 cup sour cream
¼ cup chopped fresh dill

1. Heat oil in a large saucepan over medium-high heat. Add onion and caraway; sauté until soft, about 2 minutes. Add cabbage and sauté until cabbage begins to soften, about 5 minutes.
2. Add vinegar, sugar substitute, salt, and pepper; sauté until cabbage is crisp-tender, about 3 minutes. Stir in sour cream and dill and serve right away.

TIP TIME

MAKE A CLEAN CUT

Use a ceramic or stainless-steel knife to cut cabbage; carbon steel reacts with compounds in cabbage to turn green cabbage black and red cabbage blue.

*See photo on color page 17

Sautéed Escarole, Cannellini Beans, and Tomatoes

Phases 2, 3, 4

Make sure your saucepan is as hot as possible—if not, the escarole will steam rather than sauté. If you can't find pancetta, which is cured (not smoked) pork belly, use 3 slices of bacon or an additional 2 tablespoons olive oil.

PER SERVING:
Net Carbs: 6 grams
Total Carbs: 11 grams
Fiber: 5 grams
Protein: 8 grams
Fat: 9 grams
Calories: 160

Makes: 6 (⅔-cup) servings
Active Time: 30 minutes
Total Time: 30 minutes

- 1 tablespoon plus 1 teaspoon virgin olive oil, divided
- 3 ounces pancetta, chopped (see above)
- ½ small yellow or white onion, finely chopped
- 1 clove garlic, chopped
- 1 large head escarole, cut crosswise into 1-inch strips
- ¼ teaspoon salt
- ⅛ teaspoon freshly ground black pepper
- 1 cup canned cannellini beans, drained and rinsed
- ½ cup quartered cherry tomatoes

1. Heat 1 tablespoon oil in a large skillet over very high heat. Add pancetta and sauté until well browned, about 4 minutes. Transfer to a paper-towel-lined plate to drain.
2. Spoon off and reserve about half the fat from skillet. Add half the onion to the skillet and sauté until soft, about 3 minutes. Add half the garlic and sauté until fragrant, about 30 seconds. Add half the escarole, half the salt, and half the pepper; sauté until escarole is just wilted, about 1 minute. Transfer to a medium bowl. Repeat with remaining fat, onion, garlic, escarole, salt, and pepper; transfer to bowl with reserved escarole.
3. Heat remaining teaspoon oil in skillet over high heat. Add beans and tomatoes; sauté to warm through, about 2 minutes. Return pancetta and escarole to skillet; sauté to heat through, about 1 minute. Serve hot.

TIP TIME

PRESERVE THE COLOR

Be sure to add salt to vegetables during the cooking process—it helps green vegetables maintain their vibrant color.

WEEKDAY

Swiss Chard with Pine Nuts

Phases 2, 3, 4

PER SERVING:
Net Carbs: 3 grams
Total Carbs: 4 grams
Fiber: 1 gram
Protein: 2 grams
Fat: 8 grams
Calories: 90

Makes: 6 (½-cup) servings
Active Time: 15 minutes
Total Time: 15 minutes

This classic dish combines the mellow, earthy taste of Swiss chard with sweet, crunchy pine nuts. Any chard is fine, but the colorful stems of ruby or rainbow chard look lovely against the deep green leaves.

1 (1- to 1¼-pound) bunch Swiss chard, leaves and stems separated
2 tablespoons virgin olive oil
1 clove garlic, chopped
½ teaspoon salt
¼ teaspoon freshly ground black pepper
3 tablespoons pine nuts, toasted

1. Chop chard leaves crosswise into 2-inch slices; cut stems into ½-inch pieces. Rinse thoroughly, then spin dry.
2. Heat oil in a large saucepan over high heat. Add garlic and sauté until fragrant, about 30 seconds. Add chard stems, salt and pepper; sauté until stems are almost tender, about 5 minutes. Add chard leaves and sauté until chard is completely tender, about 5 minutes. Stir in pine nuts and serve.

TIP TIME

CHARD CARE

Chard keeps for 3 to 5 days in the vegetable crisper. Look for bunches with glossy green leaves.

Variation: Swiss Chard with Pine Nuts and Golden Raisins

Phases 3, 4

Prepare Swiss Chard with Pine Nuts as above, adding 3 tablespoons golden raisins with the pine nuts.

Braised Lettuce

Phases 1, 2, 3, 4

If you think lettuce is just for salads, you've never tried braised lettuce. Popular in Victorian times, this simple and elegant side dish should never go out of fashion!

PER SERVING:
Net Carbs: 2 grams
Total Carbs: 3 grams
Fiber: 1 gram
Protein: 2 grams
Fat: 9 grams
Calories: 90

Makes: 4 servings
Active Time: 15 minutes
Total Time: 15 minutes

- 2 tablespoons butter
- 1 clove garlic, chopped
- 2 heads Boston or Bibb lettuce, halved lengthwise, rinsed well, and patted dry
- ½ cup chicken broth
- ¼ teaspoon salt
- ⅛ teaspoon freshly ground black pepper
- 2 tablespoons heavy cream

1. Melt butter in a large skillet over medium heat. Add garlic and sauté until fragrant, about 30 seconds. Add lettuce, cut side down, and cook 2 minutes. Turn lettuce over; add broth, salt, and pepper. Cover and simmer until lettuce is slightly wilted, about 3 minutes.
2. Add cream and simmer, uncovered, until liquid is reduced by half, about 5 minutes. Serve right away.

TIP TIME

THE BEST PRODUCE

Some supermarkets offer consistently better produce than others. Three signs of a good produce section are fast turnover—greens that sell quickly have much less chance of wilting—refrigerated shelves, and squeaky-cleanness. All three are a sure sign that veggies get the respect they deserve.

Variation: Braised Lettuce with Peas

Phases 3, 4

Prepare Braised Lettuce as above, adding ½ cup fresh or frozen peas with the cream. Garnish with 2 tablespoons thinly sliced mint leaves.

WEEKDAY

Green Beans with Lemon and Cumin

Phases 1, 2, 3, 4

PER SERVING:
Net Carbs: 3 grams
Total Carbs: 6 grams
Fiber: 3 grams
Protein: 1 gram
Fat: 3 grams
Calories: 50

Makes: 6 (½-cup) servings
Active Time: 20 minutes
Total Time: 25 minutes

You can also make this dish with yellow wax beans. The taste and texture are the same, although green beans are higher in folate and beta-carotene. Cumin, a spice used to make curry and chili powders, has a peppery taste; combined with lemon zest, it gives this simple dish a complex flavor.

1 pound green beans, trimmed
2 teaspoons butter
2 teaspoons extra-virgin olive oil
¾ teaspoon ground cumin
½ teaspoon salt
1 tablespoon freshly grated lemon zest
2 teaspoons freshly squeezed lemon juice
⅛ teaspoon freshly ground black pepper

1. Bring a medium pot of salted water to a boil. Add green beans and simmer until just tender, about 3 minutes. Drain; plunge beans into a large bowl of cold water to stop the cooking. Drain again.
2. Heat butter and oil in a large skillet over high heat. Add cumin and sauté until fragrant, about 15 seconds. Add beans, salt, lemon zest, lemon juice, and pepper; sauté until beans are crisp-tender and lightly browned, about 4 minutes. Serve hot.

TIP TIME

ONE POT, LESS WORK

Cut down on cleanup time by cooking the beans in a large pot. After draining the beans in a colander, wipe the pot dry and then sauté them in the same pot rather than in a skillet.

WEEKDAY

Roasted Cauliflower

Phases 2, 3, 4

Roasting sweetens and enriches the flavor of cauliflower. Cutting the florets into fan-shaped slices makes for a lovely presentation. If you like, use pale green broccoflower or a mixture of broccoli florets and cauliflower.

PER SERVING:

Net Carbs: 7 grams
Total Carbs: 11 grams
Fiber: 4 grams
Protein: 3 grams
Fat: 11 grams
Calories: 150

Makes: 4 (½-cup) servings
Active Time: 15 minutes
Total Time: 45 minutes

- 1 medium head cauliflower, broken into florets and cut into ⅓-inch slices
- 2 small yellow or white onions, cut into wedges
- 3 tablespoons virgin olive oil
- ¾ teaspoon salt, divided
- ¼ teaspoon freshly ground black pepper, divided

1. Heat oven to 450°F.
2. Combine cauliflower, onions, oil, salt, and pepper in a large jelly roll pan or shallow baking dish; toss well. Arrange in a single layer; roast, stirring occasionally, until tender and browned, about 30 minutes. Serve warm.

TIP TIME

A SPOTLESS HEAD

Unlike most vegetables, size doesn't impact the flavor of cauliflower, but be sure to choose one without brown spots.

Variation: Spicy Roasted Cauliflower

Phases 2, 3, 4

Prepare Roasted Cauliflower as above, adding 2 teaspoons ground cumin and 2 teaspoons ground coriander with the salt and pepper.

Cauliflower-Garlic Purée

Phases 2, 3, 4

PER SERVING:
Net Carbs: 4 grams
Total Carbs: 8 grams
Fiber: 4 grams
Protein: 3 grams
Fat: 9 grams
Calories: 110

Makes: 4 (½-cup) servings
Active Time: 10 minutes
Total Time: 20 minutes

Puréed cauliflower is a great low-carb alternative to mashed potatoes, but add the big taste of garlic and this dish stands on its own. Serve it with roast beef or poultry or use it to top shepherd's pie.

1 medium head cauliflower, separated into florets
4 cloves garlic
2 tablespoons butter
2 tablespoons heavy cream
Salt
Freshly ground black pepper

1. Bring a large saucepan of salted water to a boil over high heat. Add cauliflower and garlic, reduce heat to low, partially cover, and simmer until tender, about 10 minutes.
2. Drain; return cauliflower and garlic to saucepan and increase heat to medium-high. Cook, tossing, until all moisture has evaporated. Transfer to a food processor, add butter and cream, and purée. Stir in salt and pepper to taste and serve hot.

TIP TIME

THIS END UP

Cauliflower is quite perishable. Keep it cold and use within a few days. Refrigerate it with the stem end up, as condensation on the head can speed decay.

WEEKDAY

Spaghetti Squash with Cinnamon-Spice Butter

Phases 2, 3, 4

When baked to tenderness, the flesh of this squash shreds into spaghetti-like threads, hence its name. It's the easiest of winter squashes to prepare—just bake and serve. No peeling or dicing required!

PER SERVING:
Net Carbs: 6 grams
Total Carbs: 8
Fiber: 2 grams
Protein: 1 gram
Fat: 6 grams
Calories: 90

Makes: 6 (½-cup) servings
Active Time: 10 minutes
Total Time: 1 hour 10 minutes

1 (2½-pound) spaghetti squash
4 tablespoons (½ stick) butter
1½ tablespoons granular sugar substitute
¼ teaspoon ground cinnamon
¼ teaspoon ground allspice
⅛ teaspoon nutmeg
Salt
Freshly ground black pepper

1. Heat oven to 350°F.
2. Pierce squash in several places with a knife; set on a baking sheet. Bake until tender when pierced with a knife, about 1 hour.
3. Meanwhile, melt butter, sugar substitute, cinnamon, allspice. and nutmeg in a small saucepan over medium heat.
4. Cut squash in half lengthwise. Discard seeds; loosen strands with a fork and remove from the shell. Transfer to a large bowl; toss with spiced butter, then add salt and pepper to taste. Serve hot.

Variation: Spaghetti Squash with Garlic-Herb-Cheese Butter

Phases 2, 3, 4

Prepare squash as above, omitting the sugar substitute, cinnamon, allspice, and nutmeg. Instead, substitute ¼ cup grated Parmesan, 1 tablespoon chopped fresh parsley, 2 teaspoons chopped fresh oregano, and 1 clove garlic, chopped.

Sautéed Sugar Snap Peas with Mint

Phases 2, 3, 4

PER SERVING:
Net Carbs: 5 grams
Total Carbs: 8 grams
Fiber: 3 grams
Protein: 3 grams
Fat: 3 grams
Calories: 70

Makes: 8 (½-cup) servings
Active Time: 10 minutes
Total Time: 10 minutes

Sugar snaps are rounder and have larger peas than snow peas, which can also be used in this dish. In Phase 1, simply have a smaller portion.

- 2 tablespoons butter
- 1 pound sugar snap peas, strings removed
- 2 tablespoons chopped mint
- ¼ teaspoon salt
- ⅛ teaspoon freshly ground black pepper

Melt butter in large skillet over high heat. Add peas, mint, salt, and pepper; sauté until crisp-tender, about 3 minutes. Serve right away.

TIP TIME

NO STRINGS

To remove the strings on sugar snap pea pods, break off the stem end and peel back so the string comes away.

Variations: Summer Snap Pea Medley

Phases 3, 4

Prepare as above, adding 1 cup fresh or frozen corn kernels and 4 sliced scallions with the peas; sauté until almost crisp-tender, about 2 minutes. Add 2 cups halved cherry tomatoes and sauté about 1 minute more.

Sautéed Sugar Snap Peas with Bacon

Phases 2, 3, 4

In a large skillet over medium heat, cook 4 slices of bacon until crisp, about 5 minutes. Drain bacon, reserving fat. Raise heat to high, add 1 pound sugar snap peas, ⅛ teaspoon salt, and ⅛ teaspoon pepper to the bacon fat, and sauté until crisp-tender, about 3 minutes. Crumble bacon on top and serve.

Edamame Succotash

Phases 3, 4

Tender, buttery, enriched with cream, and paired with scallions, succotash made with edamame (green soybeans) is lower in carbs than the conventional dish made with lima beans. For a vegetarian version, use vegetable broth.

PER SERVING:
Net Carbs: 9
Total Carbs: 12
Fiber: 3 grams
Protein: 7 grams
Fat: 19 grams
Calories: 240

Makes: 4 (½-cup) servings
Active Time: 20 minutes
Total Time 20 minutes

WEEKDAY

- 2 tablespoons butter
- 3 scallions, thinly sliced
- 1 cup corn kernels, fresh or frozen and thawed
- 1 cup frozen, thawed shelled edamame
- ¾ cup chicken broth
- ½ cup heavy cream
- ½ teaspoon salt
- ¼ teaspoon freshly ground black pepper

1. Melt butter in medium skillet over high heat. Add scallions and corn; sauté until scallions are soft and corn is lightly browned, about 3 minutes.
2. Add edamame and broth; simmer, stirring occasionally, until corn and beans are tender and broth has evaporated, about 12 minutes. Add cream and simmer until sauce has thickened, about 4 minutes. Season with salt and pepper and serve warm.

TIP TIME

WITH AND WITHOUT PODS

You can find frozen edamame in the frozen vegetable aisle of any well-stocked supermarket year-round. They're sold both in the pod and shelled. This recipe calls for shelled edamame.

Butternut Squash Purée

Phases 3, 4

PER SERVING:
Net Carbs: 14 grams
Total Carbs: 18 grams
Fiber: 4 grams
Protein: 2 grams
Fat: 4 grams
Calories: 110

Makes: 6 (½-cup) servings
Active Time: 20 minutes
Total Time: 45 minutes

Butternut squash is widely available and easy to peel and seed, but Hubbard, delicata, or other winter squash can be substituted in this recipe.

- 1 small (2-pound) butternut squash, peeled, seeded, and cut into 1-inch cubes
- ½ small yellow or white onion, chopped
- 2 cloves garlic, chopped
- 1 cup water or chicken broth
- ¼ cup heavy cream
- Pinch ground nutmeg
- Salt
- Freshly ground black pepper

1. Combine squash, onion, garlic, and water in a large saucepan over medium-high heat; bring to a boil. Reduce heat to low, cover, and simmer until squash is tender, about 25 minutes.
2. Transfer mixture to a food processor and purée; return to saucepan. Stir in cream, nutmeg, and salt and pepper to taste; simmer over low heat to heat through. Serve warm.

TIP TIME

SQUASH TRADE-OFFS

You can find cut-up winter squash in the produce section of the supermarket, which is a time-saver, albeit with some reduction in nutrients. Cut squash will keep for a week in the fridge; a whole winter squash can be stored as long as 3 months at cool room temperature.

Variation: Lime-Cumin Butternut Squash Purée

Phases 3, 4

Prepare Butternut Squash Purée as above, replacing nutmeg with 1 teaspoon grated lime zest, 2 teaspoons fresh lime juice, and ½ teaspoon ground cumin.

Sweet Potato Pancakes

Phases 3, 4

Sweet potatoes, which are unrelated to the common white potato, are an excellent source of beta-carotene, although it's important to eat them with fat to absorb this micronutrient. Look for a sweet potato as close to one pound as possible—you'll save time peeling, and it will be easier to grate. These pancakes go well with a dollop of sour cream or a squeeze of lemon.

PER SERVING:
Net Carbs: 11 grams
Total Carbs: 14 grams
Fiber: 3 grams
Protein: 5 grams
Fat: 9 grams
Calories: 150

Makes: 8 (2-pancake) servings
Active Time: 30 minutes
Total Time: 30 minutes

- 1 pound sweet potatoes, peeled and grated
- 1 small yellow or white onion, grated
- ⅓ cup Atkins Cuisine All Purpose Baking Mix
- 2 large eggs
- 1 teaspoon salt
- ¼ cup canola oil

1. Combine sweet potatoes, onion, baking mix, eggs, and salt in a large bowl.
2. Heat oil in a large skillet over medium-high heat. Drop 2-tablespoon mounds of sweet potato mixture into pan, flattening slightly; fry in 3 to 4 batches until golden brown, about 2 minutes per side. Drain on paper towels and serve hot.

Variation: Orange-Spiced Sweet Potato Pancakes

Phases 3, 4

Prepare Sweet Potato Pancakes as above, adding 1 tablespoon grated orange zest and ½ teaspoon ground cinnamon to the sweet potato mixture.

Maple-Citrus Glazed Carrots

Phases 3, 4

PER SERVING:
Net Carbs: 3 grams
Total Carbs: 4 grams
Fiber: 1 gram
Protein: 0 grams
Fat: 4 grams
Calories: 50

Makes: 10 (½-cup) servings
Active Time: 10 minutes
Total Time: 20 minutes

To cut the active time in this recipe, use baby carrots—they don't need to be peeled, scrubbed, or cut. Just rinse and used as is. You won't reduce the total time, though, because baby carrots take longer to cook than sliced carrots: 15–20 minutes. The butter in this recipe enables your body to absorb and use the antioxidant beta-carotene in carrots.

3 tablespoons butter
1 pound carrots, cut into ¼-inch rounds
1 teaspoon ground ginger
½ teaspoon salt
⅛ teaspoon freshly ground black pepper
1 tablespoon sugar-free pancake syrup
2 teaspoons freshly grated lemon zest or 1 tablespoon freshly grated orange zest

Melt butter in large skillet over medium-high heat. Add carrots, ginger, salt, and pepper; sauté until carrots are tender and lightly browned, about 10 minutes. Stir in syrup and zest and serve.

TIP TIME

CARROT CHECK

Check the color of carrots (the bag may be striped to make them look brighter) and peek at the ends to be sure they're not cracked or split.

WEEKDAY

Roasted Root Vegetables

Phases 3, 4

Roasting root vegetables brings out their inherent sweetness. You can prepare the vegetables up to 4 hours ahead and rewarm them in a 450°F oven.

PER SERVING:
Net Carbs: 10 grams
Total Carbs: 13 grams
Fiber: 3 grams
Protein: 1 gram
Fat: 9 grams
Calories: 130

Makes: 8 (½-cup) servings
Active Time: 20 minutes
Total Time: 1 hour 5 minutes

- 3 medium carrots, peeled and cut into 1-inch chunks
- 2 medium parsnips, peeled and cut into 1-inch chunks
- 1 small rutabaga, peeled and cut into 1-inch chunks
- 1 medium white turnip, peeled and cut into 1-inch chunks
- 1 small yellow or white onion, quartered
- 5 tablespoons virgin olive oil
- 1½ teaspoons salt
- ½ teaspoon freshly ground black pepper
- 1 tablespoon chopped fresh sage
- 1 tablespoon chopped fresh thyme

1. Heat oven to 425°F.
2. Combine carrots, parsnips, rutabaga, turnip, onion, oil, salt, pepper, sage, and thyme in a large bowl. Transfer to 2 shallow roasting pans or jelly roll pans; roast, stirring every 10 minutes, until vegetables are tender and golden brown, about 45 minutes. Serve hot.

TIP TIME

FRESH IS BEST

You must wash and chop fresh herbs; their flavor is superior. Use about one-third the amount of dried herbs if necessary.

Variation: Curried Root Vegetables

Phases 3, 4

Prepare Roasted Root Vegetables as above, substituting 1 tablespoon curry powder for the sage and thyme.

Mushroom-Barley Pilaf

Phases 3, 4

PER SERVING:
Net Carbs: 7 grams
Total Carbs: 8 grams
Fiber: 1 gram
Protein: 3 grams
Fat: 5 grams
Calories: 80

Makes: 6 (¾-cup) servings
Active Time: 15 minutes
Total Time: 1 hour

To reduce cooking time significantly, soak barley overnight in cold water to cover by 2 inches. The next day, drain well before sautéing the barley, reduce broth to a total of one cup, and cook for only 15 minutes. Cremini mushrooms are darker than the common white button mushroom.

1 tablespoon butter
1 tablespoon virgin olive oil
1 large shallot, chopped
½ pound cremini mushrooms, chopped
¾ teaspoon salt
¼ teaspoon freshly ground black pepper
⅔ cup raw pearl barley
2 teaspoons fresh chopped thyme
1⅔ cups chicken broth

1. Heat butter and oil in a medium saucepan over high heat. Add shallot and sauté until soft, about 2 minutes. Add mushrooms, salt, and pepper; sauté until mushrooms are soft and light golden brown, about 5 minutes. Add barley and thyme; sauté to allow flavors to blend, about 1 minute.
2. Add broth, cover, and simmer over low heat until barley is tender, about 45 minutes. Serve hot.

Sausage, Fennel, and Leek Wild Rice Pilaf*

Phases 3, 4

Wild rice is actually not a true rice but a form of grass. As long as no additional ingredients are added, wild rice can be cooked ahead and refrigerated for up to 1 week or frozen for up to 3 months.

PER SERVING:
Net Carbs: 7 grams
Total Carbs: 8 grams
Fiber: 1 gram
Protein: 10 grams
Fat: 13 grams
Calories: 190

Makes: 6 (½-cup) servings
Active Time: 15 minutes
Total Time: 55 minutes

1 tablespoon virgin olive oil
½ pound bulk sweet or hot Italian sausage
¾ cup wild rice, rinsed
2 cups chicken broth
2 small leeks, light green and white parts only, outer layer removed
1 fennel bulb, chopped
Salt
Freshly ground black pepper

1. Heat oil in a medium saucepan over high heat. Add sausage and cook, breaking up with wooden spoon or spatula, until golden brown, about 5 minutes. Transfer sausage to a paper-towel-lined plate to drain and set aside. Spoon off all but 1 tablespoon fat.
2. Add rice to the sausage fat; stir to coat. Add broth and bring to a boil. Reduce heat to low, cover, and simmer, stirring occasionally, until half of the kernels have popped open and texture is slightly chewy, about 30 minutes.
3. Cut the leeks in half lengthwise and wash carefully in cold water to remove any dirt (see tip). Cut into ⅛-inch slices.
4. Add leeks and fennel, cover, and simmer, stirring occasionally, until vegetables are tender, about 10 minutes. Stir in sausage; season with salt and pepper to taste. Serve warm.

TIP TIME

GET OUT THE GRIT

After trimming the roots and the ends of the leaves, slit the leeks from top to bottom and rinse thoroughly, using the faucet spray attachment.

*See photo on color page 14

Chapter 8

SOUPS AND STEWS

Steaming bowls of soup and hearty stews tend to conjure up cold winter nights, with the savory dishes simmering for hours as they fill the air with soul-warming aromas. But what if you aren't home during the day? And how about those steamy summer days and evenings? Soups, stews, and braised dishes aren't just cold-weather foods. Mexico and the Louisiana bayous aren't known for their subzero wind chill factor, are they? Nonetheless, they're home to spicy mélanges such as Classic Chili con Carne and Gulf Oyster Stew.

Nor do all soups take forever to cook. Twelve of the soups and stews in this chapter can be on the table in no more than half an hour, and we've labeled those as suitable for weekdays. The remaining soup and stew recipes need no more than half an hour of active time to prepare, and are coded for the weekend. A major time-saver is that none requires you to make your own stock or broth. By using canned or Tetra-pak broth, you cut out much of the time involved in making soup from scratch. (Of course, if you prefer, use your own stock or broth in any of these recipes.)

That said, our weekend recipes do take a while to cook, but you can be doing something else around the house. By definition, stewing and braising are cooking techniques that include long simmering. They're best done with rather tough pieces of meat; as it simmers, the collagen in the tissue breaks down. The meat is tenderized and the liquid becomes rich, thick, and extremely flavorful.

SPEEDING UP THE PROCESS

But who says this kind of simmering needs to be done in a day? It's the rare stew or soup that doesn't improve if made a day or two in advance, and there's no law that says that simmering must proceed in one continuous chunk of time.

If you only have a half hour or so a night, break your stew making down over several evenings: brown the meat one night; sauté the vegetables the next, put everything together to simmer a third night, and on the fourth, either continue the simmering or add any finishes to it. Or rely on a slow cooker. You can assemble everything in the morning or the night before (and refrigerate it in the liner overnight), turn it on, and go to work, drive the kids to soccer practice, or pick up the dry cleaning while your soup or stew safely simmers all by itself.

STARTERS, MAIN DISHES, AND MORE

Our guideline for a recipe to be considered a main dish is that it include at least 16 grams of protein, so some of the soups are main dishes and others are better regarded as starters. Just check the nutritionals listed at the top of each recipe if you're unsure of which category they fall into. Or have a starter soup with a robust salad as a filling lunch. Nor is there any reason you can't have soup for breakfast if you feel like it—the Japanese regularly sip and slurp soup for the first meal of the day.

Also be sure to check for dozens more soup and stew recipes on www.atkins.com, where you'll find such old standbys as Beef Stew, Bouillabaisse, New England Clam Chowder, and Chicken Noodle Soup, along with dozens of others as diverse as Egg Drop Soup, White Gazpacho, and Guacamole Soup.

Chicken Chowder

Phases 1, 2, 3, 4

PER SERVING:
Net Carbs: 6 grams
Total Carbs: 9 grams
Fiber: 3 grams
Protein: 27 grams
Fat: 15 grams
Calories: 270

Makes: 4 (1¼-cup) servings
Active Time: 20 minutes
Total Time: 30 minutes

WEEKDAY

Rich and creamy chowder is too good to limit only to clams or fish. Chicken and cauliflower stand in for traditional clams and potatoes in our tasty rendition of the New England classic.

- 2 slices bacon, chopped
- 1 small yellow or white onion, chopped
- 1 celery rib, trimmed and thinly sliced
- 4 cups chicken broth
- 1 cup chopped cauliflower florets
- ¾ pound boneless, skinless chicken breasts, cut into ½-inch pieces
- ½ teaspoon salt
- ¼ teaspoon freshly ground black pepper
- ¼ teaspoon dried thyme
- ¼ teaspoon dried sage
- 1 tablespoon Dixie Carb Counters Thick-It-Up low-carb thickener*
- ½ cup heavy cream

1. Brown bacon in a large saucepan over medium-high heat, stirring occasionally, until just crisp, about 4 minutes. Spoon off all but 1 tablespoon of the fat and discard. Add onion and celery and sauté until soft, about 4 minutes.
2. Add broth, cauliflower, chicken, salt, pepper, thyme, and sage. Bring to a boil; reduce heat to medium, partially cover, and simmer until vegetables are just tender, about 5 minutes.
3. Whisk in thickener and simmer until soup thickens slightly, about 2 minutes. Stir in cream and simmer to heat through before serving.

Variation: Chicken-Corn Chowder

Phases 3, 4

Prepare Chicken Chowder as above, replacing cauliflower with 1 cup corn kernels (fresh or frozen); add to soup during last 5 minutes of cooking.

*Order from www.dixiediner.com.

Pork and Bok Choy Soba Soup

Phases 3, 4

Soba are traditional Japanese buckwheat noodles. Find them in the Asian section of the supermarket, along with hot chili paste.

PER SERVING:
Net Carbs: 12 grams
Total Carbs: 14 grams
Fiber: 2 grams
Protein: 17 grams
Fat: 12 grams
Calories: 230

Makes: 4 (1½-cup) servings
Active Time: 15 minutes
Total Time: 25 minutes

1 pound bone-in pork chops
¾ teaspoon salt, divided
¼ teaspoon freshly ground black pepper, divided
1 tablespoon canola oil, divided
½ teaspoon peeled and minced fresh ginger
1 clove garlic, minced
4½ cups chicken broth
1 tablespoon sugar-free hoisin sauce (see page 8)
1 (½-pound) bunch bok choy, greens and stems sliced into ½-inch pieces
2 ounces soba noodles
1 scallion, thinly sliced
½ teaspoon dark sesame oil
Hot chili paste or oil (optional)

1. Season pork with ¼ teaspoon salt and ⅛ teaspoon pepper. Heat 1½ teaspoons canola oil in a heavy-bottomed skillet over medium-high heat. Add pork and sear until browned, about 3 minutes per side. Remove from heat; let stand 5 minutes. Slice and reserve meat; discard bones.
2. Meanwhile, heat 1½ teaspoons canola oil in a heavy-bottomed saucepan over medium heat. Add ginger and garlic; sauté until fragrant and softened, about 1 minute. Add broth and hoisin sauce; bring to a boil. Add bok choy and noodles; reduce heat to low and simmer until tender, about 5 minutes. Add pork and heat through, about 1 minute; remove from heat.
3. Stir in scallion and sesame oil. Season with remaining salt and pepper; add hot chili paste to taste, if desired. Serve hot.

Variation: Vegetarian Ginger-Tofu Soba Soup

Phases 3, 4

Prepare as above, substituting 1 (10½-ounce) package firm silken tofu, cut into quarters and sliced into ¼-inch thick squares, for the pork. Increase garlic to 2 cloves and ginger to 1 teaspoon.

WEEKDAY

Thai Coconut-Shrimp Soup*

Phases 1, 2, 3, 4

PER SERVING:
Net Carbs: 6 grams
Total Carbs: 7 grams
Fiber: 1 gram
Protein: 20 grams
Fat: 17 grams
Calories: 260

Makes: 6 (1-cup) servings
Active Time: 20 minutes
Total Time: 30 minutes

WEEKDAY

Fresh ginger infuses this creamy soup with wonderful flavor. Be sure you use coconut milk, not cream of coconut. You'll find the former (along with fish sauce) in the Asian food section of most supermarkets. Cream of coconut is found with the cocktail mixers and is full of added sugar.

- 3 cups chicken broth
- 1 (13½-ounce) can unsweetened coconut milk
- 1 (1-inch) piece fresh ginger, peeled and cut into ⅛-inch slices
- 2 tablespoons fish sauce (nam pla or nuoc mam)
- 1 jalapeño, finely chopped
- 1 tablespoon freshly grated lime zest
- 1 teaspoon granular sugar substitute
- 1 pound medium shrimp, peeled and deveined
- 4 ounces button mushrooms, cut into ¼-inch slices (optional)
- 2 scallions, thinly sliced
- ¼ cup chopped fresh cilantro
- 1 tablespoon fresh lime juice

1. Combine broth, coconut milk, ginger, fish sauce, jalapeño, lime zest, and sugar substitute in a large saucepan over medium-low heat. Bring to a low boil, partially cover, and simmer for 10 minutes.
2. Add shrimp and mushrooms, if using; simmer until shrimp are cooked through, 3 to 5 minutes. Remove and discard ginger. Stir in scallions, cilantro, and lime juice and serve.

Variation: Thai Coconut-Vegetable Soup

Phases 1, 2, 3, 4

Prepare Thai Coconut-Shrimp Soup as above, replacing chicken broth with vegetable broth and substituting 1 cup shredded Napa cabbage and 8 ounces cubed firm tofu for the shrimp.

*See photo on color page 12

Chinese Hot-and-Sour Soup

Phases 1, 2, 3, 4

Rice vinegar adds a subtly sour punch to a rich, peppery broth in this Chinese classic. Be sure to use unseasoned or natural rice vinegar.

PER SERVING:
Net Carbs: 3 grams
Total Carbs: 5 grams
Fiber: 2 grams
Protein: 9 grams
Fat: 7 grams
Calories: 110

Makes: 4 (1½-cup) servings
Active Time: 20 minutes
Total Time: 20 minutes

WEEKDAY

⅓ cup unseasoned, unsweetened rice vinegar
1 tablespoon Dixie Carb Counters Thick-It-Up low-carb thickener*
1 teaspoon canola oil
1 clove garlic, finely chopped
½ cup button mushrooms, thinly sliced
4 cups chicken broth
1 (10½-ounce) package firm tofu, cut into ¼-inch dice
2 tablespoons tamari (see page 11)
½ teaspoon red pepper flakes
1 teaspoon dark (toasted) sesame oil

1. Whisk together vinegar and thickener in a small bowl; set aside.
2. Heat canola oil in a medium saucepan over medium-high heat. Add garlic and sauté until fragrant, about 30 seconds. Add mushrooms and sauté until slightly soft, about 3 minutes.
3. Add broth, tofu, tamari, and pepper flakes; cover and simmer until flavors blend, 5 to 7 minutes. Stir in vinegar mixture and simmer until soup thickens, about 1 minute. Add sesame oil just before serving.

TIP TIME

ABOUT BROTH

Canned and Tetra-pak broths and packaged bouillon cubes often contain preservatives, so read the ingredients list carefully before purchasing. Cubes tend to be saltier than liquid broths, so you may need to use a bit less salt than called for in the recipe.

*Order from www.dixiediner.com.

Creamy Cheddar Cheese Soup

Phases 1, 2, 3, 4

PER SERVING:
Net Carbs: 7 grams
Total Carbs: 9 grams
Fiber: 2 grams
Protein: 17 grams
Fat: 32 grams
Calories: 390

Makes: 4 (1-cup) servings
Active Time: 20 minutes
Total Time: 20 minutes

Low in carbs and high in protein, this basic cheese soup is a great vegetarian meal. Try using different cheeses, such as Monterey Jack, Parmesan, Gouda, or even blue cheese.

1 tablespoon butter
1 shallot, minced
2½ cups vegetable broth
1 tablespoon Dixie Carb Counters Thick-It-Up low-carb thickener*
1½ cups half-and-half
8 ounces Cheddar cheese, shredded (2 cups)
2 teaspoons paprika
½ teaspoon salt

1. Melt butter in a large saucepan over medium heat. Add shallot and sauté until soft, about 3 minutes. Add broth and bring to a simmer. Whisk in thickener; cook until mixture thickens, about 2 minutes.
2. Add half-and-half and simmer, stirring occasionally, until hot. Slowly whisk in cheese until melted and thoroughly combined. Stir in paprika and salt and serve.

TIP TIME

TOO HOT TO HANDLE

When working with jalapeños or any other hot chile, wear gloves to prevent irritation. Also be extremely careful not to touch your eyes.

Variation: Jalapeño-Cheddar Soup

Phases 1, 2, 3, 4

Prepare Cheddar Cheese Soup as above, adding one seeded and minced jalapeño with the shallot. Season with hot pepper sauce to taste just before serving.

*Order from www.dixiediner.com.

WEEKDAY

Versatile Vegetable Soup

Phases 2, 3, 4

Why spend money on canned soup when you can cook this tasty soup in less than half an hour? It's also infinitely adaptable. Swap out the vegetables for seasonal ones or your favorites. Or add leftover meat, poultry, or shellfish for a satisfying main dish suitable for Phase 1. Otherwise, limit your serving size to ¾ cup in this phase.

PER SERVING:
Net Carbs: 6 grams
Total Carbs: 8 grams
Fiber: 2 grams
Protein: 3 grams
Fat: 7 grams
Calories: 110

Makes: 4 (1½-cup) servings
Active Time: 15 minutes
Total Time: 25 minutes

2 tablespoons virgin olive oil
1 celery rib, trimmed and chopped
½ small white or yellow onion, chopped
½ teaspoon dried thyme
2 cloves garlic, sliced
1 small zucchini, cut into ¼-inch dice
½ cup chopped green beans
½ teaspoon salt
¼ teaspoon freshly ground black pepper
4 cups vegetable broth
1 large tomato, chopped
¼ cup chopped fresh parsley

1. Heat oil in a heavy-bottomed saucepan over medium-high heat. Add celery, onion, and thyme; sauté until vegetables are soft, about 5 minutes. Add garlic and sauté until fragrant, about 30 seconds.
2. Add zucchini, green beans, salt, and pepper; sauté until slightly soft, about 2 minutes Add broth and tomato; increase heat to high and bring to a boil. Reduce heat to low, cover, and simmer 10 minutes. Stir in parsley. Serve hot.

TIP TIME

NAME CHANGE

You might still hear them called "string beans," but most green beans have been bred so that they no longer have strings. Simply snap or snip off the ends before cooking.

Creamy Wild Mushroom Soup

Phases 2, 3, 4

PER SERVING:
Net Carbs: 5 grams
Total Carbs: 6 grams
Fiber: 1 gram
Protein: 5 grams
Fat: 21 grams
Calories: 230

Makes: 6 (1-cup) servings
Active Time: 30 minutes
Total Time: 30 minutes

WEEKDAY

Using wild mushrooms rather than regular button mushrooms adds great flavor to this creamy soup—try a blend of shiitake, cremini, or porcini. The sherry also adds depth of flavor, but if you prefer to avoid alcohol, replace the sherry with an additional ½ cup broth.

- 3 tablespoons butter
- ½ small yellow or white onion, coarsely chopped
- 1 clove garlic, chopped
- 1 pound mixed mushrooms, cleaned, trimmed, and sliced
- 1 teaspoon salt
- ¼ teaspoon freshly ground black pepper
- 4 cups vegetable broth
- ½ cup dry sherry
- 1 cup heavy cream

1. Melt butter in a large saucepan over high heat. Add onion and sauté until soft, about 3 minutes. Add garlic and sauté until fragrant, about 30 seconds.
2. Add mushrooms, salt, and pepper; sauté until soft and light brown, about 10 minutes. Add broth and sherry; simmer to allow flavors to blend, about 5 minutes.
3. Transfer soup to a blender. Holding down blender lid firmly with a folded kitchen towel, blend at low speed to purée (you may have to work in batches). Return soup to saucepan; return to a simmer over medium heat. Add cream and simmer, stirring constantly, until soup is thick, about 5 minutes.
4. Serve right away or refrigerate in an airtight container for up to 3 days. Reheat gently before serving.

TIP TIME

CLEANING MUSHROOMS

Rather than soaking or rinsing mushrooms in water to remove soil, which may allow them to absorb water and affect their delicate flavor, brush them off with a damp paper towel or a special mushroom brush.

Cream of Broccoli Soup

Phases 1, 2, 3, 4

This soup is quick and easy—just right as the starter for a weeknight supper, either chilled or hot off the stove. Replace the broccoli with cauliflower, or experiment with other vegetables, such as asparagus, artichokes, celery, or tomatoes. If you like, stir in 1 cup sharp Cheddar cheese after you've returned the purée to the saucepan.

PER SERVING:
Net Carbs: 3 grams
Total Carbs: 7 grams
Fiber: 4 grams
Protein: 3 grams
Fat: 17 grams
Calories: 180

Makes: 6 (1-cup) servings
Active Time: 30 minutes
Total Time: 30 minutes

WEEKDAY

- 4 cups vegetable or chicken broth
- 1 teaspoon salt
- ¼ teaspoon freshly ground black pepper
- 1 pound broccoli, cut into florets, stems peeled and cut into 1-inch pieces
- 1 tablespoon Dixie Carb Counters Thick-It-Up low-carb thickener*
- 1 cup heavy cream

1. Combine broth, salt, and pepper in a large saucepan over medium-high heat; bring to a boil. Add broccoli, reduce the heat to medium-low, and simmer until tender, about 15 minutes.
2. Transfer soup to a blender. Holding blender lid down firmly with a folded kitchen towel, blend at low speed to purée (you may have to work in batches). Return soup to saucepan; bring back to a simmer over medium-high heat. Whisk in thickener and cream; simmer, whisking occasionally, until thick and hot, about 5 minutes.
3. Serve hot or refrigerate in an airtight container for up to 3 days. Reheat before serving.

*Order from www.dixiediner.com.

Tomato Bisque

Phases 3, 4

PER SERVING:
Net Carbs: 10 grams
Total Carbs: 15 grams
Fiber: 5 grams
Protein: 7 grams
Fat: 29 grams
Calories: 330

Makes: 4 (1½-cup) servings
Active Time: 25 minutes
Total Time: 45 minutes

Bisques are thick, rich smooth soups. Traditionally, they're made with seafood, but vegetable bisques are also delicious. For the best flavor and color, use the ripest plum tomatoes you can find. When they aren't in season, canned Roma tomatoes are an acceptable substitute. To enjoy this soup in Phase 2, simply cut back slightly on the serving size.

- 2 tablespoons butter
- 1 small yellow or white onion, diced
- 3 cloves garlic, chopped
- 8 fresh ripe plum tomatoes, seeded and diced
- ¾ teaspoon salt
- ⅛ teaspoon freshly ground black pepper
- 3½ cups chicken broth
- 1 bay leaf
- 2 tablespoons Dixie Carb Counters Thick-It-Up low-carb thickener*
- 1 cup heavy cream
- ¼ cup chopped fresh basil

1. Melt butter in a medium saucepan over medium-high heat. Add onion and sauté until soft, about 3 minutes. Add garlic and sauté until fragrant, about 30 seconds.
2. Stir in tomatoes, salt, pepper, broth, and bay leaf; bring to a boil. Reduce heat to medium, cover, and simmer until tomatoes break down, about 20 minutes. Whisk in thickener.
3. Remove and discard bay leaf. Transfer soup to a blender. Holding down the blender lid with a folded kitchen towel, blend at low speed to purée (you may have to work in batches). Strain and return to saucepan. Stir in cream and basil; simmer over medium heat until heated through, about 2 minutes.

*Order from www.dixiediner.com.

Cold Roasted Tomato Soup*

Phases 2, 3, 4

This refreshing rustic soup is something like gazpacho, but because it lacks peppers and cucumbers you may find it easier to digest. Roasting the tomatoes gives them a slightly sweet, slightly smoky flavor.

PER SERVING:
Net Carbs: 9 grams
Total Carbs: 12 grams
Fiber: 3 grams
Protein: 5 grams
Fat: 8 grams
Calories: 140

Makes: 6 (1-cup) servings
Active Time: 15 minutes
Total Time: 1 hour, 45 minutes

- 3 pounds fresh plum tomatoes, halved lengthwise
- 1 small yellow or white onion, peeled and quartered
- 3 tablespoons extra-virgin olive oil
- 3 cloves garlic, peeled
- 1½ teaspoons salt
- ½ teaspoon freshly ground black pepper
- 4 cups chicken broth
- 6 tablespoons thinly sliced fresh basil

1. Heat oven to 450°F. Line a jelly roll pan with parchment paper or foil.
2. Combine tomatoes, onion, oil, garlic, salt, and pepper in a mixing bowl; toss to coat. Transfer ingredients to pan, making sure to include all of the liquid and arranging tomatoes cut side down in a single layer
3. Roast until tomato skins are puckered and browned, about 20 minutes, turning pan once halfway through. Let cool.
4. Add garlic and roasted vegetables and any juices to blender. Holding down blender lid firmly with a folded kitchen towel, blend at low speed until slightly chunky (you may have to work in batches). Add broth and pulse once to combine.
5. Refrigerate until ready to serve or at least 1 hour. Serve, topped with basil.

TIP TIME

PLUM TOMATOES

As their name implies, plum tomatoes are egg-shaped. They come in red or yellow varieties, and have a relatively thick skin, so they don't collapse when roasted. Their strong flavor also makes them ideal for roasting.

*See photo on color page 10

WEEKEND

Classic Chili con Carne

Phases 2, 3, 4

PER SERVING:
Net Carbs: 7 grams
Total Carbs: 10 grams
Fiber: 3 grams
Protein: 36 grams
Fat: 26 grams
Calories: 410

Makes: 12 (¾-cup) servings
Active Time: 15 minutes
Total Time: 1½ hours

WEEKEND

Our chili's got all the essentials and all the flavors without any excess carbs. Top it with shredded Cheddar, sour cream, or chopped parsley.

- 2 tablespoons canola oil
- 2½ pounds ground round or ground sirloin
- 2 pounds ground pork
- 1 large red bell pepper, stemmed, seeded, and chopped
- 1 large yellow or white onion, chopped
- ¼ cup chili powder
- 2 tablespoons ground cumin
- 1 teaspoon dried oregano
- 3 (14-ounce) cans diced tomatoes
- 1 cup cooked or canned pinto beans, drained
- 1 tablespoon plus 1½ teaspoons salt
- ¼ teaspoon freshly ground black pepper

1. Heat oil in a large heavy-bottomed saucepan or Dutch oven over high heat. Add beef and pork; sauté until browned, about 5 minutes.
2. Drain off all but 2 tablespoons fat. Add bell pepper, onion, chili powder, cumin, and oregano, stirring to coat meat and vegetables with spices; sauté until vegetables soften, about 5 minutes. Add tomatoes. Reduce heat to medium-low, cover, and simmer until chili gets thick and flavors blend, about 1 hour.
3. Add beans; heat through, about 3 minutes. Stir in salt and pepper and serve.

TIP TIME

CHUCK OR GROUND ROUND?

Ground beef that's 85 percent lean (sometimes called ground round) is the most versatile. Use a less fatty cut and your dish may end up dry or lacking in flavor; more fat can make it unpleasantly greasy. Ground sirloin is 80–85 percent lean and ground chuck is 75–80 percent lean.

Hungarian Goulash

Phases 1, 2, 3, 4

As with most stews, it's the long simmering that results in tender, melt-in-your-mouth chunks of meat, but once everything's in the pot, this dish requires very little attention. Low-carb noodles can soak up the delicious gravy, or you can serve the goulash on its own.

PER SERVING:
Net Carbs: 7 grams
Total Carbs: 9 grams
Fiber: 2 grams
Protein: 48 grams
Fat: 18 grams
Calories: 400

Makes: 4 (2-cup) servings
Active Time: 30 minutes
Total Time: 2 hours

- 2 slices bacon, cut into ¼-inch strips
- 1½ pounds beef chuck, cubed
- 1 teaspoon salt, divided
- ¼ teaspoon freshly ground black pepper
- 1 tablespoon virgin olive oil
- 1 large yellow or white onion, coarsely chopped
- 1 clove garlic, minced
- ¼ teaspoon caraway seeds
- 1½ tablespoons paprika, preferably Hungarian
- 3½ cups beef broth
- 1 ripe tomato, coarsely chopped
- 1 green bell pepper, stemmed, seeds and ribs removed, and cut into ½-inch strips
- ¼ cup sour cream

1. Cook bacon in a large saucepan or Dutch oven over medium-high heat until crisp, about 5 minutes. Transfer bacon to plate, leaving fat in pan.
2. Season beef with ½ teaspoon salt and the pepper. Working in batches, brown meat on all sides in pan, about 10 minutes per batch. Transfer to plate with bacon.
3. Add oil to pan. Add onion and sauté until soft, about 5 minutes. Add garlic, caraway seeds, and paprika; sauté until fragrant, about 1 minute. Stir in broth and bring to a boil; return beef and bacon to pot.
4. Reduce heat to medium-low, partially cover, and simmer until beef is beginning to become tender, about 1 hour.
5. Add tomato, bell pepper, and remaining ½ teaspoon salt; continue to simmer until vegetables are tender, about 30 minutes longer. Serve warm, garnished with sour cream.

Green Chile Pork Stew*

Phases 1, 2, 3, 4

PER SERVING:
Net Carbs: 4 grams
Total Carbs: 5 grams
Fiber: 1 gram
Protein: 32 grams
Fat: 32 grams
Calories: 450

Makes: 8 (1-cup) servings
Active Time: 15 minutes
Total Time: 2 hours 30 minutes

WEEKEND

Garnish this Southwestern favorite with sour cream, sliced black olives, sliced avocado, or grated Jack cheese. Use low-carb tortillas, if you like, to scoop up the stew.

- 2½ pounds boneless country-style pork ribs, cut into ¾-inch cubes
- 1¾ cups chicken broth, divided
- 2 medium yellow or white onions, chopped
- 4 cloves garlic, crushed
- 2 (10-ounce) cans diced tomatoes
- 2 cups canned roasted poblano chiles
- 2 teaspoons dried oregano
- 1 teaspoon ground cumin
- ¼ teaspoon salt
- ¼ cup chopped fresh cilantro
- 2 tablespoons freshly squeezed lime juice

1. Combine pork, ½ cup broth, onions, and garlic in large saucepan over medium-high heat; cook until liquid evaporates and meat begins to brown, about 45 minutes.
2. Add remaining broth, scraping up any browned bits. Add tomatoes, chiles, oregano, cumin, and salt. Reduce heat to medium-low, cover, and simmer until pork is fork-tender, about 1½ hours. Stir in cilantro and lime juice just before serving.

TIP TIME

ROASTING POBLANOS

To roast fresh poblanos, heat oven to 475°F. Place peppers on an ungreased baking sheet and roast until blackened, about 40 minutes; transfer to a paper or plastic bag. Close bag tightly; set aside until peppers are cool enough to handle, about 15 minutes. When cool, remove seeds and stems and rub off blackened peel.

*See photo on color page 11

Sea Scallops Étouffée

Phases 2, 3, 4

Étouffée (the word means "smothered" in French) is a thick, rich, and spicy Cajun stew. It's traditionally made with crawfish, but sea scallops are easier to come by if you don't live near the Big Easy.

PER SERVING:
Net Carbs: 9 grams
Total Carbs: 11 grams
Fiber: 2 grams
Protein: 21 grams
Fat: 18 grams
Calories: 290

Makes: 4 (1-cup) servings
Active Time: 15 minutes
Total Time: 40 minutes

- 6 tablespoons butter
- 2 medium yellow or white onions, chopped
- 4 celery ribs, trimmed and chopped
- 1 green bell pepper, stemmed, seeds and ribs removed, and chopped
- 1 pound sea scallops
- 2 bay leaves
- 1 cup chicken broth
- 1 teaspoon Dixie Diner's Thick-It-Up low-carb thickener*
- 1 teaspoon salt
- ¼ teaspoon cayenne, or to taste
- ¼ cup chopped fresh parsley
- 1 scallion, sliced

1. Melt butter in a large skillet over medium-high heat. Add onions, celery, and pepper; sauté until soft and slightly colored, about 10 minutes.
2. Add scallops and bay leaves; simmer until scallops lose most of their translucence, about 5 minutes (do not overcook). Add broth, thickener, salt, and cayenne; stir until sauce thickens, about 2 minutes. Stir in parsley and scallion; serve right away.

TIP TIME

THE SCOOP ON SCALLOPS

Whether you choose sea scallops (up to 1½ inches in diameter; used in this recipe), bay scallops (about ¾ inch), or calicos (up to ½ inch), they should be firm, with translucent flesh. Bay and sea scallops are sweeter than calicos. Smaller scallops require very little cooking.

*Order from www.dixiediner.com.

WEEKEND

Gulf Oyster Stew

Phases 2, 3, 4

PER SERVING:
Net Carbs: 10 grams
Total Carbs: 11 grams
Fiber: 1 gram
Protein: 8 grams
Fat: 34 grams
Calories: 370

Makes: 4 (1-cup) servings
Active Time: 15 minutes
Total Time: 40 minutes

WEEKEND

Oyster stew gets updated with the addition of mushrooms and spinach, which blend harmoniously with cream and oysters.

1 cup heavy cream
1 cup half-and-half
1½ cups chicken broth
1 cup freshly shucked oysters, liquor reserved
½ cup sliced shiitake mushrooms
½ teaspoon salt
¼ teaspoon freshly ground black pepper
Dash hot pepper sauce
1½ cups baby spinach leaves, thinly sliced
1 tablespoon butter
1 tablespoon chopped fresh tarragon

1. Combine cream, half-and-half, broth, oyster liquor, mushrooms, salt, pepper, and hot pepper sauce in a medium saucepan. Bring to just under a boil over high heat. Reduce heat to medium-low and simmer, uncovered, until reduced by about one-third, about 20 minutes.
2. Add oysters and cook until they begin to curl, about 2 minutes. Stir in spinach and cook until just wilted, about 1 minute. Remove from heat; stir in butter and tarragon until butter has melted. Serve right away.

TIP TIME

OYSTERS AHOY

Oyster shells should be tightly closed or snap shut if tapped. Shucked meat should be beige, and the broth, or liquor as it's called, should be only slightly cloudy.

Chapter 9

CHICKEN AND TURKEY ENTRÉES

Whether you're looking for a fast weeknight supper, a luncheon salad, or a holiday feast, poultry may well be your first choice. From Thai Chicken Curry and Chicken Paprikash, a Hungarian favorite, to such good old American favorites as Beer-Can Grilled Chicken or Green Goddess Grilled Chicken, poultry is always popular, versatile, and satisfying. Its comparatively bland flavor marries well with a variety of seasonings and sauces. You can also usually substitute one bird for another, making a duck curry or stuffing a few Rock Cornish hens instead of a single chicken. Poultry is equally adaptable as a substitute in virtually all pork recipes, and in lieu of beef or fish in many others.

CHICKEN CHOICES

Because there are so many forms of chicken available, it's easy to simply reach for skinless, boneless chicken breasts when you're at the supermarket. And while this particular cut has many assets—it cooks quickly, it goes with a variety of seasonings from any number of cuisines, and there's virtually no waste—like anything else, it can become boring. As the recipes in this chapter attest, other cuts are every bit as easy to prepare and as versatile; some are as quick, too. The simplest swap is to select skinless, boneless chicken thighs, which can be used in place of breasts in almost all recipes. Their richer flavor stands up well to highly seasoned dishes. You might want to save the chicken breasts for delicate Chicken Cutlets Milanese, but use the thighs in curries, stews, or fricassees.

Don't be afraid to reach for bone-in or skin-on chicken, either. Chicken parts are available by part (all drumsticks, all thighs, etc.) or as a cut-up chicken (two breasts, two thighs, two drumsticks, two wings, and the back). The skin is especially beneficial if you're broiling or grilling, as it helps to keep the meat from drying out. And although boneless meat cooks faster, cuts on the bone are often more flavorful. One of the bonuses of following the Atkins Diet is that it's fine to eat the crispy, tasty skin of chicken and other poultry. All poultry has 0 grams of Net Carbs.

BUYING POULTRY

Chicken picking is a matter of trading convenience or taste for price. Taste-wise, organic and free range usually win out over conventional birds, but you pay for those benefits. Convenience-wise, skinless, boneless cuts are easier to work with and cook faster. You pay for that, too. Here's how to decode the labels:

- *Free-range/free-roaming* chickens get access to the outdoors. Of course, this doesn't mean they use it; it just means there's a door and a yard.
- *Hormone-free and/or antibiotic-free* birds, as the names imply, have not been fed or injected with hormones and/or antibiotics, but this doesn't necessarily mean that they have been feed organic food or are free range.
- *Natural* means no artificial ingredients or colorings in feed and minimal processing.
- *Organic* chickens get organic feed and access to the outdoors, and they aren't given hormones or antibiotics.
- *Kosher* chickens are treated with salt to remove blood, giving them a distinctly salty flavor. The brining effect makes chicken hold its juices. Kosher chickens are fed a special diet, aren't given hormones, and can roam freely in an indoor area.
- *Fresh* is not a synonym for "not frozen." Fresh poultry can be stored at temperatures as low as 26°F. (Frozen birds are stored as low as 0°F.)

COOKING POULTRY

The old adage refers to having "a chicken in every pot," but it could just as easily be an oven, grill, or skillet: poultry can be grilled, broiled, stir-fried, deep-fried, braised, poached, roasted, sautéed, and even smoked. You'll find most of these techniques used in the recipes in this chapter. What you won't find are such basics as Roast Chicken and Roast Turkey, which can be found at www.atkins.com, along with Chicken and Dumplings, Chicken Cordon Bleu, Chicken Pot Pie, Oven-Fried Chicken, and dozens of other dishes.

Beer-Can Grilled Chicken

Phases 1, 2, 3, 4

Try this novel method of cooking chicken at your next barbecue. You can also cook chicken this way in the oven—just set the beer can in a roasting pan and roast the bird in a 400°F oven for about an hour.

PER SERVING:
Net Carbs: 1 gram
Total Carbs: 2 grams
Fiber: 1 gram
Protein: 49 grams
Fat: 49 grams
Calories: 680

Makes: 4 servings
Active Time: 20 minutes
Total Time: 1 hour 30 minutes

1½ teaspoons salt
½ teaspoon freshly ground black pepper
1 teaspoon paprika
1 teaspoon chili powder
¾ teaspoon dried thyme
½ teaspoon garlic powder
½ teaspoon ground cumin
1 (3½- to 4-pound) chicken
1 tablespoon virgin olive oil
1 (12-ounce) can low-carb beer

1. Combine salt, pepper, paprika, chili powder, thyme, garlic powder, and cumin in a small bowl. Pat chicken dry with paper towels. Rub inside and outside with oil and then the spice mixture.
2. Prepare a grill for indirect heat grilling and set a drip pan in the center of the floor of the grill. (A disposable aluminum cake pan works well as a drip pan.) Arrange charcoal around drip pan. Oil grill grate.
3. Open beer can; pour out about one-fourth of the beer. Holding the chicken upright, lower it onto the beer can. Stand the chicken upright on grill—the legs will support it and keep it from toppling over.
4. Cover grill and cook chicken until juices run clear when thickest part of thigh is pierced with a fork or a thermometer inserted into thigh, not touching bone, registers 170°F, about 1 to 1½ hours. Transfer chicken to a cutting board; let stand 10 minutes before carving.

TIP TIME

LOW-CARB BREW

Low-carb beer typically contains 2–7 grams of Net Carbs per 12-ounce serving (compared to 11–13 grams for regular beers). Don't assume that "lite" beer is low in carbs. Check the label to be sure.

Tarragon Braised Chicken

Phases 1, 2, 3, 4

PER SERVING:
Net Carbs: 3 grams
Total Carbs: 3 grams
Fiber: 0 grams
Protein: 34 grams
Fat: 35 grams
Calories: 480

Makes: 6 servings
Active Time: 25 minutes
Total Time: 45 minutes

WEEKEND

Chickens are traditionally cut into eight serving pieces: two breasts, two drumsticks, two thighs, and two wings. If you're armed with a sharp and sturdy knife, it's fairly simple to do, but it's easier to buy packages of cut-up chicken at your supermarket.

1 (3½- to 4-pound) chicken, cut up
¾ teaspoon salt, divided
⅛ teaspoon
1 tablespoon canola oil
2 scallions, thinly sliced
4 ounces button mushrooms, thinly sliced (1½ cups)
⅓ cup dry white wine
½ cup half-and-half
2 teaspoons Dijon mustard
1 tablespoon chopped fresh tarragon or 1 teaspoon dried
1 plum tomato, seeded and diced

1. Pat the chicken dry and season with ½ teaspoon salt and the pepper. Heat oil over medium-high heat in a large skillet with a tight-fitting lid. Add chicken; sear until golden brown, about 5 minutes each side. Transfer chicken to a plate. Spoon off all but 1 tablespoon of fat from the skillet.
2. Reduce heat to medium. Add scallions and mushrooms to skillet and sauté until mushrooms are soft, about 5 minutes. Stir in wine and let simmer 1 minute.
3. Add chicken and any juices that have accumulated on plate; reduce heat to medium-low, cover, and simmer until juices run clear when pierced with a fork, about 20 minutes.
4. Transfer chicken to a platter. Add half-and-half, mustard, tarragon, tomato, and remaining ¼ teaspoon salt to skillet. Simmer until flavors are blended and sauce is slightly thickened, about 3 minutes. Pour over chicken and serve.

Chicken Paprikash

Phases 1, 2, 3, 4

Make this hearty and satisfying dish on a cold winter night. It's traditionally served over egg noodles. Instead, substitute veggie noodles: use a vegetable peeler to cut thin lengthwise strips from zucchini or yellow squash and cook them briefly in boiling salted water.

PER SERVING:

Net Carbs: 2 grams
Total Carbs: 3 grams
Fiber: 1 gram
Protein: 34 grams
Fat: 38 grams
Calories: 500

Makes: 6 servings
Active Time: 20 minutes
Total Time: 1 hour 15 minutes

- 2 tablespoons butter
- 2 scallions, sliced
- 2 cloves garlic, thinly sliced
- ¾ teaspoon red pepper flakes
- 1½ tablespoons sweet paprika, divided
- 1 (3½- to 4-pound) chicken, cut up
- 2 cups sliced button mushrooms
- ¾ cup water
- ¾ teaspoon salt
- 1 bay leaf
- ½ cup sour cream
- 1 teaspoon Dixie Carb Counters Thick-It-Up thickener*

1. Melt butter in a large skillet or Dutch oven set over high heat. Add scallions and garlic; sauté until softened, about 2 minutes. Stir in red pepper flakes and 1 tablespoon paprika; sauté until fragrant, about 30 seconds.
2. Add chicken pieces, skin side down, and sear 3 minutes. Add mushrooms, water, salt, and bay leaf; bring to a boil. Reduce heat to low, cover, and simmer until chicken is cooked through, about 45 minutes; turn chicken halfway through.
3. Transfer chicken to a plate. Spoon off fat from sauce and discard. Remove and discard bay leaf. Increase heat to high and boil liquid until reduced to about 1 cup, about 5 minutes.
4. Remove from heat and gradually stir in sour cream, thickener, and remaining ½ tablespoon paprika. Reduce heat to medium-low and bring sauce to a simmer, stirring constantly. Return chicken to pot and simmer until heated through.

WEEKEND

*Order from www.dixiediner.com.

Poached Chicken Breasts in Mornay Sauce

Phases 1, 2, 3, 4

PER SERVING:
Net Carbs: 2 grams
Total Carbs: 3 grams
Fiber: 1 gram
Protein: 31 grams
Fat: 23 grams
Calories: 350

Makes: 6 servings
Active Time: 15 minutes
Total Time: 30 minutes

WEEKDAY

This is fast food at its elegant best. The mild Mornay sauce can also be used in a variety of gratins or soufflés. Traditionally thickened with a roux (a flour-and-fat mixture), our version uses heavy cream and low-carb thickener instead.

Sauce

1 cup heavy cream
1 cup water
½ small yellow or white onion, coarsely chopped
1 teaspoon salt
¼ teaspoon freshly ground pepper
Pinch ground nutmeg
1 tablespoon Dixie Carb Counters Thick-It-Up thickener*
½ cup grated Gruyère cheese
1 tablespoon butter

Chicken

6 boneless, skinless chicken breast halves
3 bay leaves
6 sprigs parsley
1 teaspoon salt
½ teaspoon freshly ground black pepper

1. For sauce, combine cream, water, onion, salt, pepper, and nutmeg in a small saucepan over medium heat; bring to a simmer. Remove from heat; let stand 15 minutes. Strain the cream mixture and return to the saucepan. Set aside.
2. While the sauce is standing, put chicken, bay leaf, parsley, salt, and pepper in a large saucepan; add enough cold water to cover. Bring to a boil, cover, reduce heat to medium-low, and simmer until chicken is just cooked through, about 10 minutes.
3. While chicken is simmering, place the saucepan with the sauce over medium heat. Whisk in thickener; cook until sauce thickens, about 3 minutes. Remove from heat; swirl in cheese and butter until melted.
4. Place the cooked chicken on a serving plate, patting dry any liquid with a paper towel; pour the sauce over it. Serve right away.

*Order from www.dixiediner.com.

Mushroom-Herb-Stuffed Chicken Breasts

Phases 1, 2, 3, 4

This recipe calls for flavorful shiitake mushrooms, but you can use any other variety (or combination) you'd like.

PER SERVING:
Net Carbs: 2 grams
Total Carbs: 3 grams
Fiber: 1 gram
Protein: 41 grams
Fat: 14 grams
Calories: 300

Makes: 4 servings
Active Time: 20 minutes
Total Time: 55 minutes

- 3 tablespoons butter, divided
- ½ pound fresh shiitake mushrooms, wiped clean, trimmed, and minced
- ½ small yellow or white onion, minced
- 2 cloves garlic, minced
- 2 tablespoons dry sherry
- 3 tablespoons chopped fresh parsley
- ½ teaspoon chopped fresh thyme
- ¾ teaspoon salt, divided
- ⅛ teaspoon freshly ground black pepper
- 4 bone-in chicken breast halves (about 2 pounds)

1. Heat oven to 400°F.
2. Melt 2 tablespoons butter in a large skillet over medium-high heat. Add mushrooms and onion; sauté until mushrooms have released their liquid, about 5 minutes. Stir in garlic and sherry; cook 1 minute longer. Remove from heat; stir in parsley, thyme, ½ teaspoon salt, and pepper.
3. Using a thin sharp knife, cut a pocket in the thicker part of the breast, being careful not to cut all the way through; stuff mushroom mixture into pockets.
4. Set chicken, skin side up, in a 9-by-13-inch baking pan. Melt remaining tablespoon butter and brush on chicken. Season with remaining ¼ teaspoon salt. Bake until cooked through, about 35 minutes. Serve warm.

TIP TIME

IS IT DONE YET?

To be sure a chicken breast is properly cooked, insert an instant-read meat thermometer (not touching the bone), which should read 165°F. Try not to prick the breast much, which will make the juices run out. Whole chickens must be brought to an internal temperature of 180°F.

Jerk Chicken

Phases 1, 2, 3, 4

PER SERVING:
Net Carbs: 5 grams
Total Carbs: 7 grams
Fiber: 2 grams
Protein: 34 grams
Fat: 17 grams
Calories: 320

Makes: 4 servings
Active Time: 10 minutes
Total Time: 4 hours 55 minutes

WEEKEND

This searingly hot Jamaican specialty is a favorite worldwide. The chiles and marinade are so fiery it's best to avoid contact with your skin—use plastic gloves, and wash your hands after you remove them. Offset the heat by serving with cooling Cucumber-Dill Salad (page 83).

6 scallions, sliced
2 cloves garlic, minced
3 Scotch bonnet chile peppers, seeded and minced (see tip)
¼ cup canola oil
2 tablespoons freshly squeezed lime juice
2 tablespoons ground allspice
4 teaspoons mustard powder
2 teaspoons salt
2 teaspoons granular sugar substitute
1 teaspoon ground cinnamon
4 bone-in, skin-on chicken breast halves

1. Combine scallions, garlic, peppers, oil, lime juice, allspice, mustard, salt, sugar substitute, and cinnamon in a food processor or blender; purée. Transfer to a resealable plastic bag or glass baking dish; add chicken and turn to coat. Refrigerate at least 4 hours and preferably overnight, turning once.
2. Heat oven to 450°F.
3. Line a baking sheet with foil. Remove chicken from marinade, letting excess drain off; transfer to baking sheet. Bake until just cooked through, 30–40 minutes.

TIP TIME

HEAT WAVE

Don't let the Scotch bonnet chile's small size fool you. Irregularly shaped and yellow, orange, or red, it's a close relation of the Jamaican hot chile and the habañero chile, either of which can replace it in this or any other recipe.

Chicken Cutlets Milanese

Phases 2, 3, 4

This is the classic preparation for breaded chicken cutlets, with a low-carb twist. They're great with just lemon wedges, or see the variations below for quick pan sauces.

PER SERVING:
Net Carbs: 2 grams
Total Carbs: 4 grams
Fiber: 2 grams
Protein: 30 grams
Fat: 18 grams
Calories: 300

Makes: 4 servings
Active Time: 20 minutes
Total Time: 20 minutes

¼ cup Atkins Cuisine All Purpose Baking Mix
½ teaspoon freshly ground black pepper
½ teaspoon salt
1 large egg
2 tablespoons heavy cream
8 (4-ounce) chicken cutlets
3 tablespoons virgin olive oil
1 lemon, cut into wedges

1. Combine baking mix, pepper, and salt in a shallow dish. Beat egg and cream in another shallow dish. Dip cutlets in egg wash, then in baking mix to coat. Set on waxed paper.
2. Heat 1½ tablespoons oil in a very large skillet over medium-high heat. Add 4 cutlets and sear until golden and cooked through, about 3 minutes per side. Transfer to a platter; cover loosely to keep warm. Repeat with remaining 1½ tablespoons oil and cutlets.
3. Serve with lemon wedges.

WEEKDAY

Variations: Chicken Cutlets with Lemon-Caper Sauce*

Phases 2, 3, 4

Prepare Chicken Cutlets Milanese as above through Step 2. Transfer cutlets to a heatproof platter or dish; keep warm in a 200°F oven. Spoon off any oil in pan and add 1 cup chicken broth. Bring to a simmer and cook until reduced to ¼ cup, about 7 minutes, scraping up any brown bits from the bottom of the pan. Turn off the heat and add 2 tablespoons drained capers, 2 tablespoons chopped parsley, ¼ teaspoon salt, ⅛ teaspoon freshly

*See photo on color page 16

ground black pepper, and 2 teaspoons freshly squeezed lemon juice. Add 2 tablespoons cold butter, whisking until melted. Serve cutlets with sauce on the side, omitting lemon wedges.

Chicken Cutlets Parmesan

Phases 2, 3, 4

Heat oven to 375°F. Prepare Chicken Cutlets Milanese as on the preceding page through Step 2. Transfer cutlets to a baking dish. Spoon 1½ cups low-carb (no added sugar) tomato sauce over cutlets. Top with 1¾ cups shredded mozzarella and ½ cup grated Parmesan. Bake until cheese is melted and sauce is heated through, 10 to 12 minutes. Top with 3 tablespoons slivered basil leaves and serve, omitting the lemon wedges.

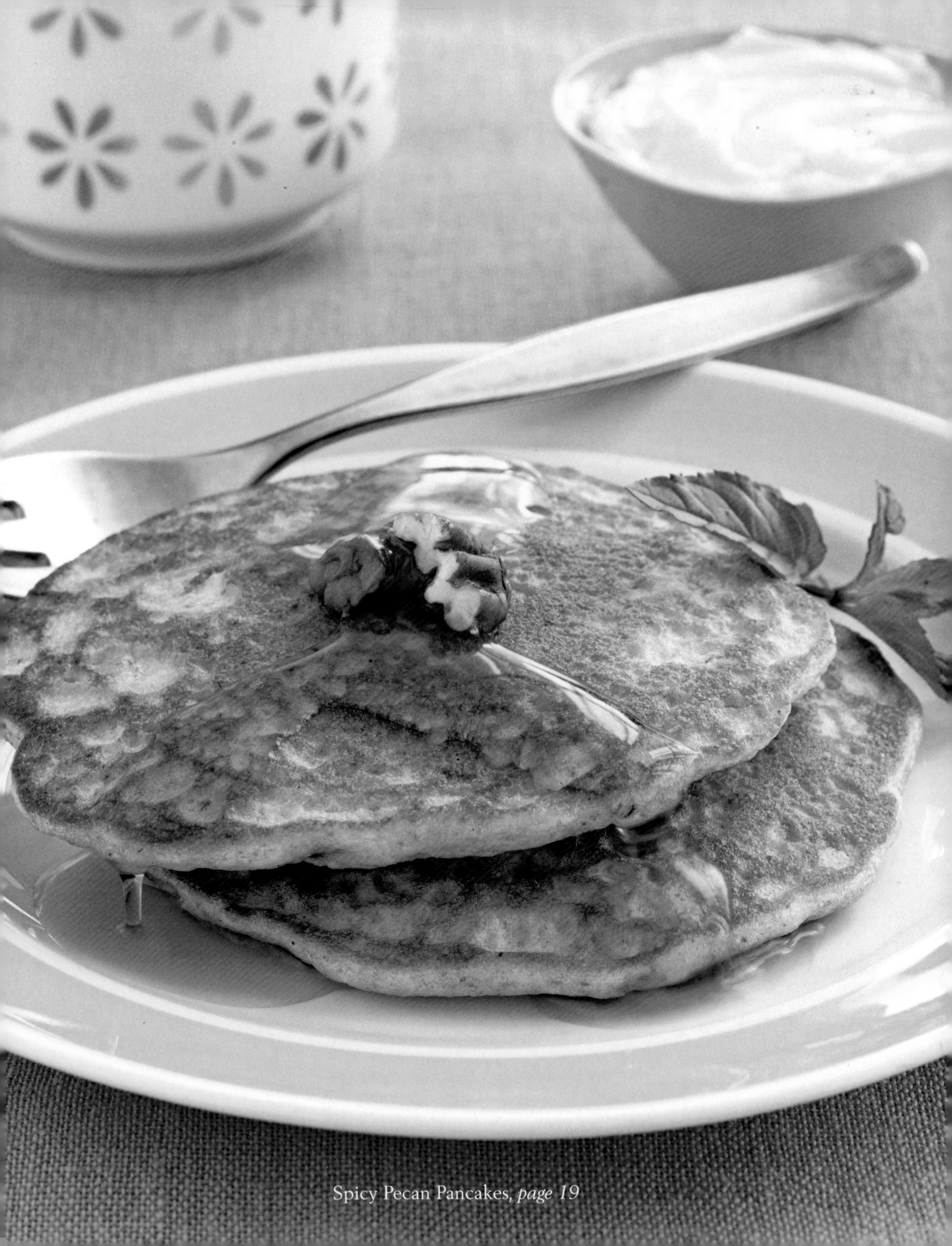

Spicy Pecan Pancakes, *page 19*

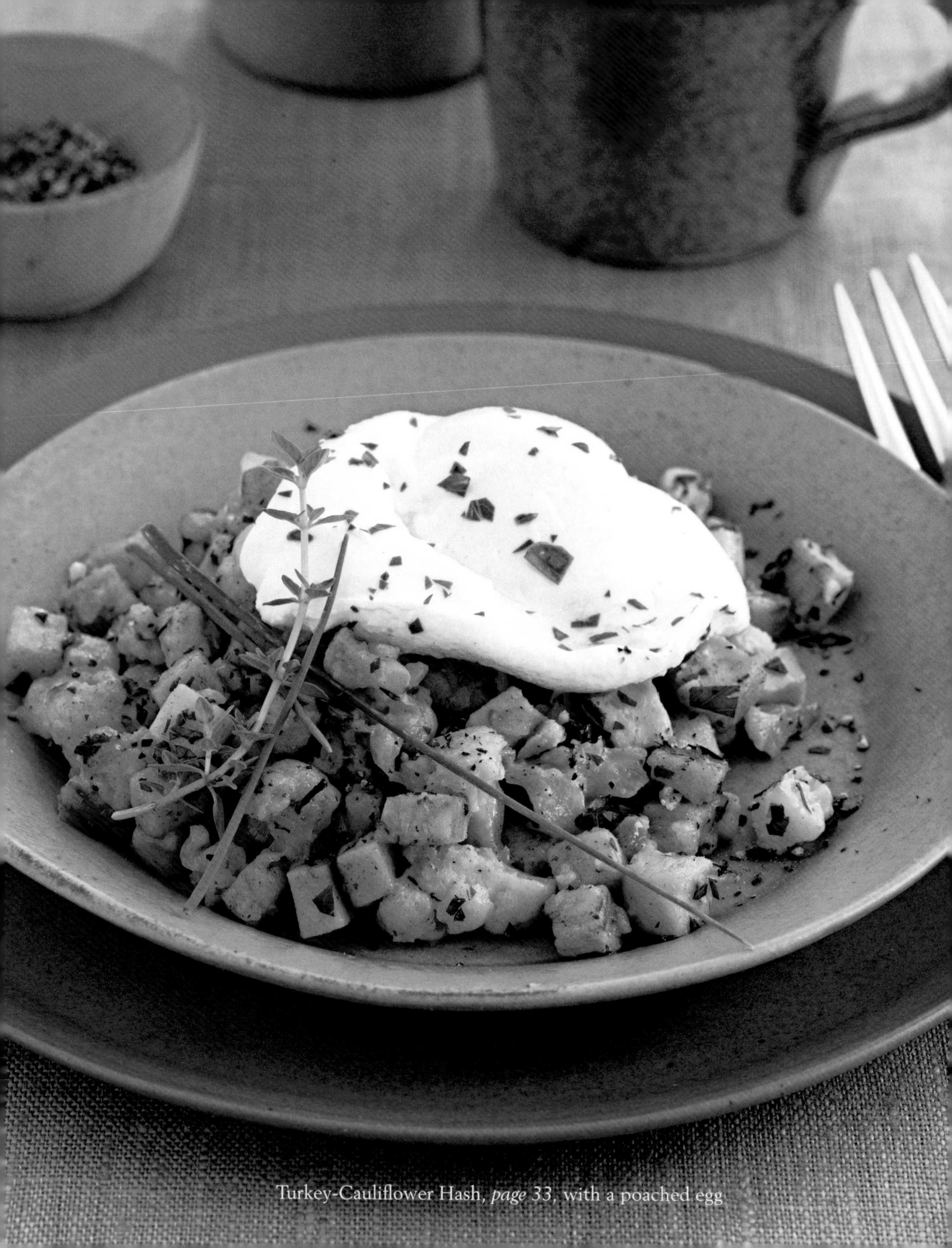

Turkey-Cauliflower Hash, *page 33*, with a poached egg

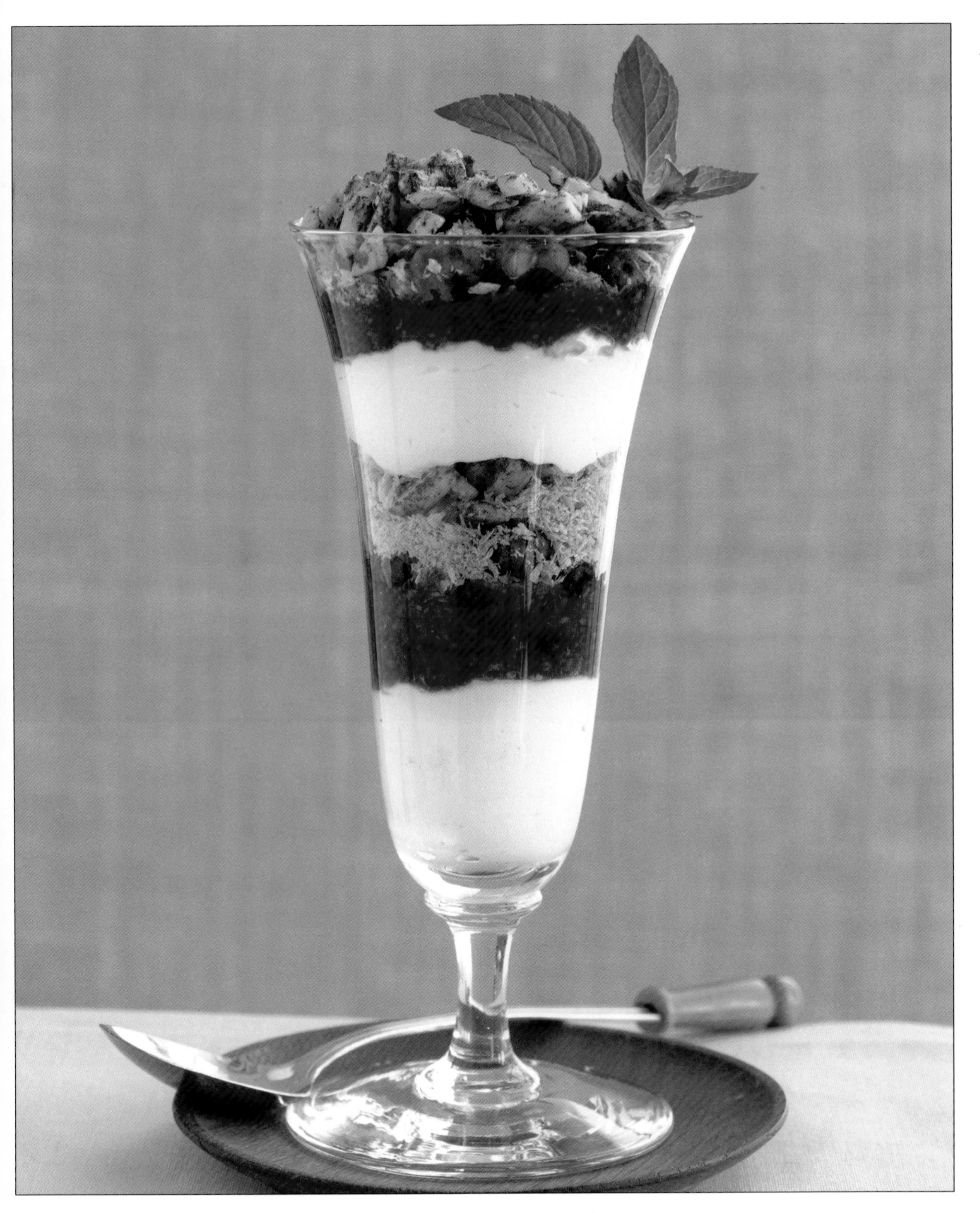

Crunchy Tropical Berry and Almond Breakfast Parfait, *page 25*

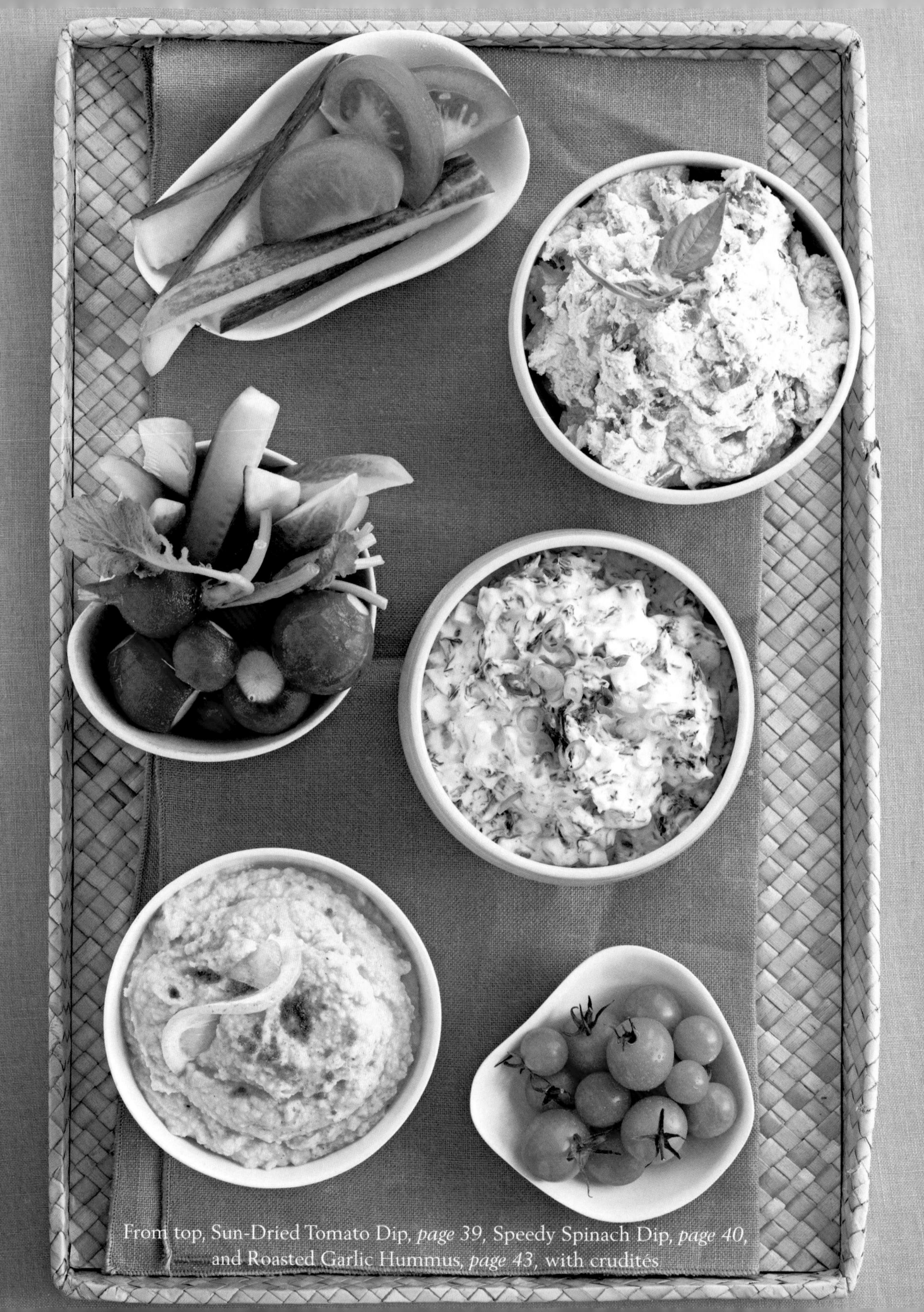

From top, Sun-Dried Tomato Dip, *page 39*, Speedy Spinach Dip, *page 40*, and Roasted Garlic Hummus, *page 43*, with crudités

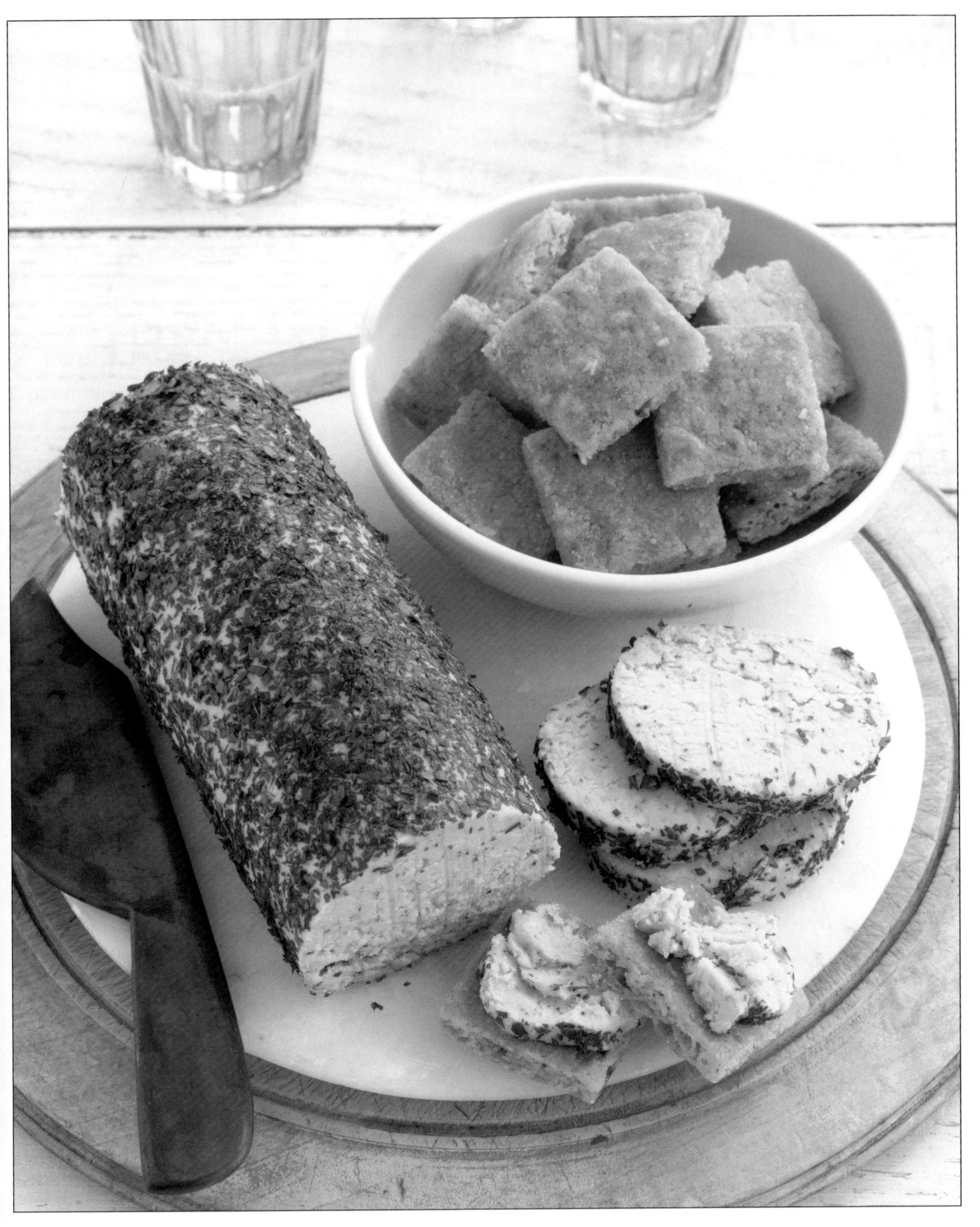

Smoky Cheese Log, *page 48*, and Chili-Cheese Crisps, *page 46*

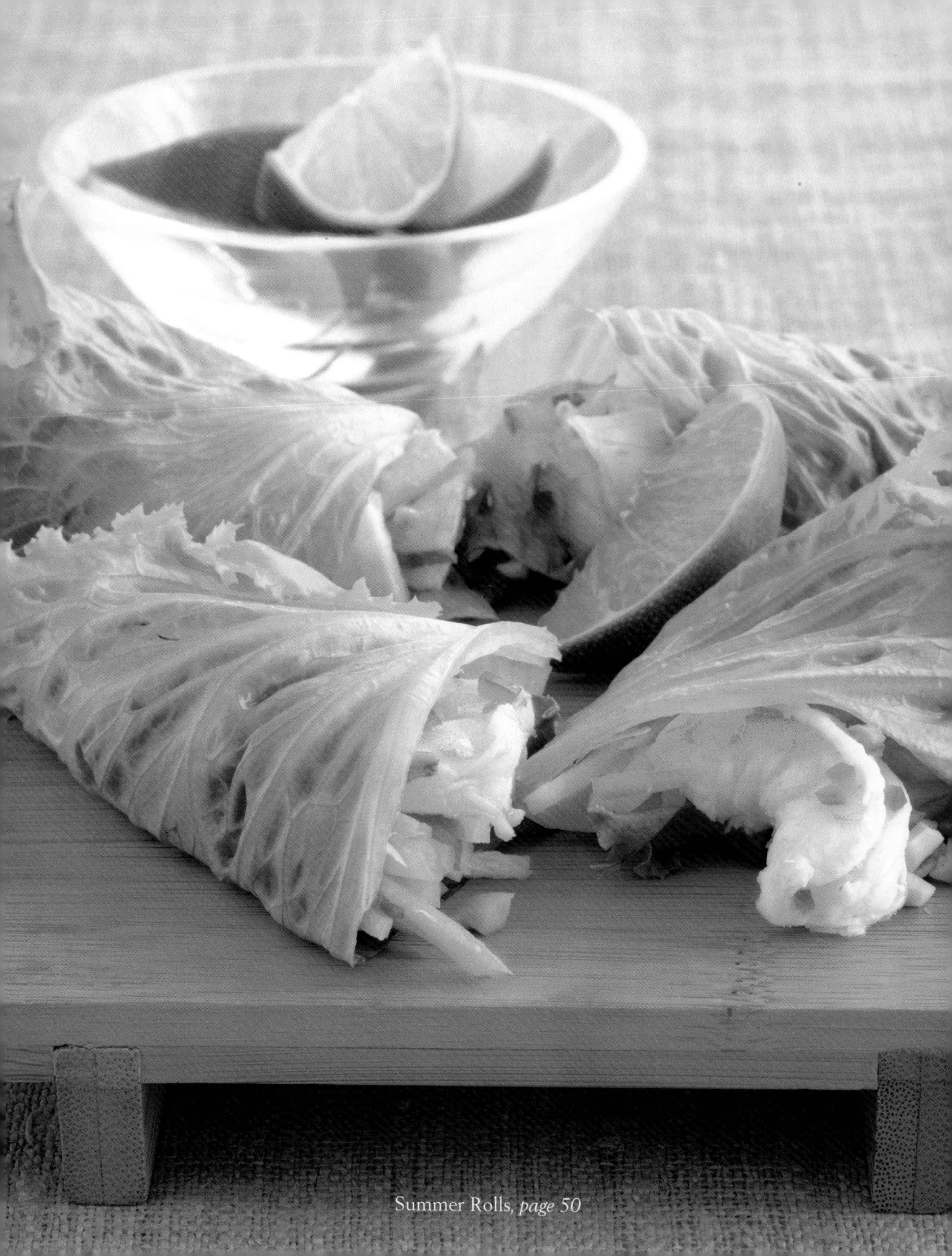
Summer Rolls, *page 50*

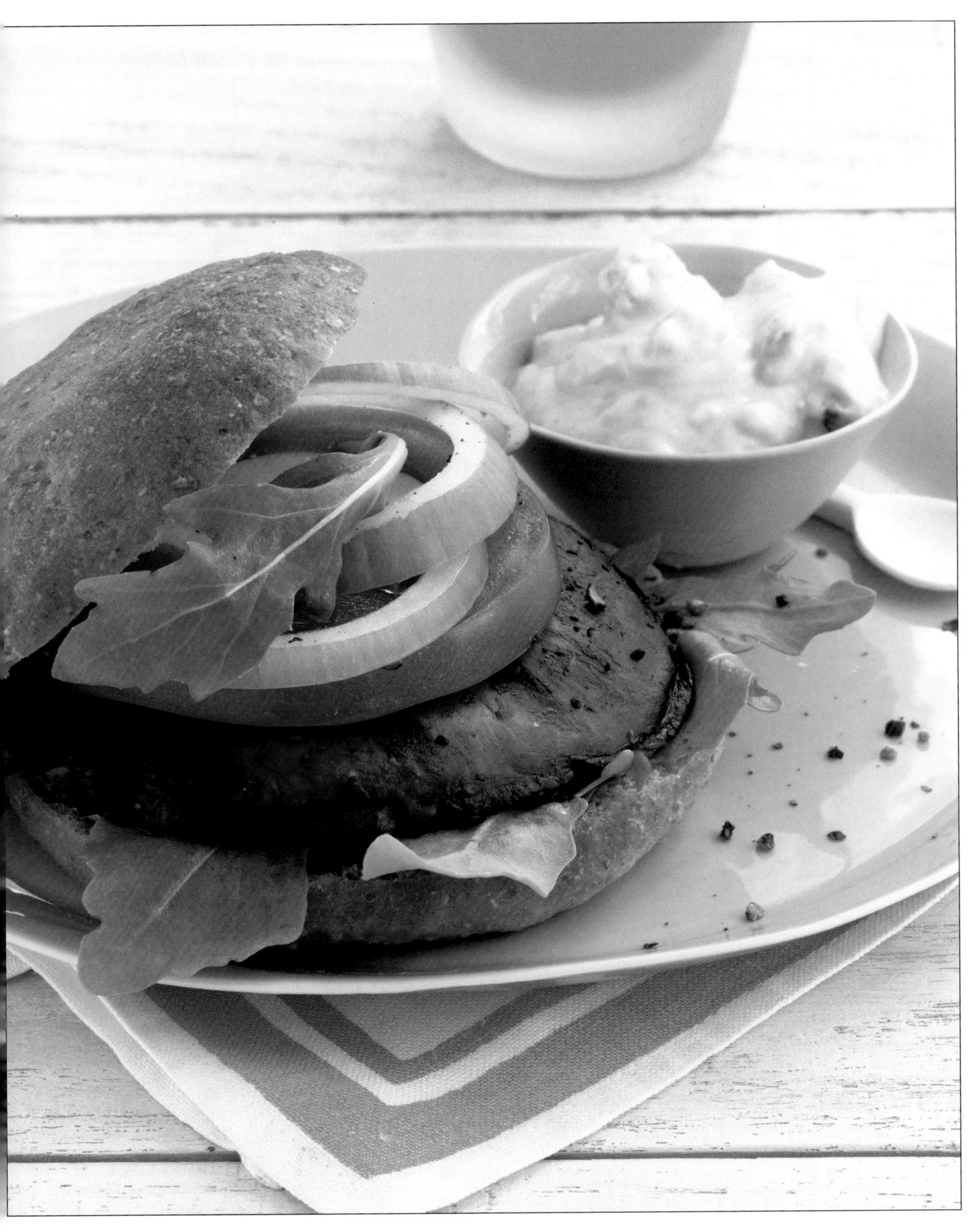

Portobello Burger with Blue Cheese Sauce, *page 65*, on Atkins Hamburger Bun, *page 60*

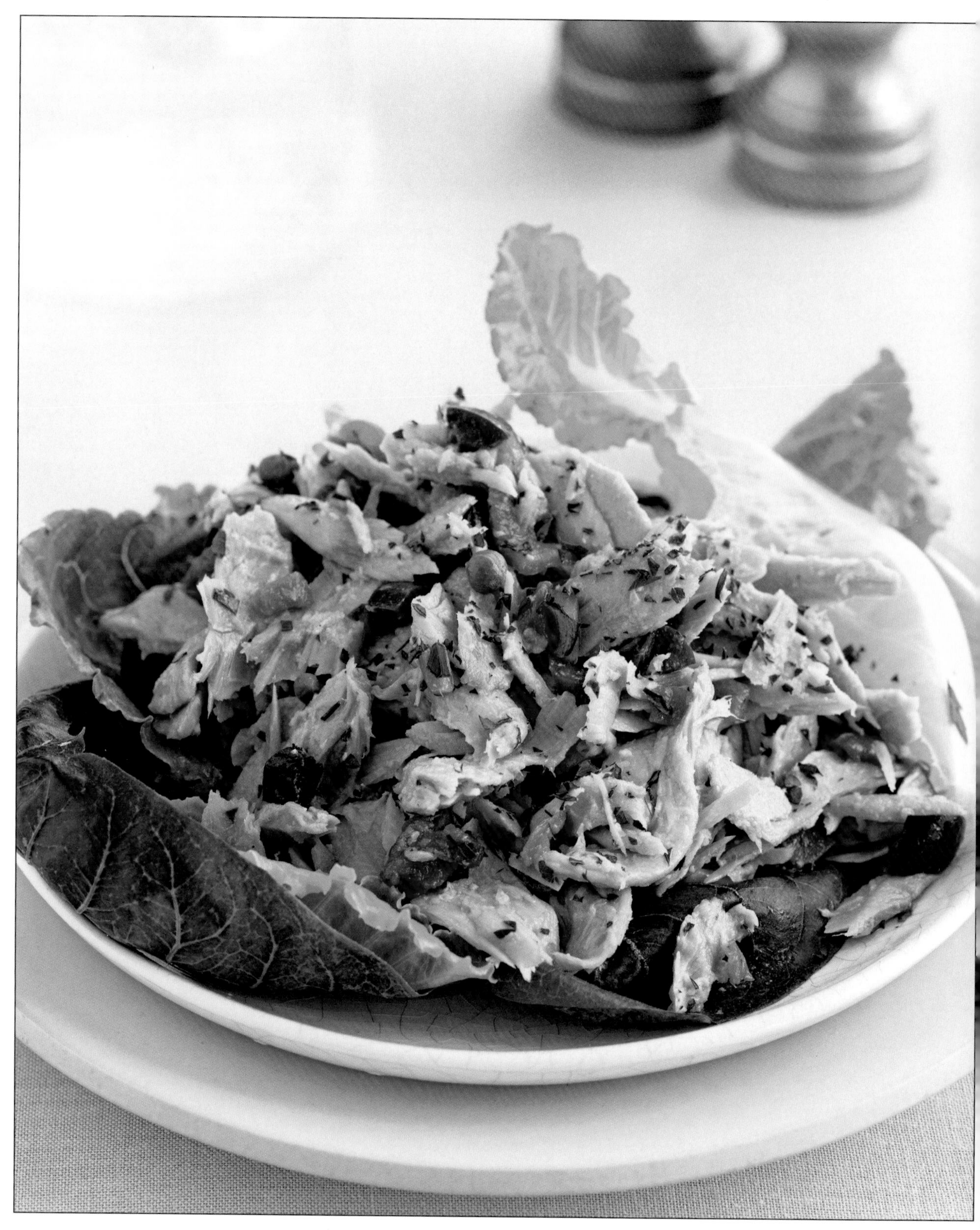

Mediterranean-Style Tuna Salad, *page 71*

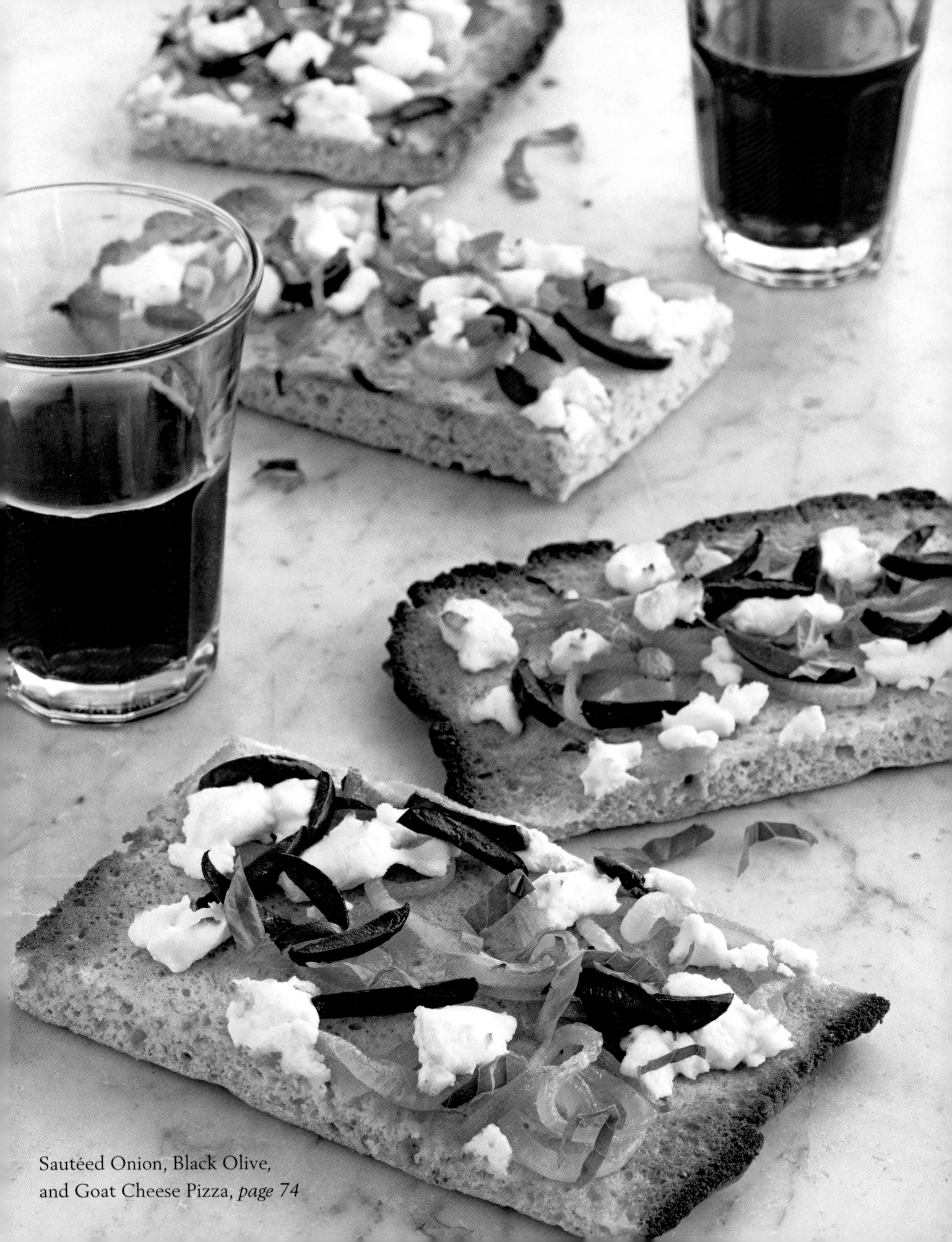

Sautéed Onion, Black Olive, and Goat Cheese Pizza, *page 74*

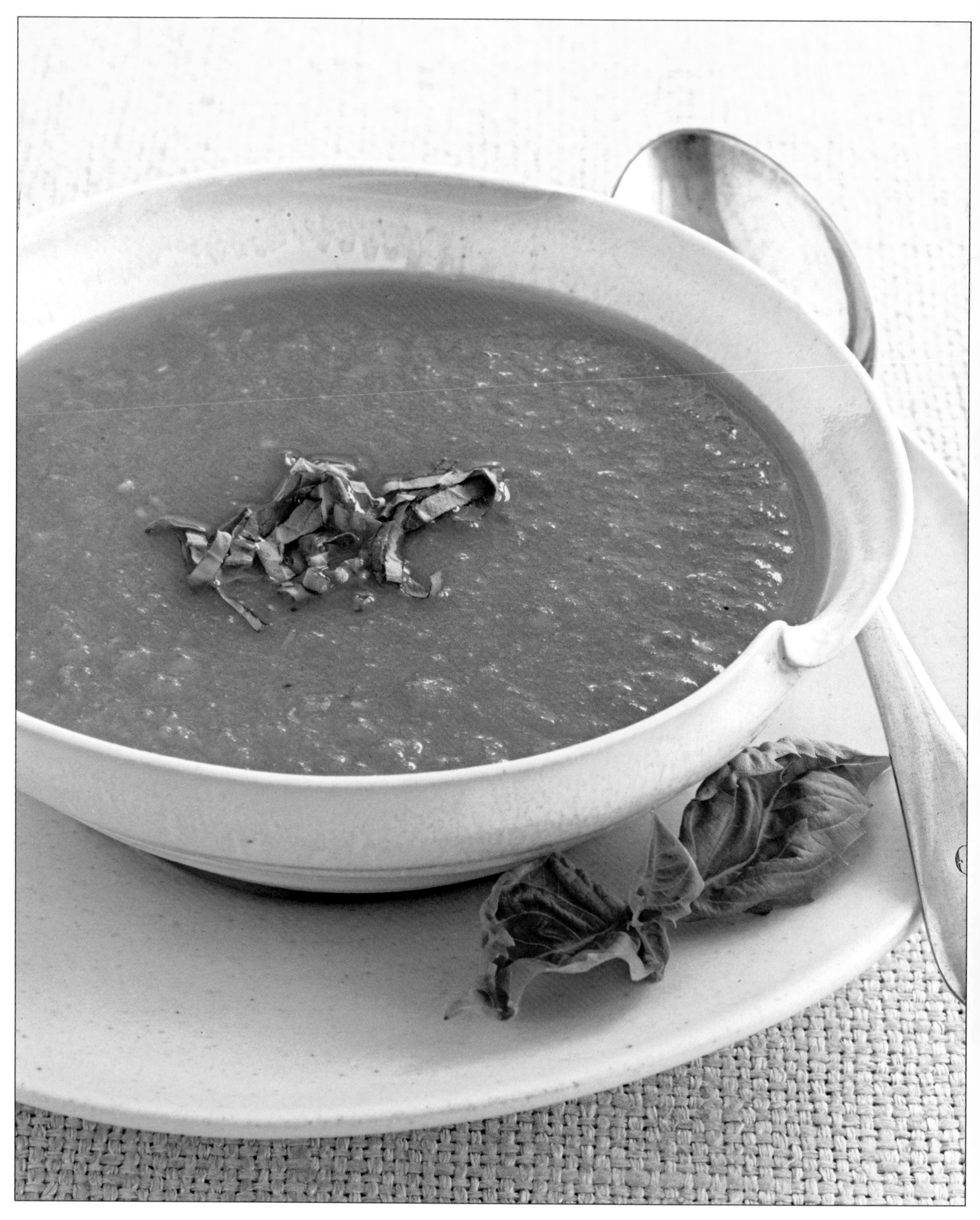

Cold Roasted Tomato Soup, *page 133*

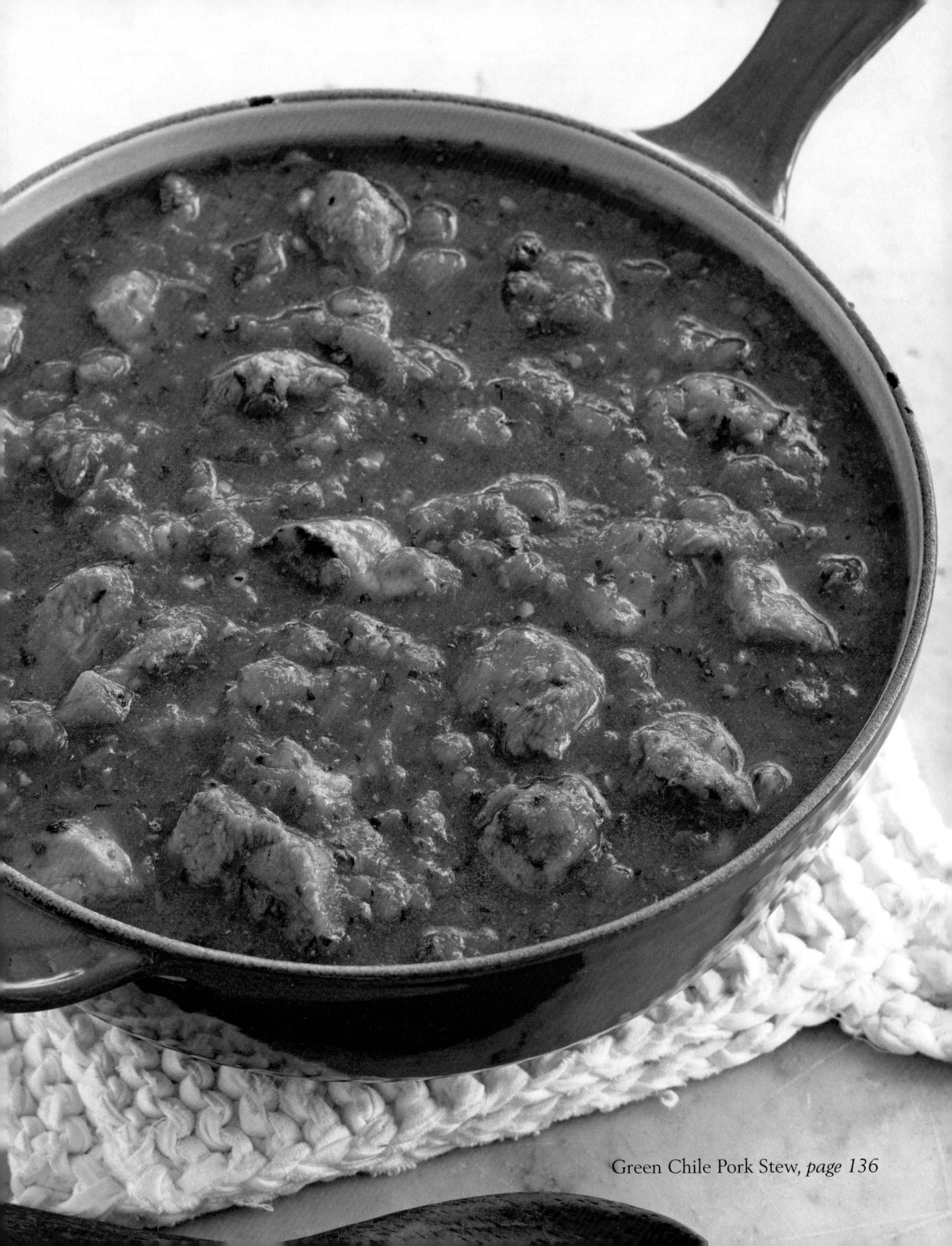

Green Chile Pork Stew, *page 136*

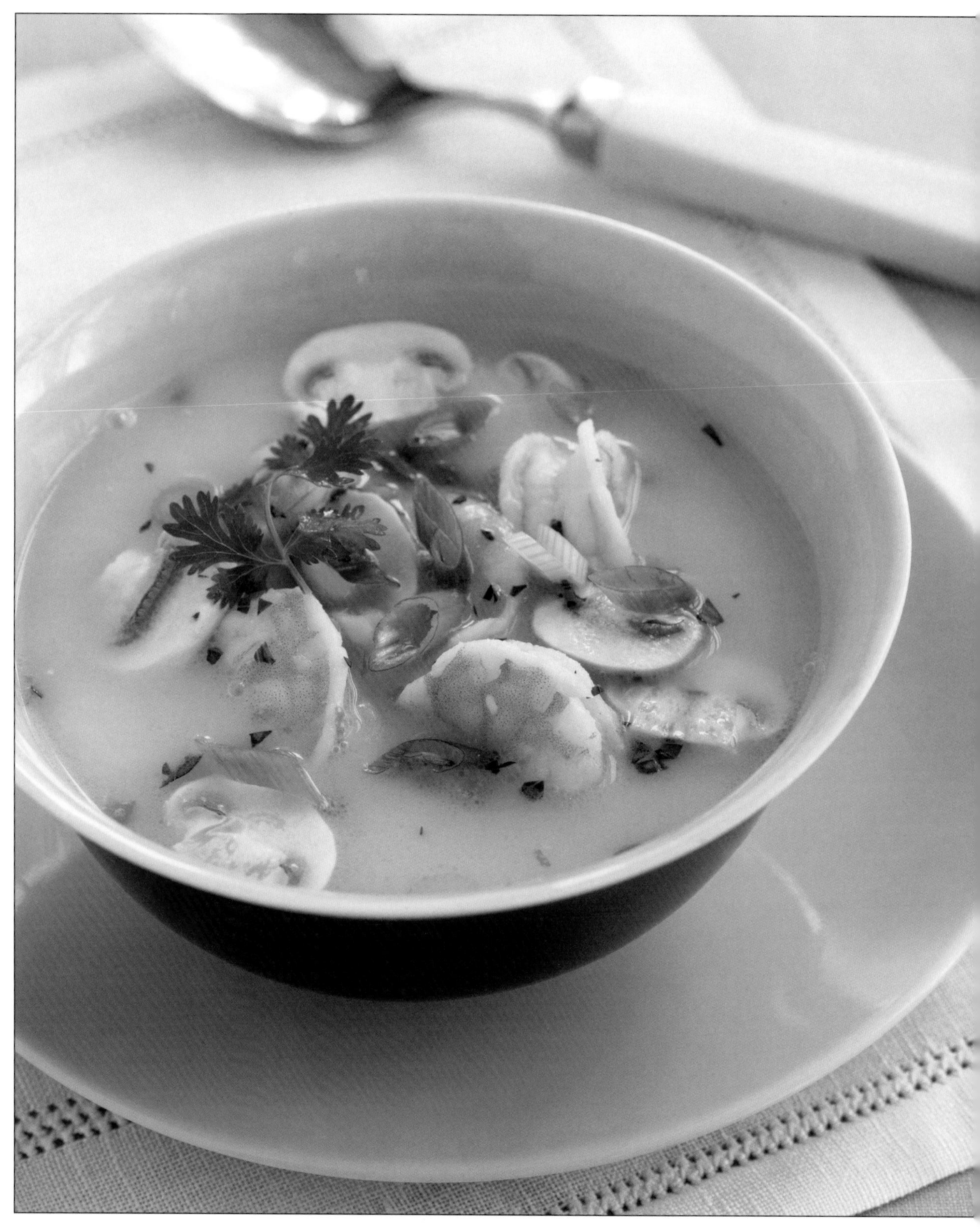

Thai Coconut-Shrimp Soup, *page 126*

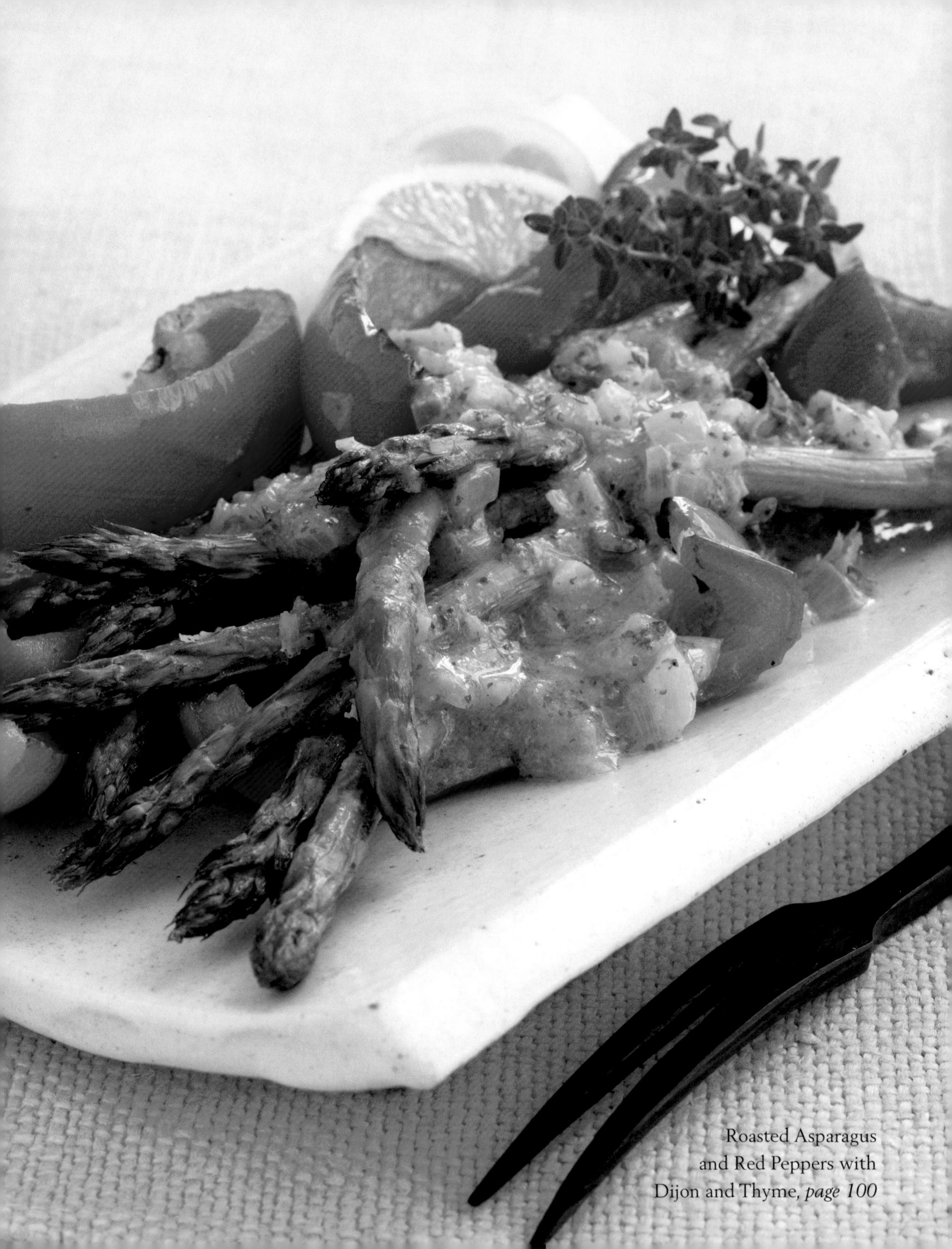

Roasted Asparagus
and Red Peppers with
Dijon and Thyme, *page 100*

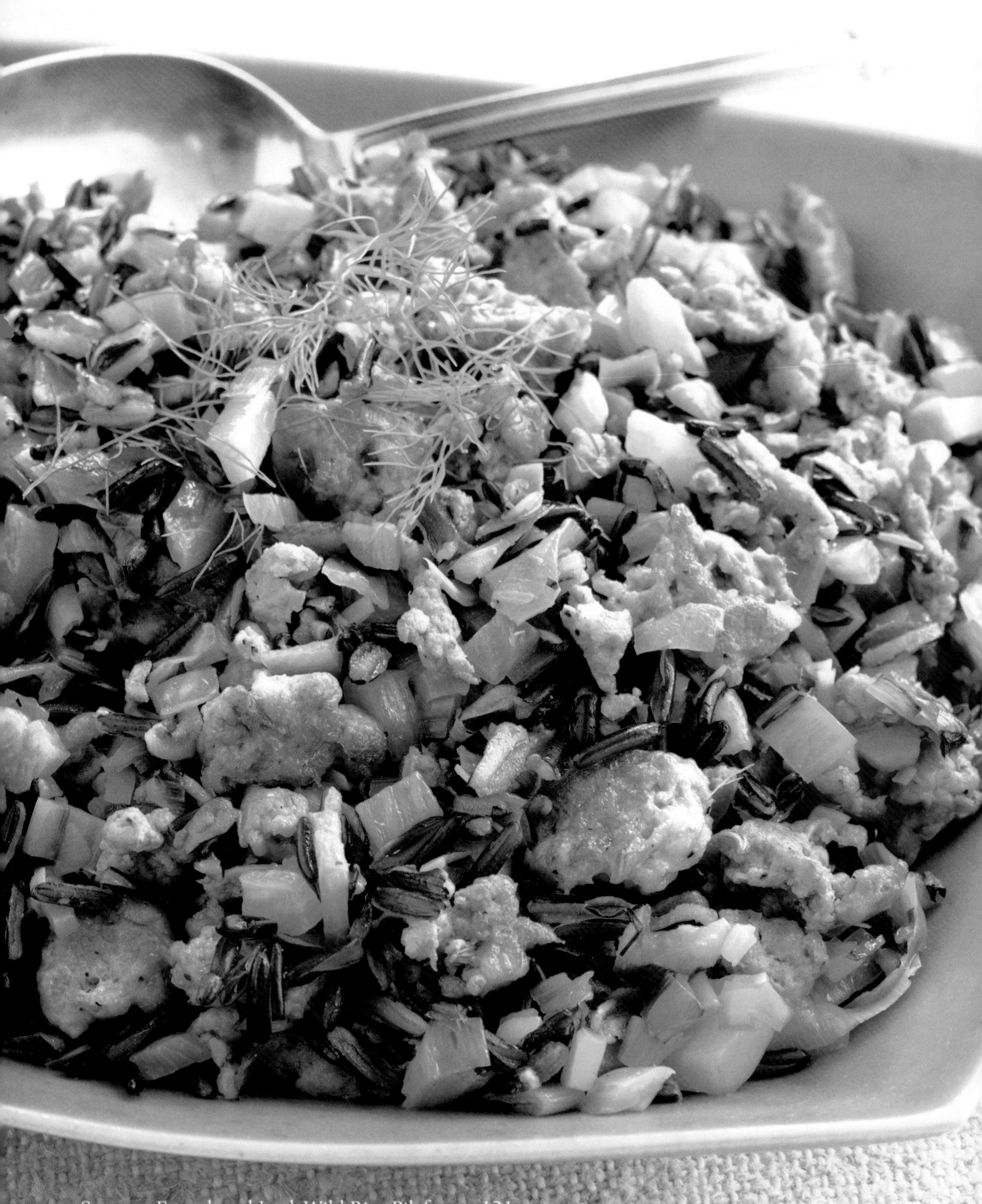
Sausage, Fennel, and Leek Wild Rice Pilaf, *page 121*

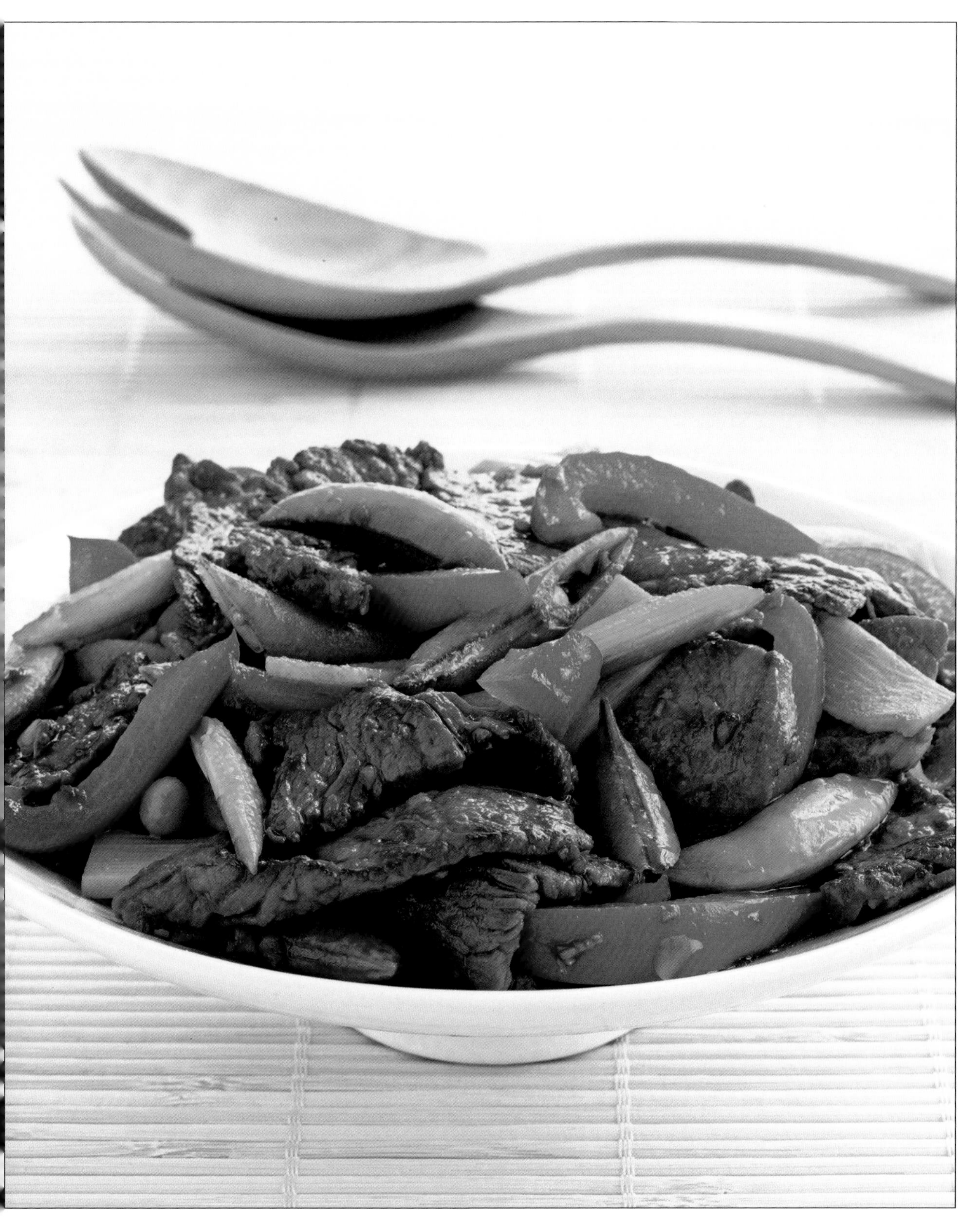

Beef and Asian Vegetable Stir-Fry, *page 163*

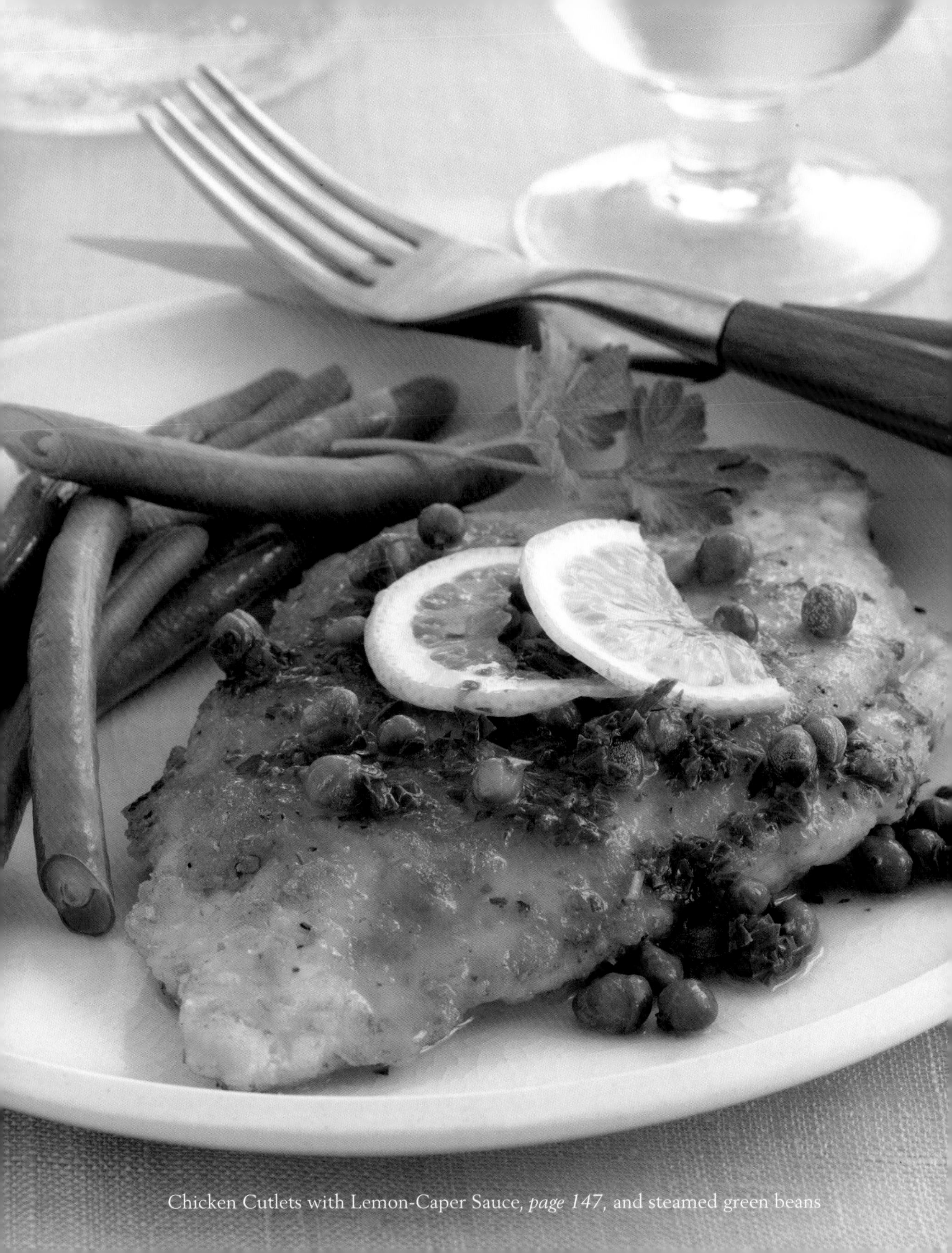

Chicken Cutlets with Lemon-Caper Sauce, *page 147,* and steamed green beans

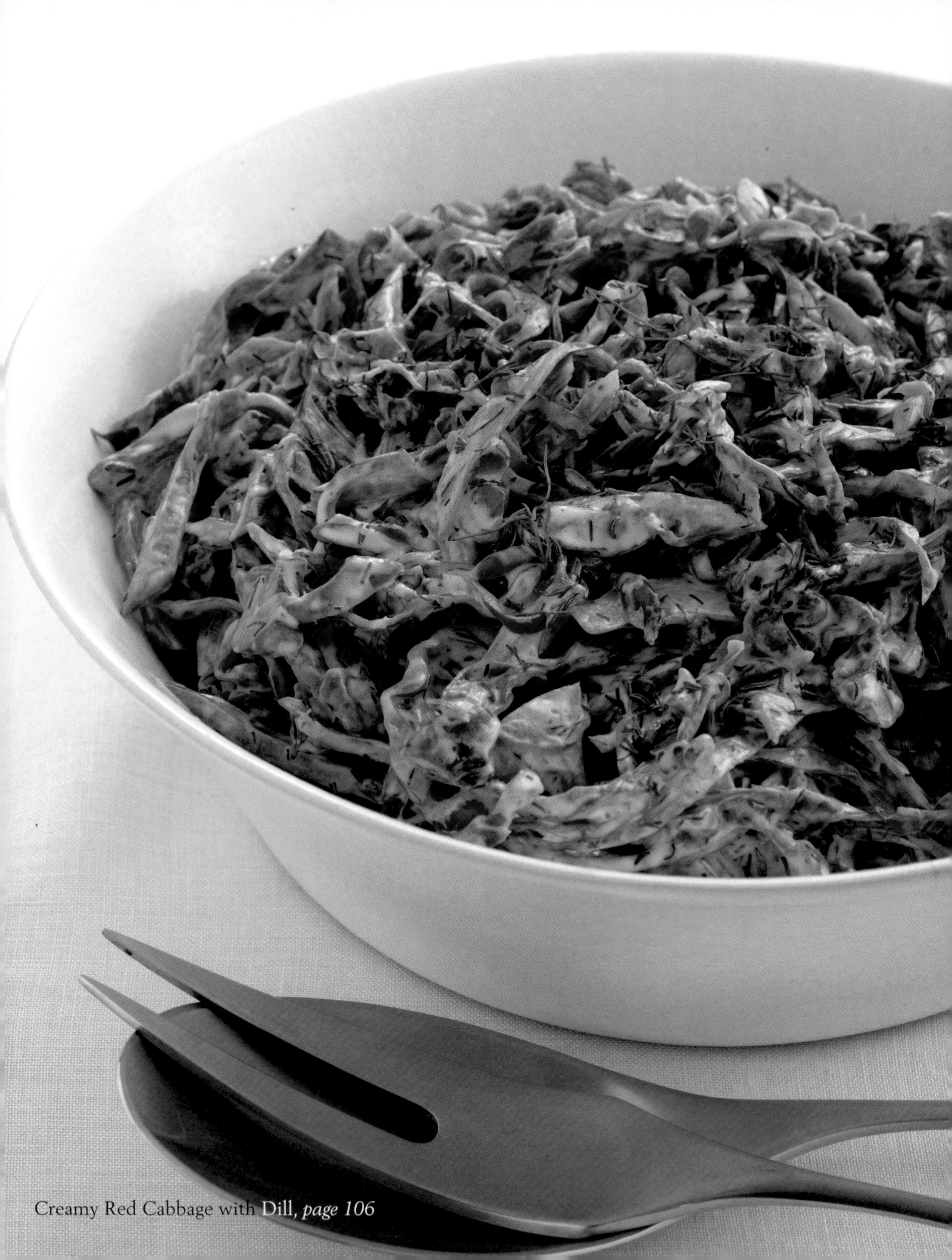

Creamy Red Cabbage with Dill, *page 106*

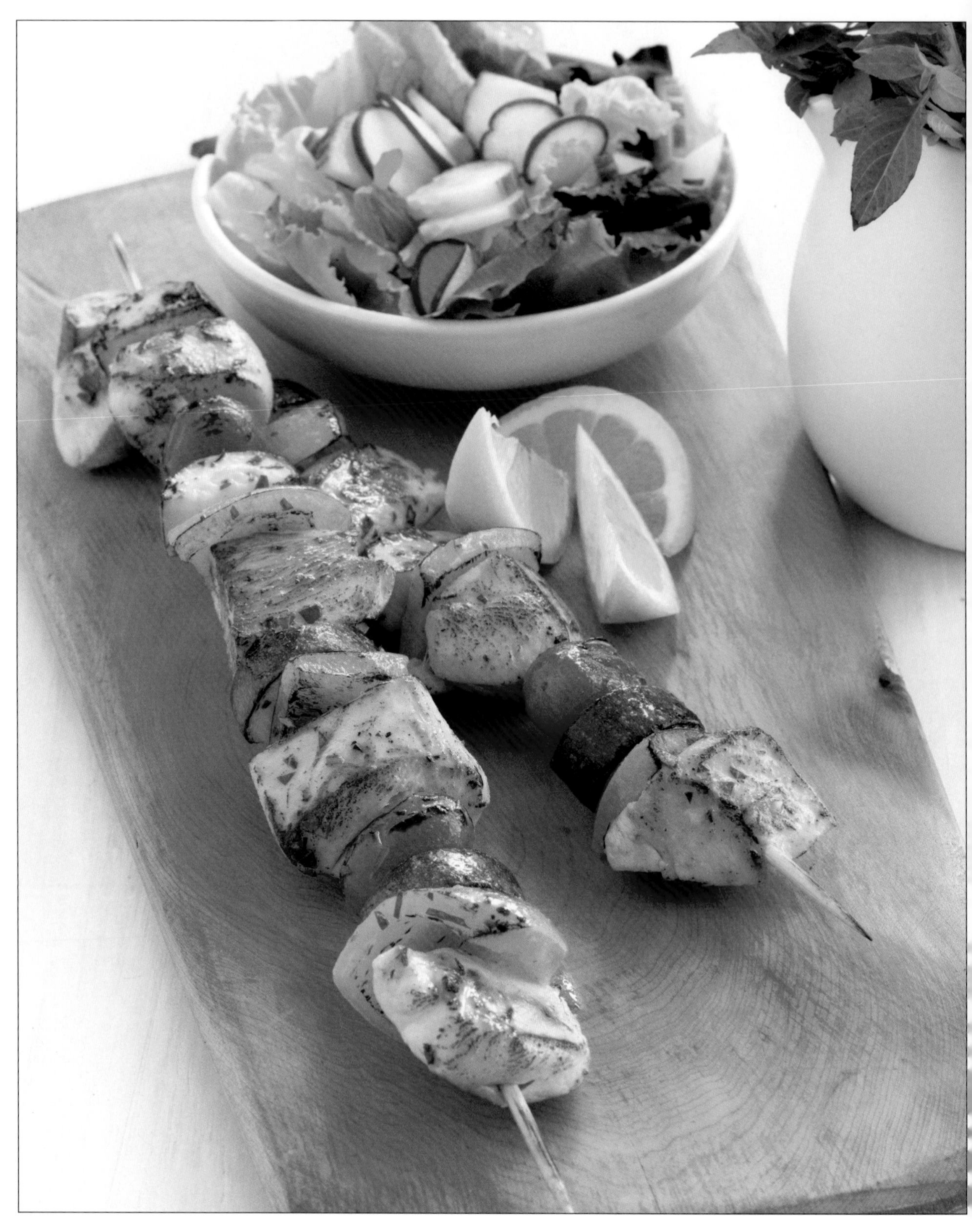

Lemon-and-Basil Chicken-Veggie Kebabs, *page 151,* with a tossed salad

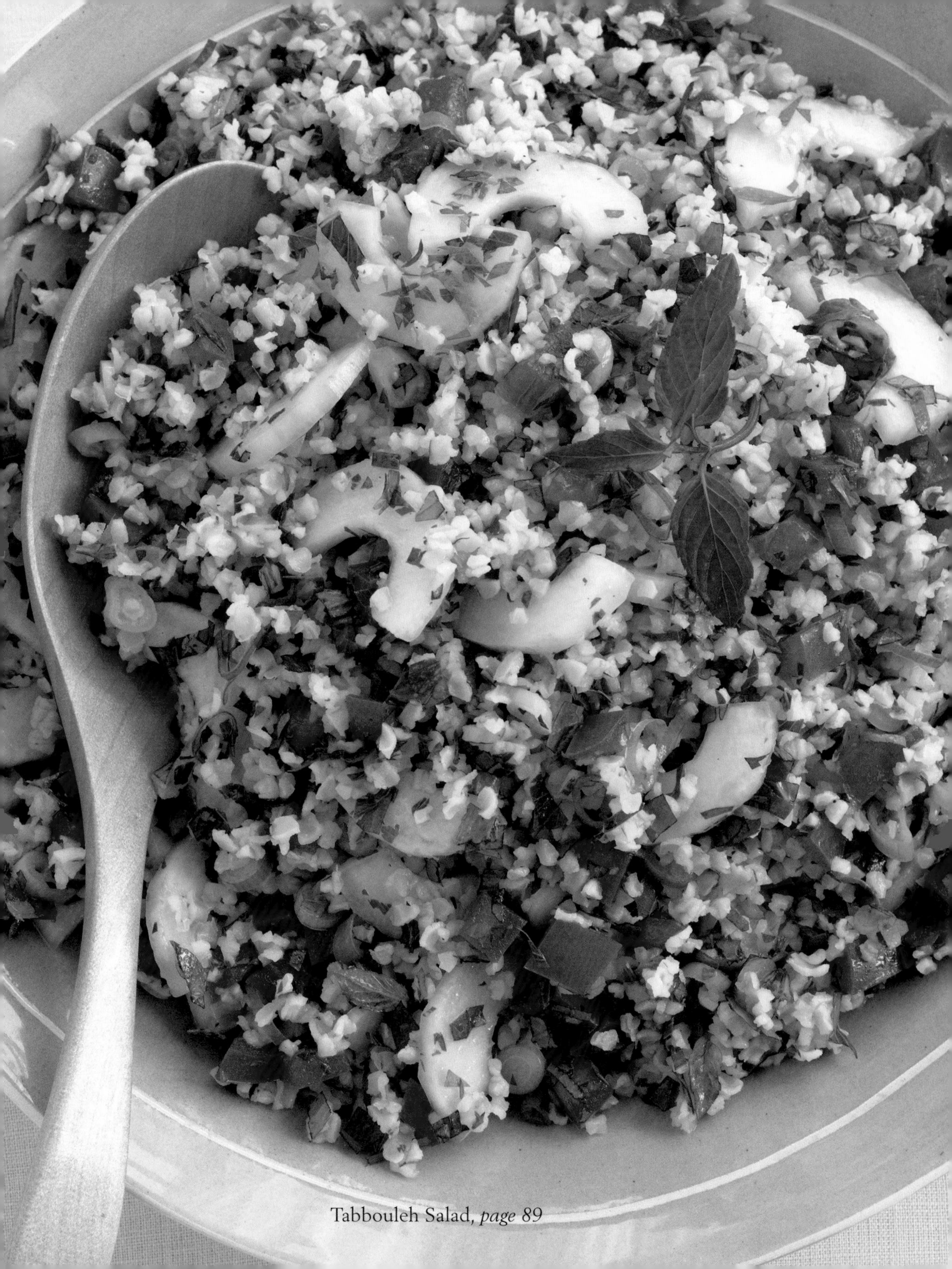
Tabbouleh Salad, *page 89*

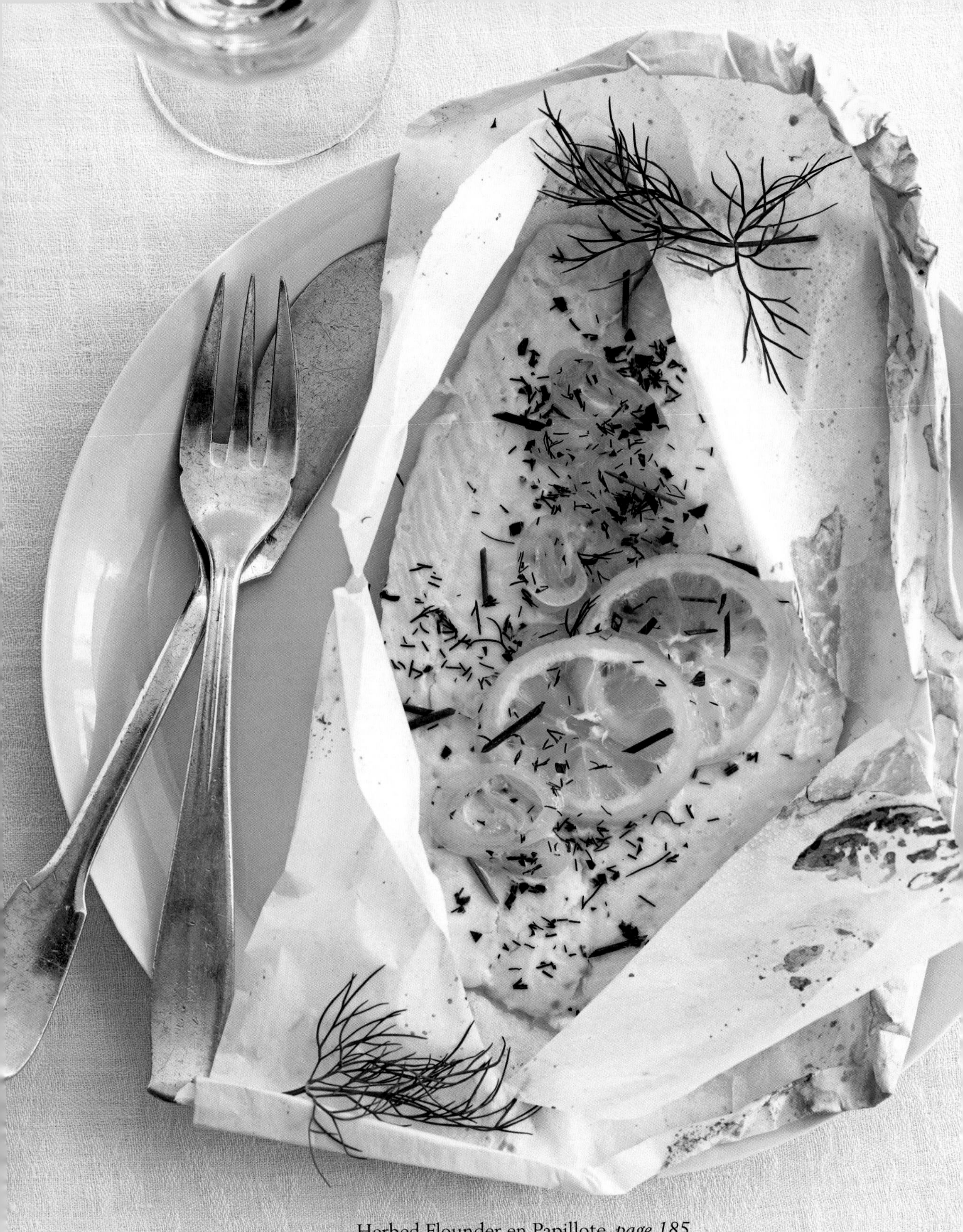

Herbed Flounder en Papillote, *page 185*

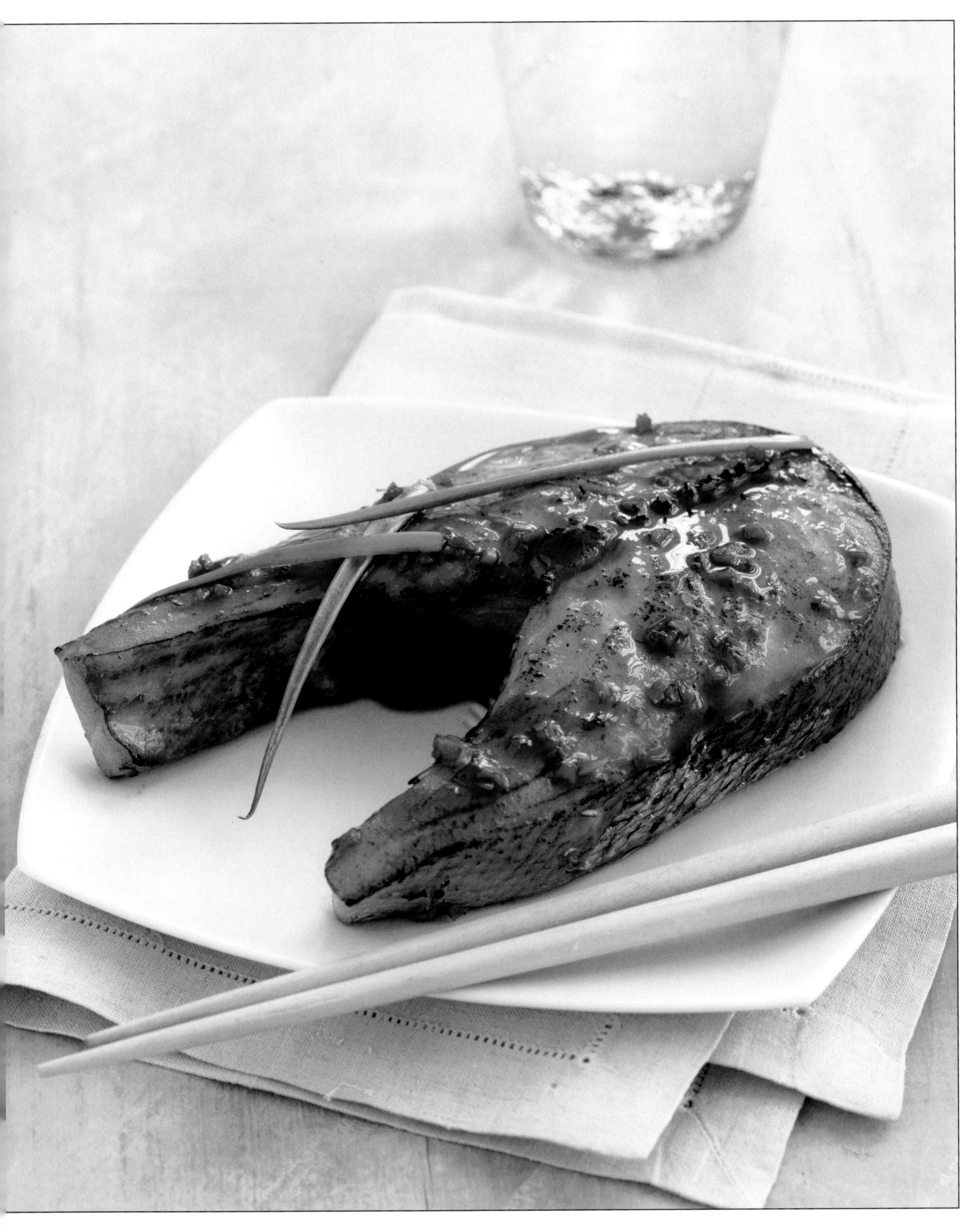

Roasted Ginger-Tamari Salmon Steaks, *page 189*

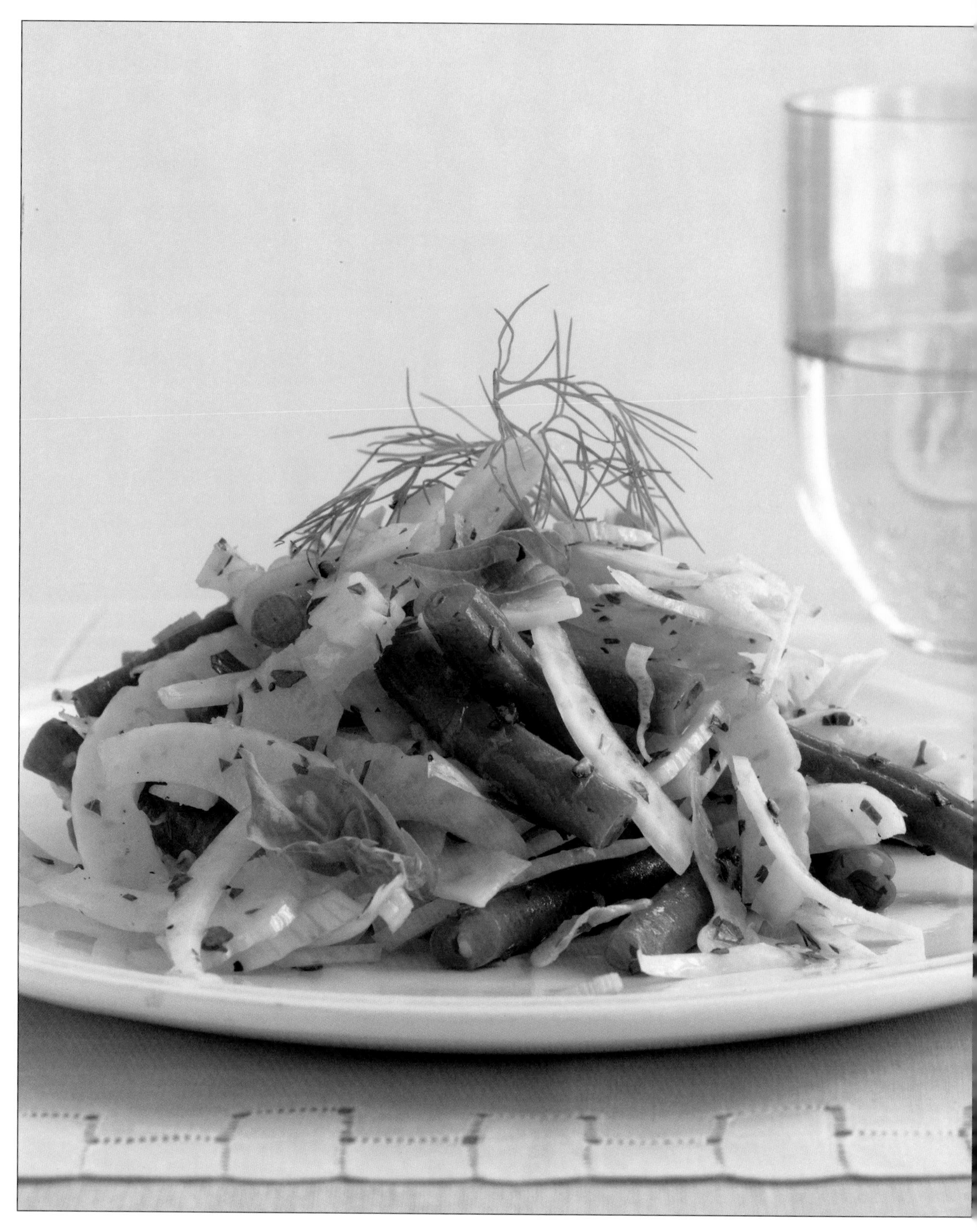

Shaved Fennel Salad with Lemon Dressing, *page 82*

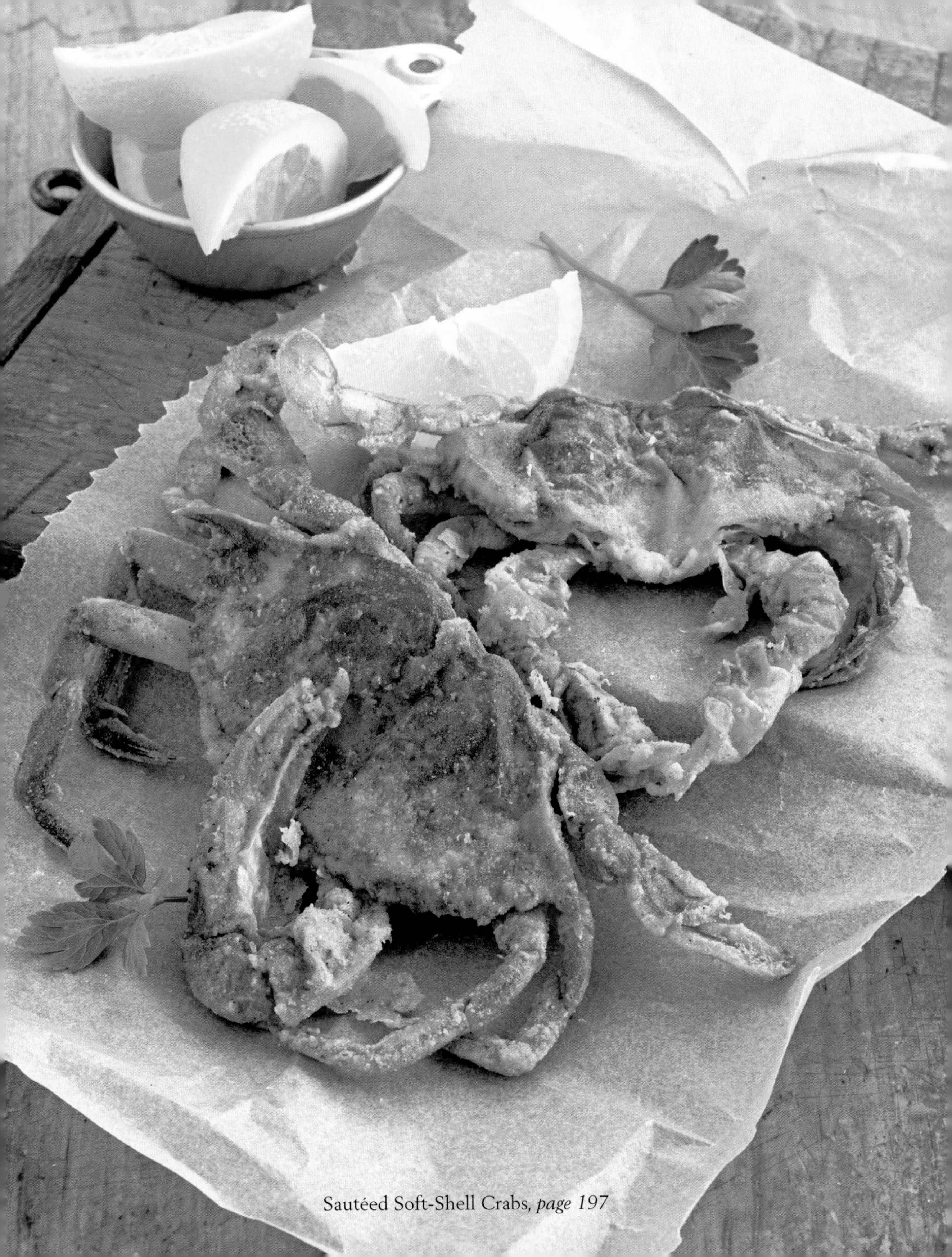

Sautéed Soft-Shell Crabs, *page 197*

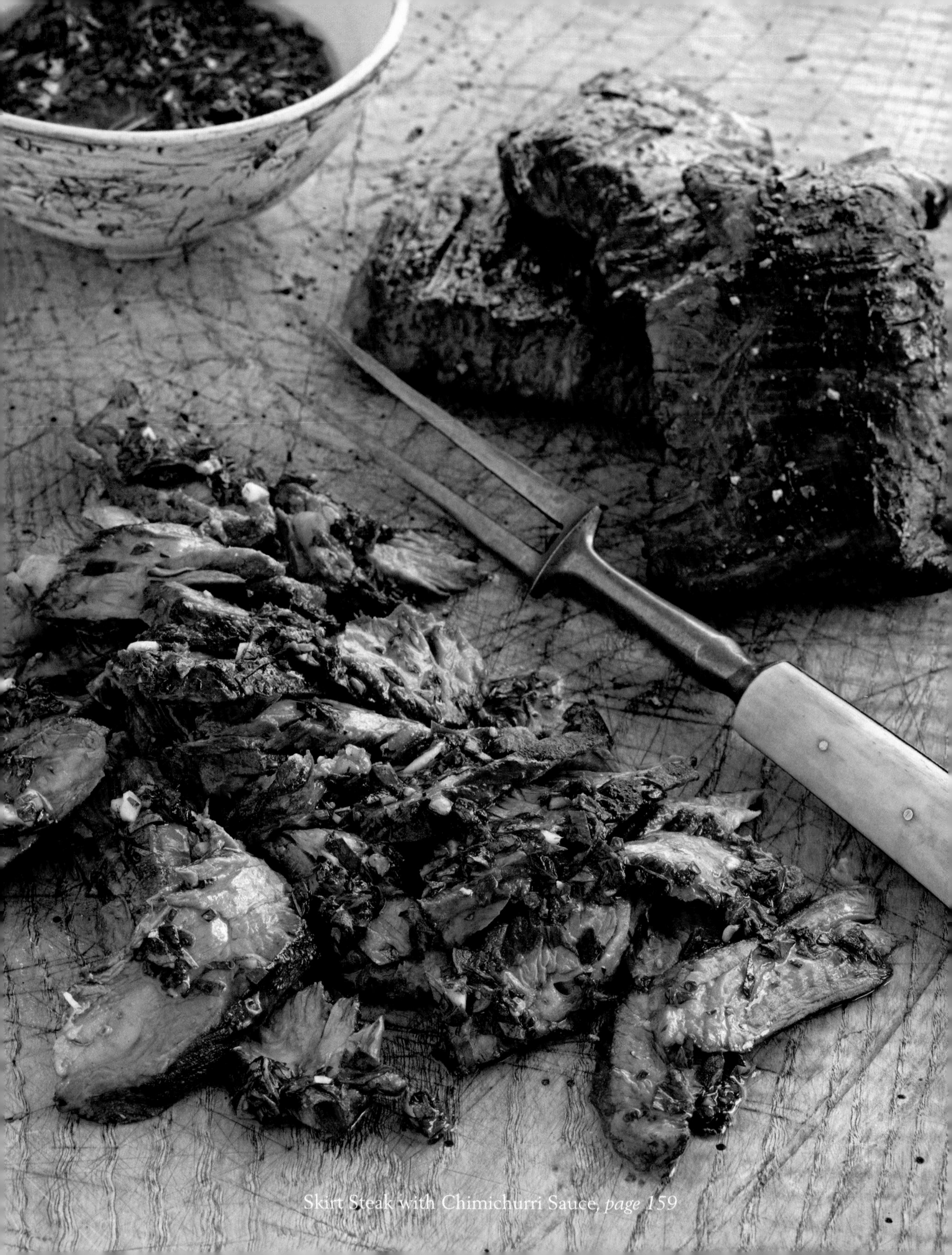

Skirt Steak with Chimichurri Sauce, *page 159*

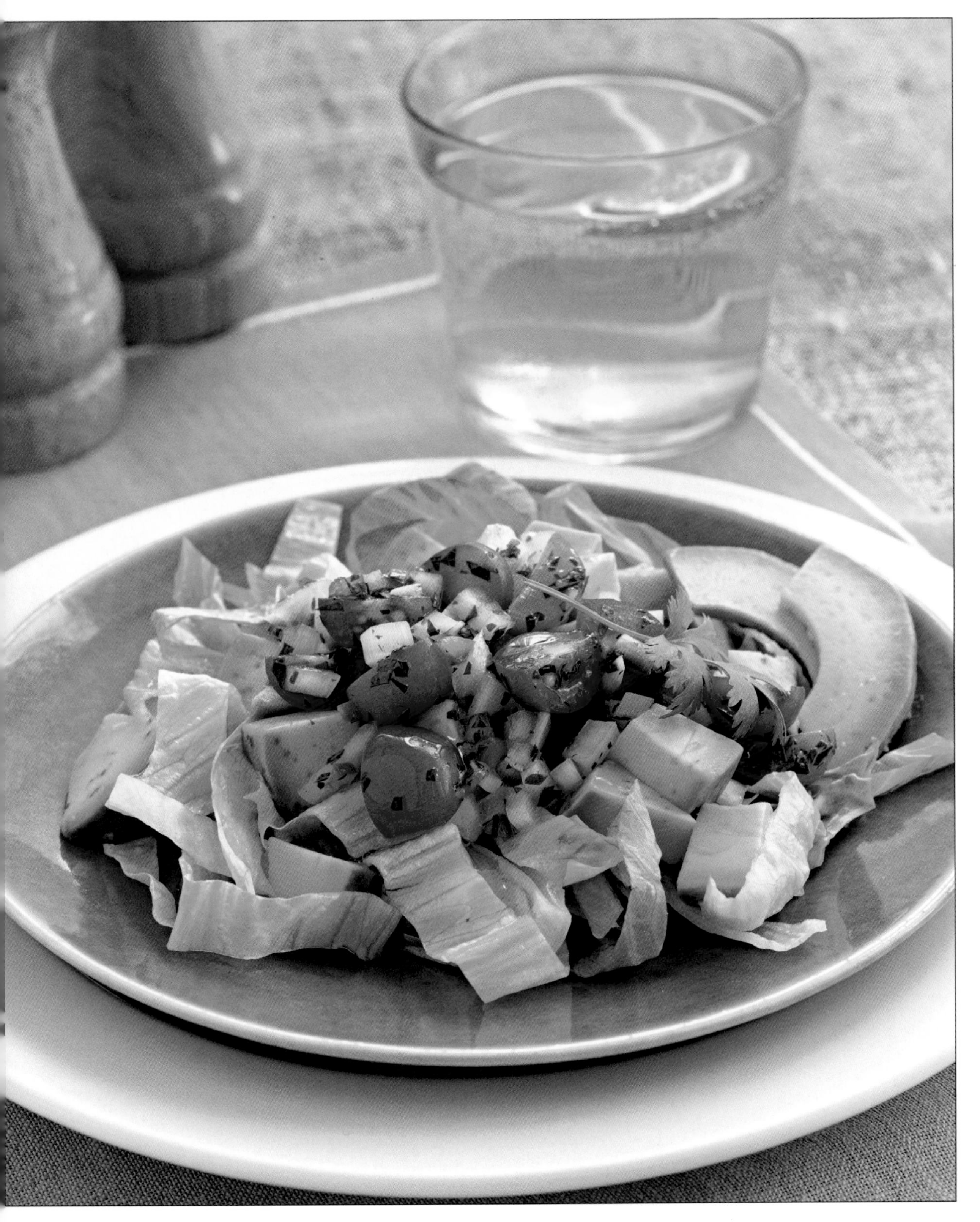

Mexican Avocado Salad, *page 80*

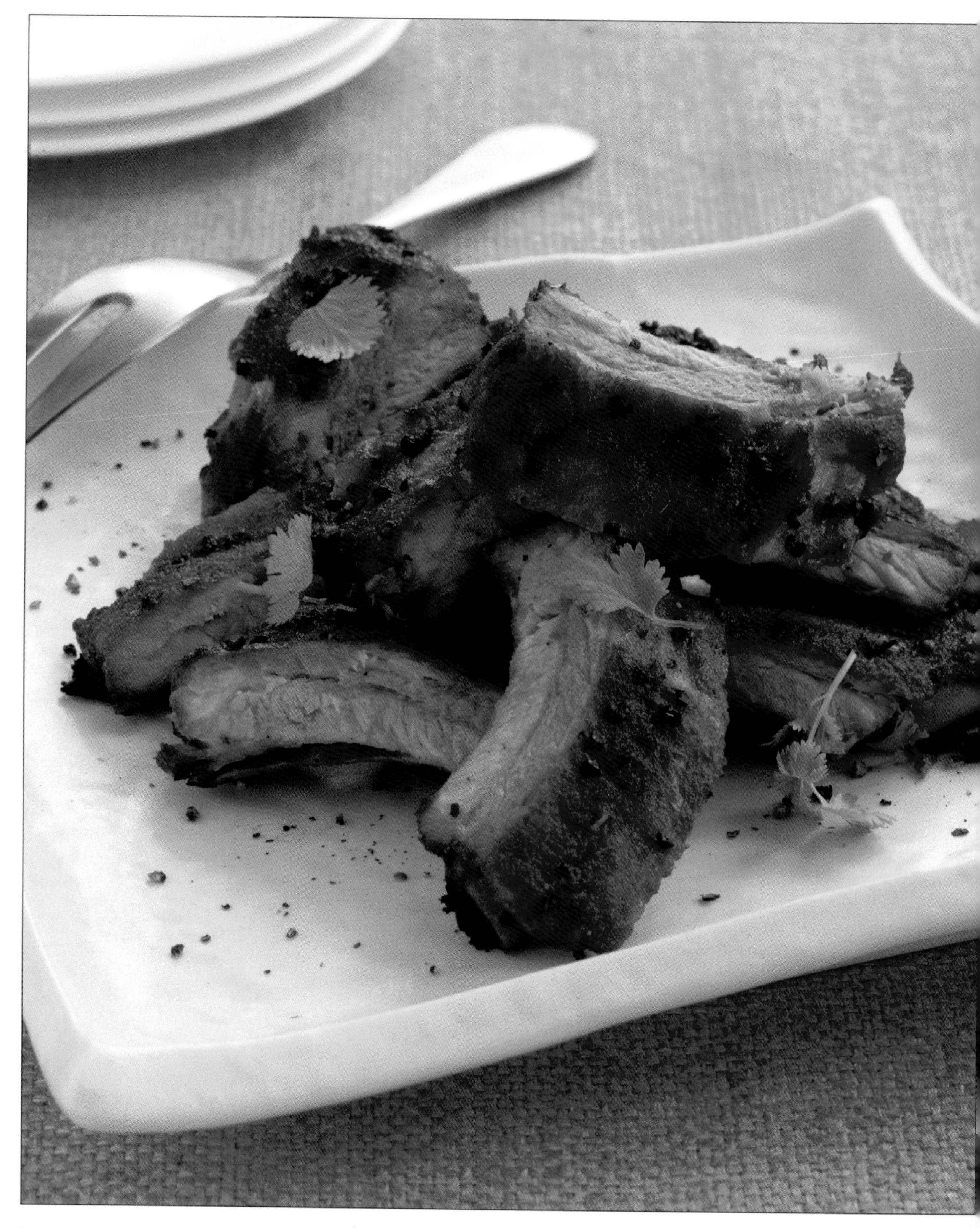

Peppery-Spicy Baby Back Ribs, *page 169*

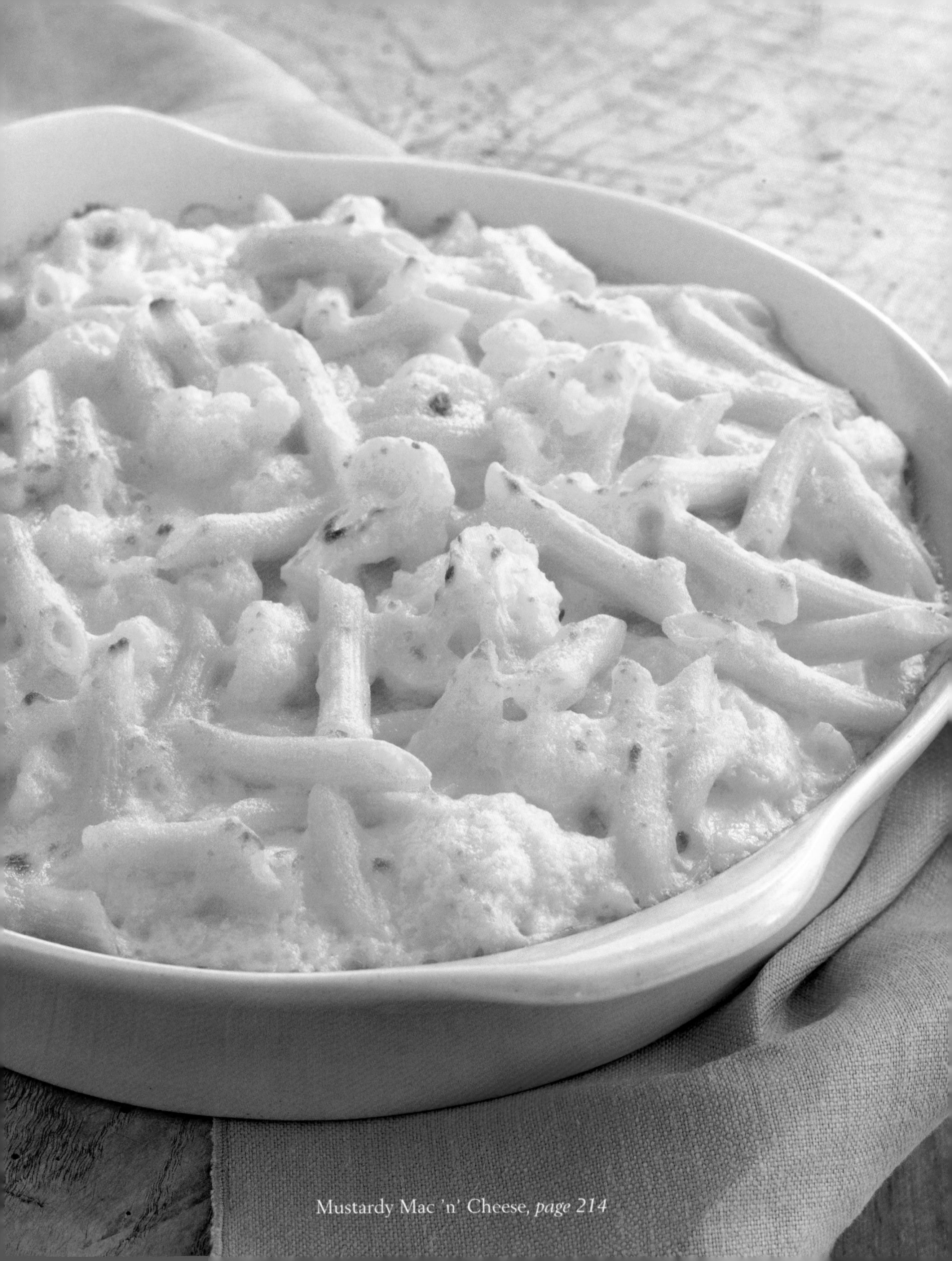

Mustardy Mac 'n' Cheese, *page 214*

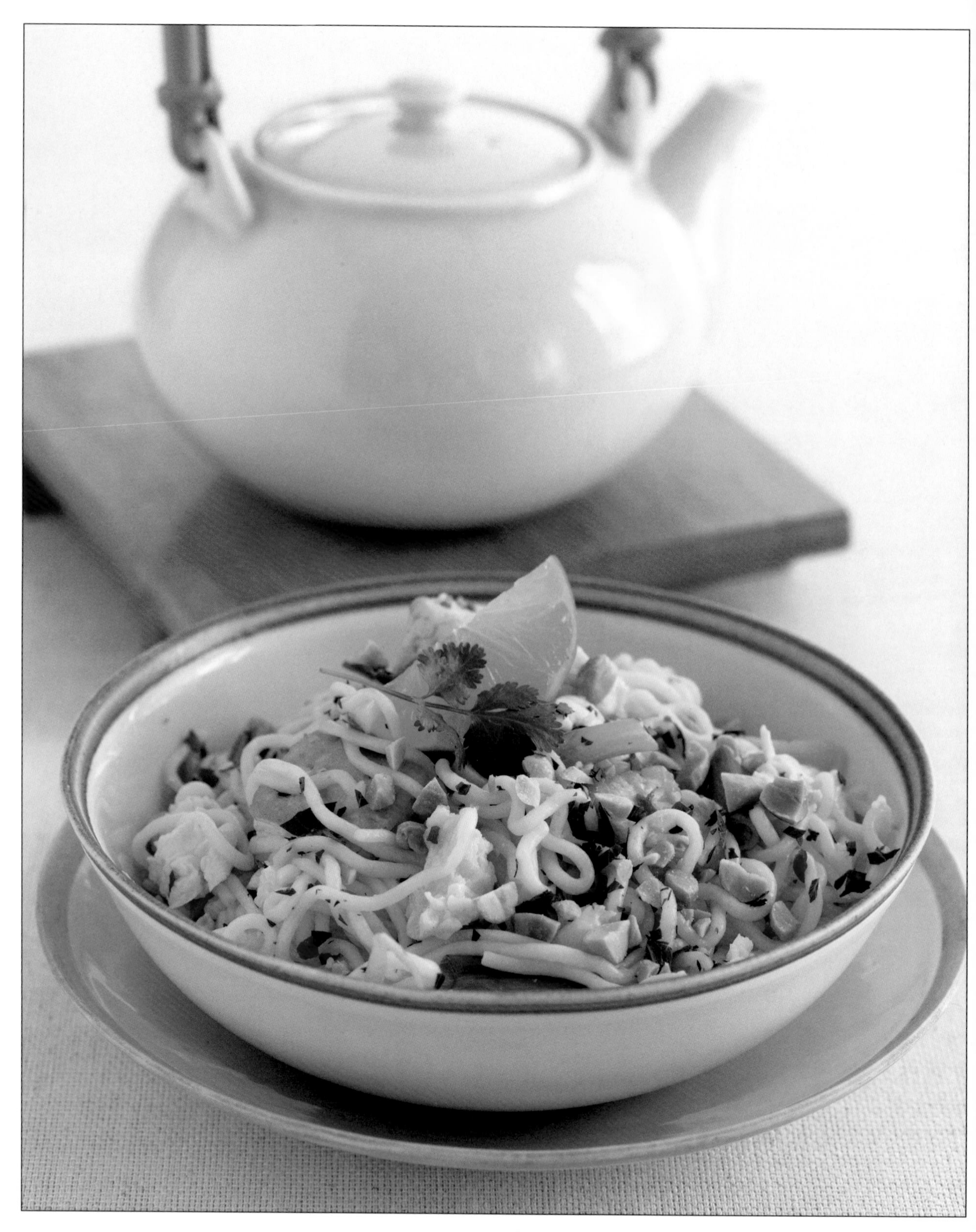

Tofu Pad Thai, *page 216*

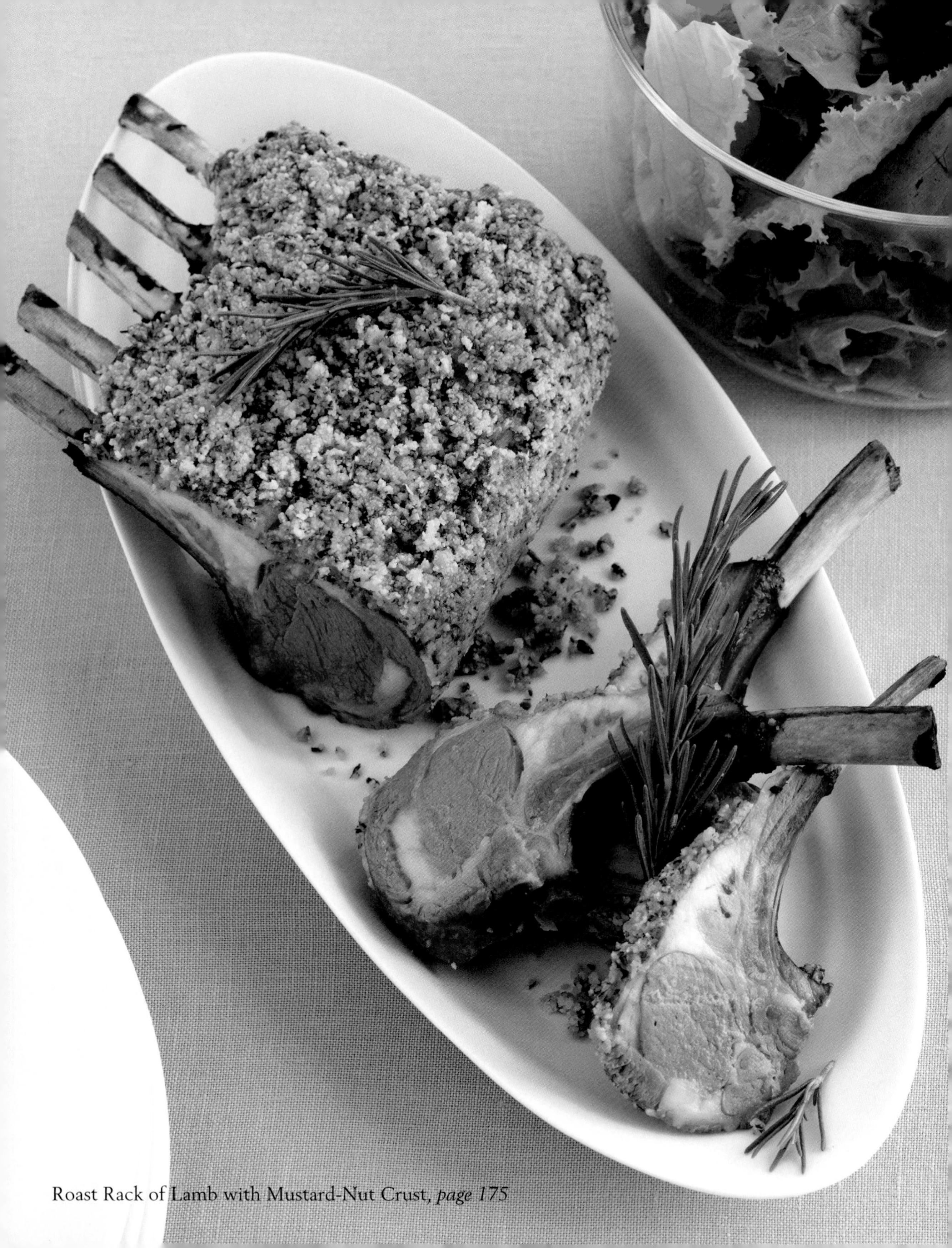

Roast Rack of Lamb with Mustard-Nut Crust, *page 175*

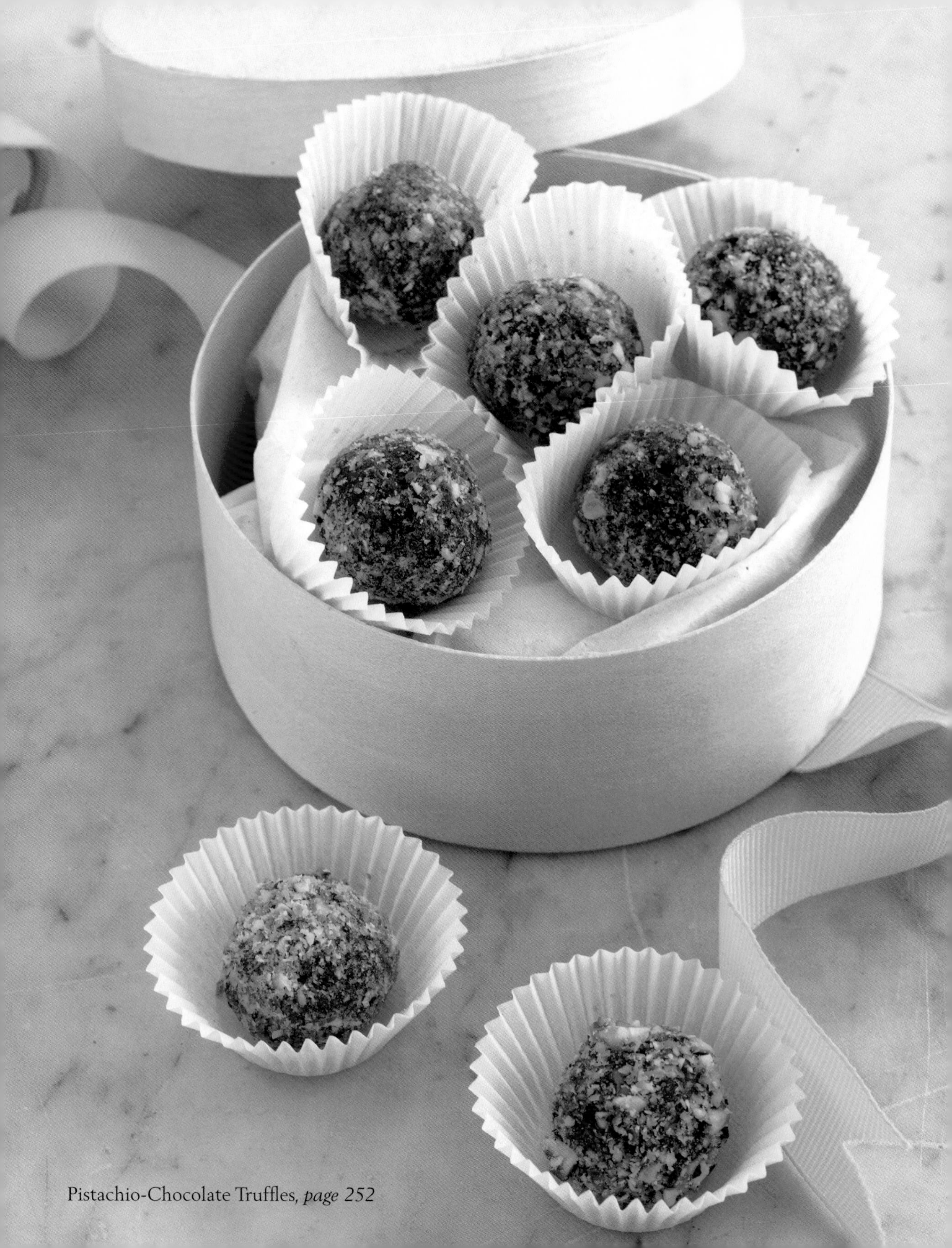

Pistachio-Chocolate Truffles, *page 252*

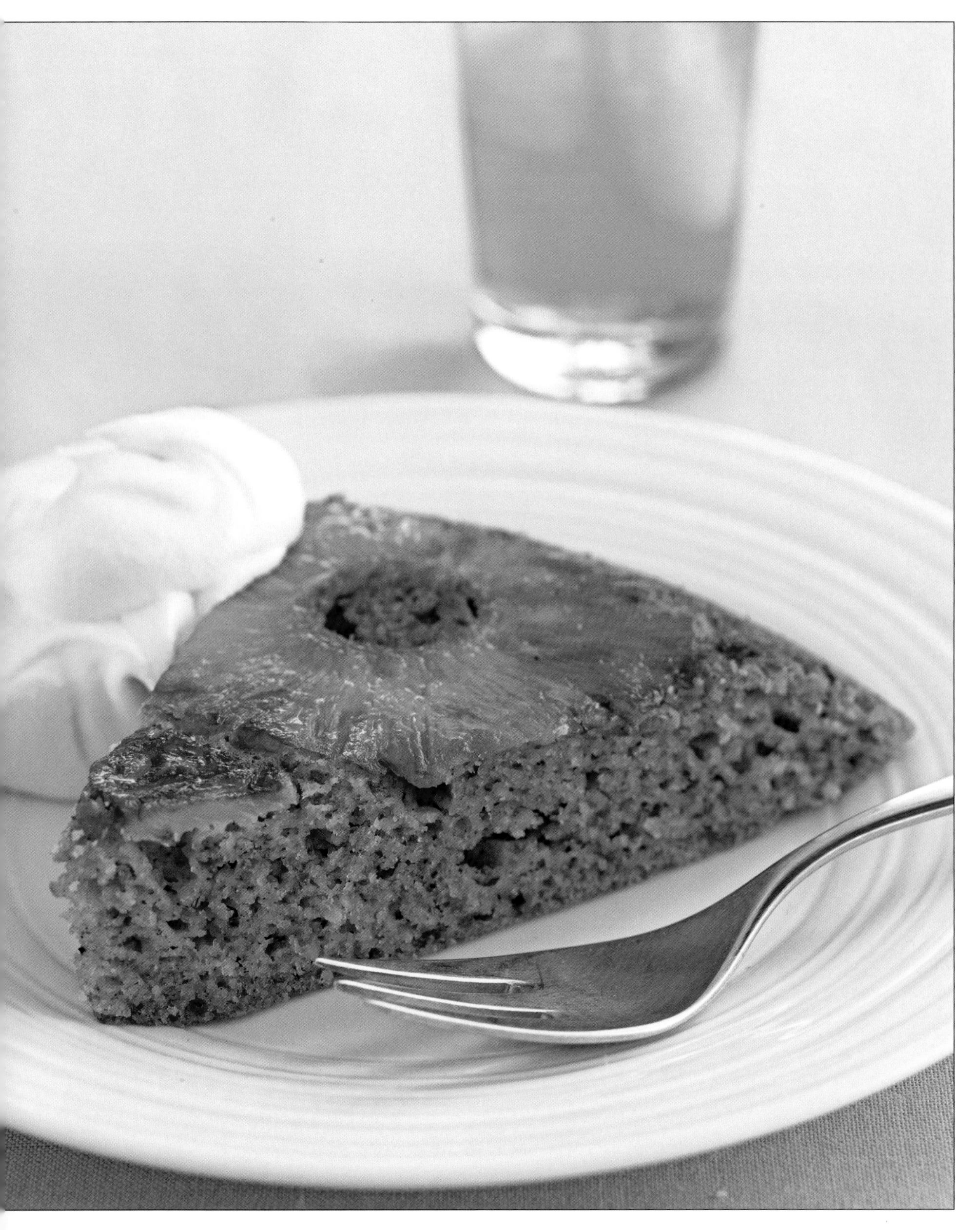

Pineapple Upside-Down Cake, *page 242,* with whipped cream

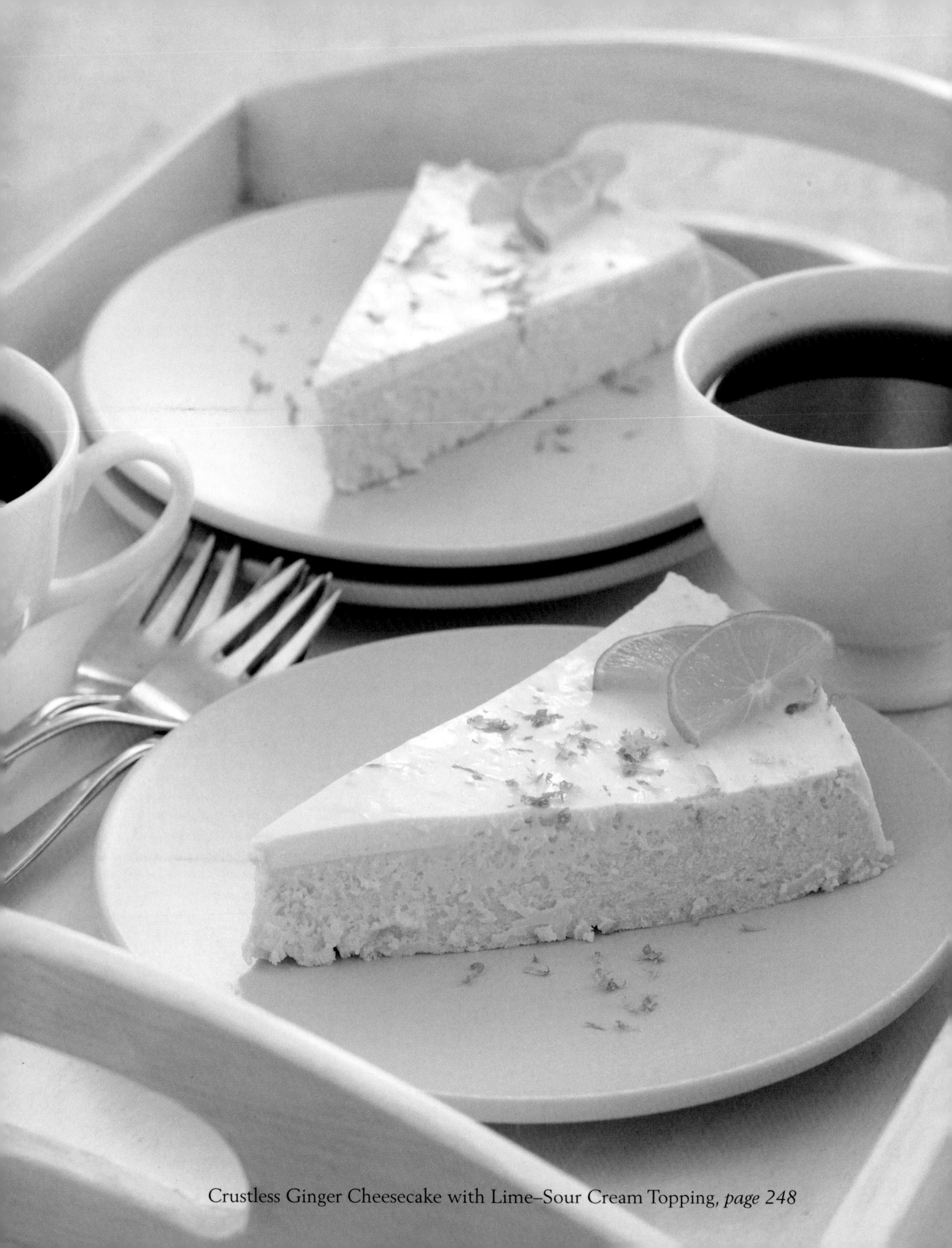

Crustless Ginger Cheesecake with Lime–Sour Cream Topping, *page 248*

Green Goddess Grilled Chicken*

Phases 1, 2, 3, 4

This flavorful marinade of fresh herbs is reminiscent of green goddess dressing, but it uses lemon juice and fresh tarragon, rather than the tarragon vinegar found in the dressing. If you wish, make an extra batch of sauce to serve with the chicken. The sauce can also be used for salad dressing or with flounder or other mild white fish.

PER SERVING:
Net Carbs: 2 grams
Total Carbs: 2 grams
Fiber: 0 grams
Protein: 53 grams
Fat: 24 grams
Calories: 450

Makes: 4 servings
Active Time: 20 minutes
Total Time: 1 hour 20 minutes

WEEKEND

- ¼ cup regular (not low-fat) mayonnaise
- 2 tablespoons extra-virgin olive oil
- 3 tablespoons freshly squeezed lemon juice
- 2 tablespoons minced fresh parsley
- 1 large scallion, thinly sliced
- 1 tablespoon minced fresh tarragon
- 1 small clove garlic, minced
- 1 teaspoon salt
- 1 teaspoon granular sugar substitute
- ½ teaspoon freshly ground black pepper
- 1½ pounds boneless, skinless chicken breast halves, each split in half horizontally

1. Combine mayonnaise, oil, lemon juice, parsley, scallion, tarragon, garlic, salt, sugar substitute, and pepper in a gallon-size resealable plastic bag. Add chicken, seal bag, and shake to coat. Refrigerate 1 hour.
2. Heat a charcoal or gas grill to medium or heat a grill pan.
3. Remove chicken from marinade and shake off any excess. Grill chicken, turning occasionally, until just cooked through, about 7 minutes.

TIP TIME

ONE BREAST OR TWO?

When a recipe calls for a chicken breast, what does it really mean? A whole breast is heart-shaped and weighs 6–10 ounces; most so-called chicken breasts sold in the supermarket are actually halves.

*See photo on the front cover

Classic Chicken Fricassee

Phases 1, 2, 3, 4

PER SERVING:
Net Carbs: 3 grams
Total Carbs: 3 grams
Fiber: 0 grams
Protein: 52 grams
Fat: 20 grams
Calories: 410

Makes: 6 servings
Active Time: 25 minutes
Total Time: 1 hour 10 minutes

WEEKEND

A fricassee is a poultry dish that's seared and then simmered slowly in less liquid than is normally used for a stew. The traditional addition of cream at the end makes the dish a bit more elegant.

3 tablespoons butter
4 pounds bone-in chicken parts
1 medium yellow or white onion, finely chopped
1 celery rib, trimmed and finely chopped
¼ teaspoon dried thyme
¼ teaspoon dried marjoram
1 clove garlic, minced
1½ cups chicken broth
½ cup heavy cream
¾ teaspoon salt
¼ teaspoon freshly ground black pepper

1. Melt butter in a large, heavy saucepan over medium-high heat. Add chicken and brown evenly on all sides, about 10 minutes.
2. Reduce heat to medium. Add onion, celery, thyme, and marjoram; sauté until vegetables are soft, about 6 minutes. Add garlic and sauté until fragrant, about 30 seconds.
3. Add broth; increase heat to high and bring to a boil. Reduce heat to medium-low, cover, and simmer until chicken is tender, about 45 minutes.
4. Transfer chicken to platter. Stir cream into saucepan; increase heat to medium and simmer until sauce thickens slightly, about 10 minutes. Add salt and pepper. Pour over chicken and serve.

Lemon-and-Basil Chicken-Veggie Kebabs*

Phases 1, 2, 3, 4

Full of fresh flavor and quick to prepare (most of the time the chicken is marinating), this entrée pairs well with greens—try Sautéed Greens with Pecans (page 101), Sautéed Baby Bok Choy with Garlic and Lemon Zest (page 104), Swiss Chard with Pine Nuts (page 108)—or a simple tossed salad.

PER SERVING:
Net Carbs: 7 grams
Total Carbs: 9 grams
Fiber: 2 grams
Protein: 41 grams
Fat: 17 grams
Calories: 360

Makes: 4 servings
Active Time: 30 minutes
Total Time: 2 hours 35 minutes

WEEKEND

- ⅓ cup virgin olive oil
- 3 tablespoons freshly squeezed lemon juice
- 1 tablespoon freshly grated lemon zest
- 2 cloves garlic, minced
- 1 tablespoon Dijon mustard
- 1½ teaspoons salt
- ¾ teaspoon freshly ground black pepper
- ⅓ cup chopped fresh basil
- 1½ pounds boneless, skinless chicken breasts, cut into 1-inch cubes
- 1 yellow or orange bell pepper, cut into 1-inch pieces
- 2 small zucchini, split lengthwise and cut into ½-inch-thick slices
- 16 small cherry tomatoes

- 8 (12-inch) bamboo skewers

1. Combine oil, lemon juice, lemon zest, garlic, mustard, salt, pepper, and basil in a large bowl. Stir in chicken, bell pepper, zucchini, and tomatoes. Cover and refrigerate 2 hours.
2. After chicken and vegetables have been marinating for 1½ hours, soak skewers in water for 30 minutes.
3. Meanwhile, prepare a charcoal or gas grill for high-heat cooking or heat a grill pan until very hot.
4. Thread chicken and vegetables onto skewers. Grill, turning occasionally, until chicken is nicely marked and cooked through, about 10 minutes. Serve right away.

*See photo on color page 18

Thai Chicken Curry

Phases 1, 2, 3, 4

PER SERVING:
Net Carbs: 6 grams
Total Carbs: 8 grams
Fiber: 2 grams
Protein: 40 grams
Fat: 20 grams
Calories: 370

Makes: 4 servings
Active Time: 25 minutes
Total Time: 25 minutes

WEEKDAY

Thai food relies on a combination of herbs and seasons for its subtle flavor. With a full complement of vegetables, this dish is a meal in itself. However, if you prefer, serve it over tofu shirataki noodles and top with chopped peanuts. Or, if your carb threshold is high enough, serve over brown rice. If you use a jalapeño, use all or some of the seeds—they provide the heat.

- 1½ pounds boneless, skinless chicken breasts, cut into 1-inch cubes
- 2 teaspoons curry powder
- 1 clove garlic, minced
- 1 tablespoon canola oil
- 2 cups sliced button mushrooms
- 2 scallions, sliced
- 1 cup canned unsweetened coconut milk
- 1 small Thai bird chile, seeded and chopped, or 1 jalapeño, chopped
- 2 teaspoons tamari (see page 11)
- 1½ teaspoons fish sauce (nam pla or nuoc mam)
- 1 tablespoon peeled and grated fresh ginger
- 1 teaspoon freshly grated lime zest
- 6 ounces green beans, cut into 1-inch pieces (1½ cups)
- ¼ cup fresh cilantro, coarsely chopped
- 2 teaspoons freshly squeezed lime juice

1. Combine chicken, curry powder, and garlic in a bowl; toss to coat. Heat oil in a large nonstick skillet over medium-high heat. Scrape in chicken and seasonings; sauté until golden, about 5 minutes. Stir in mushrooms, scallions, coconut milk, chile, fish sauce, ginger, and lime zest. Reduce heat to medium-low and simmer until chicken is cooked through, about 10 minutes.
2. Meanwhile, bring a small saucepan of water to boil. Add green beans and cook until crisp-tender, about 4 minutes. Drain. Stir into chicken and simmer until beans are coated with sauce, about 1 minute.
3. Remove from heat and stir in cilantro and lime juice. Serve in shallow bowls.

Chicken and Apple Sausage Patties

Phases 3, 4

A savory sausage mixture formed into patties makes a great breakfast, lunch, or dinner dish. Add the sugar substitute only if your apples are especially tart. Use ground chicken, not ground chicken breast, which will be too dry and not hold its shape. If you're in Phase 3 or 4 you could serve the burger on an Atkins Hamburger Bun (page 60) if you wish.

PER SERVING:
Net Carbs: 6 grams
Total Carbs: 7 grams
Fiber: 1 gram
Protein: 20 grams
Fat: 20 grams
Calories: 280

Makes: 4 (2-patty) servings
Active Time: 20 minutes
Total Time: 25 minutes

- 3 tablespoons canola oil, divided
- 1 medium Granny Smith apple, cored, peeled, and diced
- 1 medium shallot, minced
- 1 scallion, minced
- 1 teaspoon salt
- ¼ teaspoon freshly ground black pepper
- ¾ teaspoon dried sage
- ½ teaspoon dried thyme
- ⅛ teaspoon ground allspice
- 1 tablespoon Worcestershire sauce
- ½ teaspoon granular sugar substitute (optional)
- 1 pound ground chicken

1. Heat 2 tablespoons oil in a medium skillet over medium heat. Add apple, shallot, and scallion; sauté until tender, about 3 minutes. Transfer to a medium bowl. Add salt, pepper, sage, thyme, allspice, Worcestershire sauce, sugar substitute (if using), and chicken. Stir until well blended. Form into 8 patties, using ¼ cup per patty.
2. Heat remaining tablespoon oil in a large skillet. Working in batches if necessary, cook, turning once, until golden brown and chicken is no longer pink, about 3 minutes per side.

TIP TIME

TALKING TURKEY

This recipe would be equally tasty using ground turkey, which is usually found already ground in the supermarket, in place of ground chicken.

WEEKDAY

Grilled Turkey Cutlets with Thyme

Phases 1, 2, 3, 4

PER SERVING:
Net Carbs: 1 gram
Total Carbs: 2 grams
Fiber: 1 gram
Protein: 42 grams
Fat: 5 grams
Calories: 220

Makes: 4 servings
Active Time: 20 minutes
Total Time: 20 minutes

WEEKDAY

Turkey cutlets cook quickly, making them a great choice for speedy suppers. Take this very basic recipe and dress it up as you please. Serve alongside Roasted Cauliflower (page 111) or Creamy Red Cabbage with Dill (page 106).

4 (6-ounce) turkey cutlets
1 tablespoon virgin olive oil
2 teaspoons fresh thyme, chopped, or ½ teaspoon dried
½ teaspoon garlic powder
½ teaspoon paprika
½ teaspoon salt
½ teaspoon freshly ground black pepper
1 lemon, cut into wedges

1. Heat a gas or charcoal grill to high. Brush cutlets on both sides with oil; season with thyme, garlic powder, paprika, salt, and pepper.
2. Grill cutlets until cooked through, about 3 minutes per side. Serve immediately with lemon wedges on the side.

Variation: Pan-Seared Turkey Cutlets

Phases 1, 2, 3, 4

Prepare Grilled Turkey Cutlets as above, but instead of using a grill, heat 2 more tablespoons olive oil in a very large nonstick skillet over high heat. When very hot, add seasoned cutlets; sear until cooked through, about 3 minutes per side. Serve with lemon wedges.

Mexican-Style Turkey Meatloaf

Phases 2, 3, 4

Lighter than all-beef or beef-and-pork loaves, turkey meatloaf has a finer texture and more delicate flavor, but it's just as satisfying. Our recipe uses ground almonds rather than bread crumbs to keep carbs in check.

PER SERVING:

Net Carbs: 7 grams
Total Carbs: 10 grams
Fiber: 3 grams
Protein: 33 grams
Fat: 27 grams
Calories: 410

Makes: 6 servings
Active Time: 20 minutes
Total Time: 1 hour 25 minutes

Olive oil cooking spray
1 cup almond meal (see page 11)
2 pounds ground turkey
1 medium green bell pepper, stemmed, ribs and seeds removed, and finely chopped
1 small yellow or white onion, minced
¼ cup heavy cream
¼ cup chopped fresh parsley
3 tablespoons Worcestershire sauce
2 large eggs, beaten
1 tablespoon chopped fresh oregano, or 1 teaspoon dried
1 clove garlic, minced
1 teaspoon salt
½ teaspoon freshly ground black pepper
1 teaspoon ground cumin
1 tablespoon chili powder
6 tablespoons no-sugar-added tomato salsa

1. Heat oven to 350°F. Mist a 5-by-9-inch loaf pan with cooking spray.
2. In a large bowl, mix together almond meal, turkey, bell pepper, onion, cream, parsley, Worcestershire sauce, eggs, oregano, garlic, salt, pepper, cumin, and chili powder. Gently mix with hands until incorporated; transfer to loaf pan.
3. Spread salsa evenly over loaf; bake until cooked through, about 1 hour. Let stand 5 minutes before slicing.

TIP TIME

THE RIGHT SALSA

Fresh salsa from the dairy section is tastier—and less likely to include added sugar or corn syrup than canned or bottled types.

Chapter 10

BEEF, PORK, LAMB, AND VEAL ENTRÉES

"What's for dinner?" For a lot of us, the preferred answer to this question is meat. Whether beef, lamb, pork, or veal, meat is often the centerpiece of our meals and our primary source of protein, whether we choose a simple grilled steak, succulent pork chops, savory lamb kebabs, or elegant veal roast. And since uncooked, unseasoned meat, with the exception of some sausages, contains no carbohydrates, meat is a natural component of the Atkins Diet.

There's an overwhelming selection of cuts at the supermarket. Which meat you choose will dictate how you cook it—of course you'll cook a roast differently from a steak, but even steaks can vary considerably in tenderness and how they should be prepared. For example, some cuts are better marinated, as the acids in marinades help to tenderize the meat, but marinating can ruin others. (Marinating also adds flavor.) Likewise, some roasts should be braised or pot-roasted, not roasted in the usual sense.

COOKING TECHNIQUES

Most often, meat is browned, a complex process that creates hundreds of flavor compounds. Even stews and braises often begin with the meat being browned to intensify the flavors. The timing may differ depending on whether you're cooking beef, lamb, pork, or veal, but the basic techniques are the same. The recipes that follow employ these cooking methods. Some, such as stir-frying and grilling, lend themselves to speedy weeknight meals. Others, such as roasting and pot-roasting, may be better suited for the weekend. However, none of these recipes take more than 30 minutes of active time.

RIGHT-SIZE SERVINGS

Aim for 4–6 ounces of protein per meal. Although you don't need to worry about weighing foods or counting calories when you're following a low-carb lifestyle, it's still wise to pay attention to portion sizes. Filling up on too much meat, for instance, could mean that you don't get enough of other important nutrients. Depending upon how much fat is in the cut and any other protein sources in a recipe, start with about 5–8 ounces of raw meat per person—that is, buy 1¼–2 pounds of boneless meat to serve four people.

DON'T FEAR FAT

Depending on the cut, you may wish to cut off some of the fat before you cook meat, but don't remove it all—fat provides flavor and can help to keep the meat moist while it's cooking. This is especially important with lean cuts that have little marbling, or fat, within the muscle. Marbling appears as white lines throughout the meat. Rib cuts have more marbling than sirloin, for example, so it's okay to trim more of the external fat from a rib eye than from a sirloin steak.

MEAT 101

High in protein, iron, and vitamin B_{12}, beef is available in an almost endless variety, as well as being by far the most popular form of protein in the United States. When you select beef, look for bright- to deep-red meat (vacuum-sealed beef may look burgundy or purple). Any fat should be creamy white, not yellow or grayish.

Pork today is much leaner than it was twenty or thirty years ago, so choose carefully to be sure you get meat that's flavorful and juicy, rather than bland or dry. Lean pork should be cooked quickly so it doesn't toughen. Most pork is so tender it doesn't need to be braised or pot-roasted to become tender, but some cuts of pork can be braised or stewed with delicious results. Avoid meat that's pale pink or gray; reach for reddish-pink cuts instead. Pork should feel firm, not soft (press or squeeze it through the plastic wrap). Any fat on the meat should be creamy white.

It's a pity that the average American eats only about a pound of lamb per year, but that can probably be attributed to its higher cost and a slightly gamy flavor that some find too assertive. To recognize the appeal of lamb, trim off most of the fat, which is responsible for the gamy taste, and you'll find a wonderfully mild, versatile meat that marries perfectly with strong seasonings such as garlic, lemon, rosemary, mustard, and spices common to Indian and Moroccan cooking. Lamb is high in iron, protein, zinc, and several of the B vitamins. Choose reddish-pink cuts with pearly white fat. Dark red or purple meat and yellow fat are signs of older animals.

Like lamb, veal is not often consumed in the United States. High in protein and B vitamins, it's lower in fat and saturated fat than beef, mostly because it has very little marbling, or fat inside the muscle. Its mildness means it takes well to garlic, herbs, and other savory seasonings. All veal is quite tender, although range-fed veal tends to be redder than stall-raised veal. Don't buy veal that is dark red or whitish pink. The former is on the old side, the latter will lack flavor. Fat should be white, ivory, or pale yellow, and the meat should be slightly moist but not mushy when you press it.

MORE FOR MEAT LOVERS

Eagle-eyed readers will note the absence of classics such as hamburgers, sirloin steaks, Beef Stroganoff, Meatloaf, Brisket, Lamb Curry, Osso Bucco, and Crown Roast of Pork in this chapter. Not to worry: these favorites all appear, along with hundreds of other meaty delights, at www.atkins.com.

Florentine-Style Porterhouse Steak

Phases 1, 2, 3, 4

PER SERVING:
Net Carbs: 1 gram
Total Carbs: 1 gram
Fiber: 0 grams
Protein: 41 grams
Fat: 36 grams
Calories: 503

Makes 4 servings
Active Time: 10 minutes
Total Time: 25 minutes

Bistecca fiorentina is one of Italy's most famous beef dishes. Like all simple dishes, it benefits from using the best ingredients: buy aged steak if you can (its flavor is deeper and it shrinks less in cooking) and use a good-quality, fruity olive oil. Coarse sea salt is an integral part of this dish; if you don't have it, use kosher salt or about half as much regular table salt.

1 (1½-pound) porterhouse steak, 1½ inches thick
3 teaspoons extra-virgin olive oil, divided
1 clove garlic, cut in half
3 rosemary sprigs
3 thyme sprigs
1½ teaspoons coarse sea salt or kosher salt
¼ teaspoon coarsely ground black pepper

1. Rub the steak with 1 teaspoon oil, then rub it all over with the cut sides of the garlic; discard garlic. Rub steak again with 1 rosemary sprig and 1 thyme sprig; discard herbs. Season steak on both sides with salt and pepper; set aside.
2. Prepare a high-heat grill or set a grill pan or large cast-iron skillet over high heat. When very hot, add steak and grill or sear until done to taste, 4 to 5 minutes per side for medium-rare.
3. Transfer steak to a cutting board and let stand 5 minutes. With a sharp knife, cut around the bone so that you have 2 pieces of meat. Trim off any fat. Thinly slice steak and transfer to a platter. Surround with the remaining rosemary sprigs and thyme sprigs. Drizzle steak with the remaining 2 teaspoons olive oil and serve.

Skirt Steak with Chimichurri Sauce*

Phases 1, 2, 3, 4

In Argentina, beef is often served with chimichurri, a spicy, garlicky sauce. If the steak is less than ½ inch thick, adjust the cooking time accordingly.

PER SERVING:
Net Carbs: 2 grams
Total Carbs: 3 grams
Fiber: 1 gram
Protein: 37 grams
Fat: 32 grams
Calories: 450

Makes: 4 servings
Active Time: 25 minutes
Total Time: 30 minutes

Sauce
¼ cup extra-virgin olive oil
2 cups fresh parsley, finely chopped
3 tablespoons fresh oregano, finely chopped
2 tablespoons red wine vinegar
2 cloves garlic, minced
½ teaspoon red pepper flakes
½ teaspoon salt
¼ teaspoon freshly ground black pepper

Steak
1½ pounds skirt steak, ½-inch thick, trimmed of fat and cut into 4 equal pieces
1 tablespoon virgin olive oil
½ teaspoon salt
½ teaspoon freshly ground black pepper

1. For the sauce, mix oil, parsley, oregano, vinegar, garlic, red pepper flakes, salt, and pepper in a bowl; set aside.
2. For the steak, heat a large heavy skillet over high heat until very hot. Brush steak with oil and season with salt and pepper. Add steak to pan, reduce heat to medium-high, and sear until done to taste, about 3 minutes per side for medium-rare.
3. Transfer steak to a cutting board and let stand 5 minutes. Thinly slice across the grain. Stir sauce again and serve steak with sauce on the side.

TIP TIME

SALT FIRST

Salting before cooking allows the salt to combine with released juices to form a crust that accentuates flavors.

*See photo on color page 24

Bistro Flank Steak

Phases 1, 2, 3, 4

PER SERVING:
Net Carbs: 0 grams
Total Carbs: 0 grams
Fiber: 0 grams
Protein: 42 grams
Fat: 13 grams
Calories: 300

Makes: 6 servings
Active Time: 25 minutes
Total Time: 4 hours 35 minutes

WEEKEND

Red wine, rosemary, and garlic make a zesty marinade that infuses this classic dish with flavor. Flank steak lends itself well to marinating and grilling, but it should be cooked rare or medium-rare to keep it from getting tough.

- ½ cup dry red wine, such as merlot, Chianti or cabernet
- 1 tablespoon chopped fresh rosemary, or 1½ teaspoons dried
- 2 tablespoons extra-virgin olive oil
- 1 tablespoon Dijon mustard
- 1 tablespoon red wine vinegar
- ½ teaspoon granular sugar substitute
- 1 tablespoon Worcestershire sauce
- 2 large cloves garlic, chopped
- 1 (2-pound) flank steak
- ¾ teaspoon salt
- ½ teaspoon freshly ground black pepper

1. Combine wine, rosemary, oil, mustard, vinegar, sugar substitute, Worcestershire sauce, and garlic in a large resealable plastic bag. Seal bag and knead to mix marinade. Add steak, reseal bag, and turn to coat. Refrigerate for at least 4 hours, but preferably overnight.
2. Prepare a medium-high-heat grill; oil grill rack.
3. Remove steak from marinade and season on both sides with salt and pepper. Discard the marinade or boil it for 3–4 minutes to serve with steak.
4. Grill steak until done to taste, about 5 minutes per side for medium-rare. Transfer steak to a cutting board and let stand 10 minutes. Thinly slice steak diagonally across the grain.

TIP TIME

ALCOHOL ON ATKINS

Although you shouldn't drink alcohol in Phase 1 of Atkins, it's fine to eat food that's been marinated in wine. The heat burns off the alcohol, so it doesn't interfere with your body burning fat for energy.

Mushroom-Smothered Minute Steak

Phases 1, 2, 3, 4

Minute steak, also called cube steak, is a tenderized, thinly sliced piece of round beef. A simple mushroom sauce is the perfect complement.

- 1½ pounds minute steaks (4 steaks)
- ¾ teaspoon salt, divided
- ¼ teaspoon freshly ground black pepper, divided
- 3 tablespoons butter, divided
- 3 tablespoons virgin olive oil, divided
- 12 ounces button mushrooms, wiped clean, trimmed, and sliced
- 1 small yellow or white onion, sliced
- ½ cup beef broth
- 1 tablespoon freshly squeezed lemon juice
- 1 teaspoon paprika
- 3 tablespoons chopped fresh parsley

PER SERVING:
Net Carbs: 5 grams
Total Carbs: 6 grams
Fiber: 1 gram
Protein: 24 grams
Fat: 36 grams
Calories: 440

Makes: 4 servings
Active Time: 30 minutes
Total Time: 30 minutes

1. Season steaks with ¼ teaspoon salt and ⅛ teaspoon pepper. Heat 1 tablespoon butter and 1 tablespoon oil in large nonstick skillet over high heat. Add 2 steaks and sear until just cooked through, about 3 minutes per side. Transfer to plate and keep warm. Repeat with other steaks.
2. Heat remaining 2 tablespoons butter and 2 tablespoons oil in the skillet over high heat. Add mushrooms and onion; sauté until golden, about 8 minutes. Add broth, any accumulated juices from the steaks, lemon juice, paprika, remaining ½ teaspoon salt, and remaining ⅛ teaspoon pepper. Cook until sauce thickens slightly, about 3 minutes.
3. Pour sauce over steaks, sprinkle with parsley, and serve hot.

TIP TIME

A CUT BY ANY NAME

The names of meat cuts vary in different parts of the country. Once you find a cut that you like, look for it by shape and size rather than by name.

Chicken-Fried Steak

Phases 2, 3, 4

PER SERVING:
Net Carbs: 4 grams
Total Carbs: 8 grams
Fiber: 4 grams
Protein: 37 grams
Fat: 38 grams
Calories: 520

Makes: 6 servings
Active Time: 20 minutes
Total Time: 20 minutes

WEEKDAY

A quick bath in buttermilk and a coating of seasoned low-carb baking mix makes these steaks crunchy on the outside and super-tender on the inside—just like great southern fried chicken. Be sure to pat the steaks dry before coating them so they become nice and crunchy.

- 1 cup Atkins Cuisine All Purpose Baking Mix
- 1 teaspoon garlic powder
- 1 teaspoon paprika
- 1½ teaspoons salt, divided
- ½ teaspoon freshly ground black pepper
- 2 large eggs
- ½ cup buttermilk
- ¾ cups canola oil
- 1½ pounds London broil, cut into ¼-inch slices and patted dry
- 1 tablespoon fresh chopped parsley
- 1 lemon, cut in wedges

1. Whisk baking mix, garlic powder, paprika, 1 teaspoon salt, and pepper in a shallow bowl. Whisk eggs, buttermilk, and ½ teaspoon salt in another shallow bowl.
2. Heat oil in a large, heavy skillet over medium-high heat until very hot. Dredge steaks in seasoned baking mix and shake off excess. Dip in egg wash, shake off excess, and dredge again in baking mix. Fry steaks in 2 batches until golden brown, turning once, about 3 minutes per side.
3. Transfer to a warm platter and garnish with parsley and lemon wedges.

Variation: Chicken-Fried Steak with Cream Sauce

Phases 2, 3, 4

Follow directions above, but omit lemon. After Step 2, pour off all but 1 tablespoon oil. Return skillet to medium-high heat; add ½ cup heavy cream, ¼ cup cold water, ¼ teaspoon salt, and ½ teaspoon pepper. Bring to a boil, scraping up brown bits from bottom of pan and cooking until slightly thickened, about 5 minutes. Serve steaks with sauce on the side.

Beef and Asian Vegetable Stir-Fry*

Phases 2, 3, 4

Shake the meat to remove excess liquid when you remove it from the marinade, but don't wipe it dry or you'll mute the flavors of the finished dish. However, too much liquid will cause the oil to spatter, so shake the meat well.

PER SERVING:
Net Carbs: 10 grams
Total Carbs: 13 grams
Fiber: 3 grams
Protein: 30 grams
Fat: 15 grams
Calories: 310

Makes: 4 (1-cup) servings
Active Time: 20 minutes
Total Time: 3 hours 20 minutes

- 1 pound sirloin steak, cut into ¼-inch-thick strips
- ⅓ cup tamari (see page 11)
- 1 tablespoon unsweetened rice wine or dry sherry
- 2 cloves garlic, minced
- 1 teaspoon peeled, minced ginger
- 1 teaspoon sugar substitute
- 3 tablespoons canola oil
- 1 medium red bell pepper, cored, seeded, and sliced
- 1 (8-ounce) can bamboo shoots, drained
- 8 ounces sugar snap peas, strings removed and halved diagonally
- 2 scallions, sliced on the diagonal in 1-inch pieces
- 1½ teaspoons dark (toasted) sesame oil

1. Combine steak, tamari, wine, garlic, ginger, and sugar substitute in a resealable plastic bag. Refrigerate for at least 3 and up to 12 hours.
2. Remove meat from marinade, shaking off extra liquid; reserve marinade.
3. Heat oil in a wok or large skillet over high heat until oil shimmers. Add meat and stir-fry until slightly colored, about 1 minute. Add bell peppers and stir-fry for 3 minutes. Add bamboo shoots and peas and stir-fry until just soft, about 1 minute. Add scallions and stir-fry 1 minute longer. Transfer beef and vegetables to serving bowl.
4. Add reserved marinade to wok; boil until slightly thickened, 3–4 minutes. Remove from heat; stir in sesame oil. Pour sauce over meat and vegetables and serve.

WEEKEND

*See photo on color page 15

Greek Meatballs

Phases 2, 3, 4

PER SERVING:
Net Carbs: 2 grams
Total Carbs: 4 grams
Fiber: 2 grams
Protein: 41 grams
Fat: 29 grams
Calories: 450

Makes: 4 (6-meatball) servings
Active Time: 10 minutes
Total Time: 30 minutes

WEEKDAY

Using a "meatloaf blend" of equal parts of ground beef, pork, and veal, makes especially moist, juicy meatballs. Serve them with no-added-sugar tomato sauce over low-carb pasta, tofu shirataki noodles, or grated raw zucchini.

Olive oil cooking spray
½ cup almond meal (see page 11)
1½ pounds ground meatloaf blend (see note above)
¼ cup grated Parmesan
2 large eggs, lightly beaten
2 tablespoons chopped fresh dill
1 clove garlic, chopped
¾ teaspoon dried mint
½ teaspoon dried oregano
¼ teaspoon ground cinnamon
1 teaspoon salt
½ teaspoon freshly ground black pepper

1. Heat oven to 425°F. Line a baking sheet with foil; lightly mist with cooking spray.
2. Combine almond meal, meat, cheese, eggs, dill, garlic, mint, oregano, cinnamon, salt, and pepper; mix gently with hands.
3. Moisten your hands (this helps prevent mixture from sticking); shape mixture into 1½-inch balls and set on prepared baking sheet. Bake until lightly browned and cooked through, about 20 minutes.

Variation: Sautéed Cocktail Meatballs

Phases 2, 3, 4

Prepare Greek Meatballs as above, shaping meat mixture into 1-inch balls. Heat 2 tablespoons olive oil in a large nonstick skillet over medium-high heat. Add half the meatballs; cook, turning frequently, until browned on all sides and cooked through, about 8 minutes. Repeat with 2 more tablespoons olive oil and remaining meatballs. Serve with toothpicks as an appetizer.

Roasted Pork Tenderloin with Maple-Mustard Sauce

Phases 1, 2, 3, 4

Pork tenderloin is a small, tender muscle that roasts quickly for an easy but elegant main course. A high temperature ensures quick roasting to maintain natural tenderness.

PER SERVING:
Net Carbs: 3 grams
Total Carbs: 3 grams
Fiber: 0 grams
Protein: 48 grams
Fat: 14 grams
Calories: 360

Makes: 4 servings
Active Time: 20 minutes
Total Time: 40 minutes

- 2 (1-pound) pork tenderloins
- 1 tablespoon virgin olive oil
- 1 teaspoon salt
- 1 teaspoon freshly ground black pepper
- 2 cloves garlic, chopped
- 1 tablespoon minced fresh sage
- ½ cup chicken broth
- ½ cup white wine
- 2 tablespoons Dijon mustard
- 2 teaspoons sugar-free pancake syrup
- 2 tablespoons cold butter, cut into cubes

1. Heat oven to 450°F.
2. Pat tenderloins dry with paper towels. Combine oil, salt, pepper, garlic, and sage in a small bowl; rub paste over tenderloins and set them in a shallow roasting pan. Roast until done to taste, about 20 minutes for medium (an instant-read thermometer inserted into the center of the loin will register 145°F). Transfer to a cutting board and let stand while you prepare the sauce.
3. Set pan over medium-high heat on range top. Add broth, wine, mustard, and pancake syrup; cook and stir, scraping up brown bits from bottom of pan, until reduced by half, about 10 minutes. Turn off heat; add butter and swirl pan to melt. Slice tenderloin and serve with sauce.

Cheese-Stuffed Pork Roast

Phases 2, 3, 4

PER SERVING:
Net Carbs: 3 grams
Total Carbs: 4 grams
Fiber: 1 gram
Protein: 49 grams
Fat: 29 grams
Calories: 500

Makes: 8 servings
Active Time: 30 minutes
Total Time: 1 hour 35 minutes

WEEKEND

A simple pork roast becomes a Sunday-dinner special with a spinach, cheese, and walnut filling. Pan juices, boosted with white wine and chicken broth, make a flavorful gravy. Be sure to squeeze all the water out of the spinach so the stuffing will hold together. This dish is acceptable after the first two weeks in Phase 1.

- 2 ounces defrosted and drained chopped frozen spinach (⅓ cup)
- 2 (5.2-ounce) packages Laughing Cow or other herb-and-garlic-flavored spreadable cheese
- ½ cup finely chopped walnuts
- 1 teaspoon chopped fresh thyme
- ¾ teaspoon salt, divided
- ¼ teaspoon freshly ground black pepper, divided
- 4-pound center cut pork loin roast
- 1 tablespoon virgin olive oil
- 1½ teaspoons Dixie Carb Counters Thick-It-Up low-carb thickener*
- ¾ cup dry white wine
- ¾ cup chicken broth

1. Heat oven to 450°F.
2. Combine spinach, cheese, walnuts, thyme, ¼ teaspoon salt, and ⅛ teaspoon pepper in a medium bowl. Set aside.
3. Slice pork loin almost in half crosswise, taking care not to cut all the way through. Open up like a book and lay loin flat. Spoon stuffing along bottom half of loin. Fold loin closed, covering stuffing. Use kitchen twine to tie roast together. Brush top and sides of roast with oil and season with remaining ½ teaspoon salt and ⅛ teaspoon pepper
4. Set roast on a rack in a shallow roasting pan. Transfer to oven, reduce temperature to 350°F, and roast until done to taste, about 55 minutes for medium (an instant-read thermometer inserted into the center of the roast will register 155°F). Transfer roast to cutting board and let stand 10 minutes.

*Order from www.dixiediner.com.

5. Meanwhile, strain pan drippings and discard excess fat. Return drippings to pan. Add thickener, wine, and broth to pan juices and cook over medium heat, stirring constantly, until mixture bubbles and thickens, about 5 minutes. Season with salt and pepper to taste. Remove twine from roast and cut into ½-inch slices; serve with pan sauce.

Variation: Sausage-Stuffed Pork Roast

Phases 1, 2, 3, 4

Prepare Cheese-Stuffed Pork Loin as on the preceding page, omitting the cheese stuffing. Instead, spread entire interior of roast with 3 tablespoons Dijon mustard; place an 8-ounce straight piece of smoked sausage, of appropriate length, on bottom half of roast. Roll up and tie.

Sweet-and-Sour Pork Chops with Cabbage

Phases 3, 4

PER SERVING:
Net Carbs: 9 grams
Total Carbs: 12 grams
Fiber: 3 grams
Protein: 36 grams
Fat: 19 grams
Calories: 360

Makes: 4 servings
Active Time: 30 minutes
Total Time: 30 minutes

This German-style dish makes a hearty dinner, perfect for a chilly autumn evening. To make this suitable for Phase 2, replace the apricot jam with 2 tablespoons sugar-free pancake syrup. To make it suitable for Phase 1, also have your chop with a slightly smaller serving of cabbage.

1 teaspoon dried sage, crumbled
½ teaspoon salt, divided
¼ teaspoon dried thyme
¼ teaspoon freshly ground black pepper
4 (4- to 5-ounce) boneless pork loin chops, ¾-inch thick
2 tablespoons canola oil
2 slices bacon, diced
1 small (1-pound) red cabbage, cored and thinly sliced
1 medium yellow or white onion, thinly sliced
¼ cup cider vinegar
2 tablespoons no-sugar-added apricot jam

1. Combine sage, ¼ teaspoon salt, thyme, and pepper in a small bowl; season chops on both sides. Heat oil in a large skillet over high heat; sear chops until no longer pink inside, about 4 minutes per side. Transfer to a platter and cover loosely to keep warm.
2. Add bacon to skillet; reduce heat to medium-high and cook until crisp, about 3 minutes. Add cabbage and onion; reduce heat to medium-low and sauté until wilted, about 15 minutes Add vinegar, jam, and remaining ¼ teaspoon salt; simmer until liquid has evaporated, stirring to scrape up any brown bits from bottom of skillet. Spoon cabbage around chops and serve.

Variation: Sweet-and-Sour Bratwurst with Cabbage

Phases 3, 4

Prepare Pork Chops with Cabbage as above, substituting an equivalent amount of bratwurst or another sausage for the pork chops and adding 1 teaspoon caraway seed with the cabbage and onion.

Peppery-Spicy Baby Back Ribs*

Phases 1, 2, 3, 4

Baby back ribs are meatier than spareribs and the slabs are shorter. These tender ribs sport a crust of spice rub that complements the succulent pork, rather than a syrupy glaze. Instead of baking the ribs, you can also cook them on a charcoal or gas grill. Set foil-wrapped ribs on the side of grill away from the flame; cover the grill and cook until very tender, about 1 hour, keeping the heat at 350–400°F if possible.

PER SERVING:
Net Carbs: 2 grams
Total Carbs: 3 grams
Fiber: 1 gram
Protein: 37 grams
Fat: 54 grams
Calories: 660

Makes: 6 servings
Active Time: 15 minutes
Total Time: 2 hours 25 minutes

1 tablespoon paprika
1½ teaspoons garlic powder
1½ teaspoons onion powder
1½ teaspoons white pepper
1½ teaspoons black freshly ground black pepper
1½ teaspoons chili powder
1½ teaspoons ground cumin
1½ teaspoons cayenne
1 teaspoon salt
1 tablespoon granular sugar substitute
2 (1½- to 2-pound) slabs baby-back pork ribs

1. Heat oven to 250°F. Combine paprika, garlic powder, onion powder, white pepper, black pepper, chili powder, cumin, cayenne, salt, and sugar substitute in a bowl. Rub ribs evenly with spices, wrap each rack in foil, and set on jelly roll pans. Bake 2 hours.
2. Carefully remove ribs from foil, draining off liquid. Increase temperature to 450°F; roast until browned, about 10 minutes.
3. Cut ribs between bones and serve.

WEEKEND

*See photo on color page 26

Chinese Sweet-and-Sour Pork

Phases 3, 4

PER SERVING:
Net Carbs: 13 grams
Total Carbs: 18 grams
Fiber: 5 grams
Protein: 41 grams
Fat: 19 grams
Calories: 410

Makes: 4 (1½-cup) servings
Active Time: 25 minutes
Total Time: 25 minutes

WEEKDAY

Stir-fried colorful peppers, pineapple, and tender pork cloaked in a sweet sauce made with low-carb hoisin sauce—you can easily make this restaurant classic at home. Be sure to use fresh pineapple rather than canned, which is swimming in sugar syrup. To save time, purchase cut-up pineapple in the produce section. Instead of rice, serve this dish over shredded lettuce.

- 3 tablespoons canola oil
- 1½ pounds pork tenderloin, cubed
- 1 small yellow or white onion, coarsely chopped
- 1 red bell pepper, stemmed, seeds and ribs removed, and cut into ¾-inch squares
- 1 green bell pepper, stemmed, seeds and ribs removed, and cut into ¾-inch squares
- 1 clove garlic, finely chopped
- ½ medium fresh pineapple, cubed (1½ cups)
- 2 tablespoons tamari
- ½ cup low-carb hoisin sauce (see page 8)
- 1 tablespoon chili sauce
- ½ teaspoon dark (toasted) sesame oil
- 6 cups shredded romaine lettuce
- 3 tablespoons sesame seeds, toasted

1. Heat oil in a large skillet or wok over very high heat. Add pork and stir-fry until browned on all sides, about 2 minutes.
2. Add onion and bell peppers; sauté until just soft, about 3 minutes. Add garlic and sauté until fragrant, about 30 seconds. Add pineapple, tamari, hoisin sauce, and chili sauce; cook until sauce thickens, about 3 minutes.
3. Remove from heat; stir in sesame oil. Serve over lettuce and garnish with sesame seeds.

Slow-Cooked Pork Shoulder

Phases 1, 2, 3, 4

Fork-tender describes this melt-in-your-mouth pork full of old-fashioned flavor. This method makes perfect pork for barbecue sandwiches, burritos, or enchiladas. If you don't have beef broth, use chicken broth.

PER SERVING:
Net Carbs: 1 gram
Total Carbs: 1 gram
Fiber: 0 grams
Protein: 43 grams
Fat: 30 grams
Calories: 460

Makes: 8 servings
Active Time: 5 minutes
Total Time: 3 hours 15 minutes

1 boneless butt (shoulder) pork roast, about 4 pounds
½ cup beef broth
2 tablespoons tamari (see page 11)
½ teaspoon hot pepper sauce
2 tablespoons red wine or cider vinegar
2 tablespoons sugar-free pancake syrup
1 teaspoon ground cumin

1. Heat oven to 325°F. Set pork in a casserole or Dutch oven with a lid. Combine broth, tamari, hot pepper sauce, vinegar, syrup, and cumin; pour over pork. Cover and bake until fork-tender, about 3 hours.
2. Let stand for 10 minutes before chopping or shredding, and serve.

TIP TIME

WATCH THE CLOCK

Roasting times for meat are approximate. Check the roast a few minutes before the time you expect it to be done to prevent overcooking. Remove it when the temperature is a few degrees below what is specified (or what the meat thermometer calls for); the meat will continue to cook as it stands before carving.

Sautéed Italian Sausage with Fennel

Phases 1, 2, 3, 4

PER SERVING:
Net Carbs: 6 grams
Total Carbs: 9 grams
Fiber: 3 grams
Protein: 25 grams
Fat: 64 grams
Calories: 710

Makes: 4 servings
Active Time: 25 minutes
Total Time: 25 minutes

Savory Italian sausage topped with fennel makes a very satisfying entrée. Use Italian sausage that's sweet, hot, or a combination of both to make this dish distinctive.

- 3 tablespoons olive oil, divided
- 1½ pounds (about 8 links) Italian sausage
- 1 medium onion, sliced
- 2 heads fennel, cored, fronds removed, and sliced thin
- 2 tablespoons red wine vinegar
- 2 cloves garlic, chopped
- 1 teaspoon dried oregano, crushed
- ¼ teaspoon salt
- ⅛ teaspoon freshly ground black pepper

1. Heat 1 tablespoon oil in a large skillet over medium heat. Add sausages and cook until browned and no longer pink inside, about 7 minutes per side. Transfer to platter and cover loosely with foil to keep warm.
2. Heat remaining 2 tablespoons oil over medium-high heat. Add onion, cover, and cook, stirring occasionally, until slightly soft, about 3 minutes. Add fennel and cook for 1 more minute. Stir in vinegar, garlic, oregano, salt, and pepper. Cover and cook until vegetables are very tender, about 5 minutes.
3. Top sausages with sautéed vegetables and serve.

TIP TIME

CHECK FOR CARBS

Sausages are made by grinding meats with fat, spices, seasonings, and perhaps fillers before (typically) being stuffed into casings. Depending on the fillers and seasonings, sausages can include carbohydrates. The Nutrition Facts panel will provide information on packaged sausages. If you buy them freshly made, ask the butcher about fillers and seasonings.

Mustard-Bourbon Glazed Ham

Phases 3, 4

Everyone loves ham, and this super-easy one is dressed for company with a piquant glaze steeped in the sweet scent of bourbon. A spiral ham is not just precooked; it's also been presliced in one continuous spiral cut around the ham, so all the slices are the same thickness.

PER SERVING:
Net Carbs: 4 grams
Total Carbs: 4 grams
Fiber: 0 grams
Protein: 59 grams
Fat: 24 grams
Calories: 490

Makes: 12 servings
Active Time: 15 minutes
Total Time: 1 hour 40 minutes

- 1 (7-pound) fully cooked smoked spiral-sliced boneless ham
- ½ cup no-sugar-added apricot jam
- ¼ cup Dijon mustard
- ¼ cup bourbon
- 2 tablespoons butter

1. Position rack in bottom third of oven and heat to 350°F.
2. Place ham on a rack in a shallow roasting pan; cover loosely with foil, and bake for 1½ hours.
3. Meanwhile, stir together jam, mustard, bourbon, and butter in a medium saucepan; bring to a boil over medium-high heat. Cook, stirring, 5 minutes. Remove from heat and set aside.
4. Reduce oven temperature to 300°F. Pour glaze over ham and continue to roast, uncovered, until a thermometer inserted into the thickest part registers 140°F, 15–30 minutes longer; baste often with pan drippings. Transfer ham to a platter; let stand 10 minutes before serving.

TIP TIME

CHOOSE SMOKED OR FRESH

Hams are cuts from the hindquarters of the hog; they're most often cured or smoked, but you'll also find fresh ham in supermarkets. Fresh ham may also be called pork leg or leg of pork.

Lamb, Zucchini, Mushroom, and Tomato Kebabs

Phases 2, 3, 4

PER SERVING:
Net Carbs: 10 grams
Total Carbs: 13 grams
Fiber: 3 grams
Protein: 40 grams
Fat: 38 grams
Calories: 530

Makes: 4 (3-skewer) servings
Active Time: 30 minutes
Total Time: 4 hours

WEEKEND

Kids of all ages love kebabs for the colorful variety and textures of the ingredients and the casual mood eating skewered food evokes. Feel free to substitute other vegetables such as bell peppers, eggplant, or yellow squash. Tabbouleh Salad (page 89) is a natural accompaniment. If you're in Phase 1, eat the lamb but cut back on the vegetables a bit to stay at 7 grams of Net Carbs.

½ cup virgin olive oil
2 cloves garlic, minced
2 tablespoons freshly grated lemon zest
2 teaspoons chopped fresh thyme, or ¾ teaspoon dried
1½ pounds boneless leg of lamb, cut into 24 (1-inch) cubes
2 medium zucchini, trimmed, each cut crosswise into 12 pieces
24 button or cremini mushrooms, trimmed and wiped clean
24 cherry tomatoes
4 scallions, cut on the diagonal in 2-inch pieces
Olive oil cooking spray
¾ teaspoon salt
½ teaspoon freshly ground black pepper

12 (10-inch) bamboo skewers or metal skewers

1. Combine oil, garlic, lemon zest, thyme, and lamb in a resealable plastic bag. Shake and turn bag to coat meat. Refrigerate for at least 3 hours, but preferably overnight.
2. During last hour of marinating time, add zucchini and mushrooms to the bag; turn to coat.
3. Meanwhile, soak bamboo skewers in warm water for ½ hour, if using.
4. Heat a grill or grill pan to very hot. Mist grill rack or pan with cooking spray. Thread meat and vegetables onto the skewers, alternating to vary colors and shapes; season with salt and pepper.
5. Grill skewers on all sides until done to taste, about 5 minutes for medium-rare. Serve right away.

Roast Rack of Lamb with Mustard-Nut Crust*

Phases 2, 3, 4

Tender, flavorful rack of lamb makes a beautiful presentation at a festive occasion. Racks are usually frenched, meaning that the meat along the bone is scraped off. If you're less concerned with a classic appearance and want a little more meat, ask your butcher not to trim between the ribs.

PER SERVING:
Net Carbs: 2 grams
Total Carbs: 4 grams
Fiber: 2 grams
Protein: 30 grams
Fat: 20 grams
Calories: 320

Makes: 4 servings
Active Time: 20 minutes
Total Time: 45 minutes

- 1 (8-rib) rack of lamb, frenched (about 1 to 1½ pounds)
- ½ teaspoon salt
- ¼ teaspoon freshly ground black pepper
- 1 tablespoon virgin olive oil
- 2 tablespoons butter
- 1 clove garlic, minced
- ¼ cup almond meal (see page 11)
- 2 tablespoons minced fresh parsley
- 2 teaspoons minced fresh rosemary
- 2 teaspoons minced fresh thyme
- ¼ cup coarse-grain mustard

1. Heat oven to 400°F. Season lamb with salt and pepper.
2. Heat oil in large ovenproof skillet over high heat. Sear lamb until browned, about 4 minutes per side.
3. Meanwhile, melt butter in a small skillet over medium-high heat. Add garlic and sauté until fragrant, about 30 seconds. Add almond meal; cook until butter is absorbed. Stir in parsley, rosemary, and thyme.
4. Brush fat side of rack of lamb evenly with mustard; pat with almond meal mixture. Roast in skillet, almond meal side up, until done to taste, about 20 minutes for rare (an instant-read thermometer inserted into thickest part of lamb, not touching bone, should register 140°F).
5. Let the roast stand 5 minutes before slicing between the ribs and serving.

*See photo on color page 29

Yogurt-Marinated Butterflied Leg of Lamb

Phases 2, 3, 4

PER SERVING:
Net Carbs: 3 grams
Total Carbs: 3 grams
Fiber: 0 grams
Protein: 38 grams
Fat: 31 grams
Calories: 460

Makes: 10 servings
Active Time: 15 minutes
Total Time: 5 hours

WEEKEND

Leg of lamb with the bones removed—referred to as "butterflied"—is a quick-cooking cut. Marinating the lamb in a mixture of yogurt and spices intensifies flavors and tenderizes the meat. Because the marinade is discarded, this recipe is suitable for Phase 1 if you omit the yogurt sauce. We've broiled the lamb, but it also works well on the grill.

- 3 cups plain unsweetened whole-milk yogurt, preferably Greek yogurt
- ¼ cup chopped fresh mint
- ¼ cup chopped fresh cilantro
- 4 small scallions, thinly sliced
- 1 tablespoon chopped fresh ginger
- 1 small clove garlic, minced
- 1 teaspoon salt
- ½ teaspoon freshly ground black pepper
- 1 butterflied leg of lamb, trimmed (about 4 pounds)

1. Combine yogurt, mint, cilantro, scallions, ginger, garlic, salt, and pepper in a large resealable plastic bag; seal bag and knead to mix thoroughly. Reserve 1 cup separately to serve with lamb. Add lamb to the remaining marinade, seal bag, and refrigerate for at least 4 hours or overnight.
2. Set an oven rack about 5 inches from the broiler element. Heat the broiler to high. Line a broiler pan with foil; cover with a broiler rack and brush lightly with oil.
3. Remove lamb from marinade and pat dry; discard used marinade. Place lamb on broiler rack and broil for 15 minutes. Turn over and continue to broil until done to taste, about 15 minutes longer for medium-rare (an instant-read thermometer inserted into thickest part of lamb, not touching bone, should register 135°F).
4. Let stand 15 minutes before carving. Serve with reserved yogurt sauce.

Variation: Butterflied Leg of Lamb with Moroccan Herb Paste

Phases 1, 2, 3, 4

Prepare Yogurt-Marinated Butterflied Leg of Lamb as on the preceding page, replacing yogurt marinade with ½ cup virgin olive oil, ½ cup freshly squeezed lemon juice, ¼ cup finely chopped parsley, 1 teaspoon ground cumin, and 1 teaspoon ground coriander, whisked together in a bowl. Pour two-thirds of paste over lamb and reserve the remainder to serve alongside.

TIP TIME

LUSCIOUS LEFTOVERS

Leftover lamb lends itself well to both cold and hot dishes. Top a salad of arugula, cherry tomatoes, and feta cheese with cubs of leftover lamb and add a zesty dressing. Or sauté onion and garlic until golden, then add curry powder, cumin, cinnamon, and salt and cook until very aromatic. Add lamb, some broth, and canned diced tomatoes and cook until the lamb is tender.

Veal Provençal

Phases 2, 3, 4

PER SERVING:
Net Carbs: 8 grams
Total Carbs: 9 grams
Fiber: 1 gram
Protein: 25 grams
Fat: 29 grams
Calories: 390

Makes: 4 servings
Active Time: 30 minutes
Total Time: 30 minutes

WEEKDAY

Scaloppini is Italian for a thin scallop of meat that's usually dredged in flour before being sautéed. In Phase 1, cut back slightly on the vegetables.

- 1¼ pounds veal scaloppini (4 cutlets, each ¼-inch thick)
- ½ teaspoon salt, divided
- ¼ teaspoon freshly ground black pepper
- 1 medium leek, light green and white parts only, outer layer removed
- 3 tablespoons virgin olive oil, divided
- 1 orange or yellow bell pepper, trimmed, seeded, and sliced
- 2 large cloves garlic, minced
- 1 (14½-ounce) can diced tomatoes in juice
- ½ cup mixed green and black olives, pitted and quartered
- ½ teaspoon chopped fresh thyme or ¼ teaspoon dried
- ½ cup loosely packed fresh basil, chopped
- 2 tablespoons butter

1. Season veal with ¼ teaspoon salt and the pepper.
2. Cut leeks in half lengthwise and wash carefully in cold water to remove any dirt. Cut into ⅛-inch slices.
3. Heat 2 tablespoons oil in large nonstick skillet over medium-high heat. Add half of the veal; sear until lightly browned and just cooked through, about 1 minute per side. Transfer to a platter; repeat with remaining veal. Keep warm.
4. Heat remaining tablespoon oil in skillet; add leek, bell pepper, and garlic. Sauté until vegetables soften, about 3 minutes. Stir in tomatoes with juice, olives, thyme, and remaining ¼ teaspoon salt. Bring to a boil. Reduce heat to medium and simmer until sauce thickens, about 8 minutes, adding any juices that have accumulated from the veal.
5. Return veal to skillet, turning to coat with sauce and heat through, about 2 minutes. Transfer cutlets to plates. Add basil and butter to sauce and stir until butter melts, about 1 minute. Spoon sauce over veal and serve.

Veal Marsala

Phases 1, 2, 3, 4

There's a reason that some recipes are classics. You'll appreciate this when you taste these tender slices of veal, sauced with sweet Marsala wine. Purists might claim that this dish shouldn't include mushrooms, but we think they add a nice touch.

PER SERVING:
Net Carbs: 7 grams
Total Carbs: 8 grams
Fiber: 1 gram
Protein: 26 grams
Fat: 26 grams
Calories: 400

Makes: 4 servings
Active Time: 30 minutes
Total Time: 30 minutes

2 tablespoons butter, divided
10 ounces button mushrooms, trimmed, wiped dry, and sliced
1¼ pounds veal scaloppini (4 cutlets, each ¼–⅛ inch thick)
¾ teaspoon salt
½ teaspoon freshly ground black pepper
2 tablespoons virgin olive oil, divided
¾ cup chicken broth
½ cup dry Marsala wine
½ teaspoon granular sugar substitute (optional)
1 tablespoon freshly squeezed lemon juice

1. Heat butter in a large skillet over medium-high heat. Add mushrooms and sauté until browned, about 8 minutes. Remove from heat.
2. Meanwhile, season veal with salt and pepper. Heat half of the oil in another large skillet over high heat. Add half of the veal; sear until lightly browned and just cooked through, about 1 minute per side. Transfer to a platter; repeat with remaining oil and veal.
3. Add broth, wine and sugar substitute to skillet; bring to a boil and cook, scraping up brown bits from bottom of pan, until liquid has reduced by half, about 5 minutes. Reduce heat to low; stir in lemon juice and mushrooms. Return veal to skillet; cook to heat through, about 30 seconds. Return to platter; serve right away.

WEEKDAY

Fontina-and-Prosciutto-Stuffed Veal Chops

Phases 1, 2, 3, 4

PER SERVING:
Net Carbs: 1 gram
Total Carbs: 1 gram
Fiber: 0 grams
Protein: 48 grams
Fat: 25 grams
Calories: 440

Makes: 4 servings
Active Time: 25 minutes
Total Time: 25 minutes

Fontina cheese is made in several European countries as well as in the United States. For this dish, choose Italian fontina—it's a bit sharper in flavor and drier in texture, and it pairs beautifully with prosciutto.

2 ounces fontina cheese, shredded (½ cup)
1 ounce prosciutto, chopped
¼ cup chopped fresh basil
4 (8-ounce) veal rib chops
¾ teaspoon salt
½ teaspoon freshly ground black pepper

1. Combine cheese, prosciutto, and basil in a small bowl.
2. Cut a horizontal pocket in each chop. Season chops inside and out with salt and pepper. Fill with cheese mixture; secure opening with toothpicks.
3. Prepare a medium-high-heat grill or heat a grill pan until very hot. Grill chops until they are browned and just lose their pink color throughout, about 5 minutes per side. Serve hot.

TIP TIME

THE SKINNY ON PROSCIUTTO

You've probably encountered prosciutto as an appetizer sliced thin and served with melon or figs. *Prosciutto* is Italian for "ham," and ham from Parma, Italy, is the original prosciutto. Today the term is used more broadly for ham that's been seasoned, salt-cured (but not smoked), air-dried, and then pressed, creating a firm, dense texture. Find it in Italian specialty stores or many supermarkets.

WEEKDAY

Chapter 11

FISH AND SHELLFISH ENTRÉES

All fish, but especially fatty fish, provide a host of nutritional benefits. Fatty species are an excellent source of omega-3 fats, which can protect against heart disease and high blood pressure and reduce levels of triglycerides. Most fish are high in protein, B vitamins (particularly B_{12}), and minerals such as zinc and selenium; they also provide varying degrees of the fat-soluble vitamins A, D, and E.

These benefits are only enhanced by the fact that fish (although not all shellfish) contains no carbohydrates. Fish and shellfish have yet another virtue: if you're after a speedy supper, you'll have to look hard to find something faster than fish. Unless you're roasting a whole fish or lobster, most recipes can be on the table in about 30 minutes. We recommend you have fish or shellfish two or three times a week.

THE DIFFERENCE BETWEEN FAT AND LEAN

Both Jack Spratt and his wife would enjoy fish. Fish can be categorized in several ways, but for nutritional and culinary purposes, "lean" and "fatty" are more important than the distinctions between freshwater and saltwater fish, or between round fish and flatfish. Lean fish typically have white flesh and are exceptionally low in fat. Fatty fish tend to have darker flesh and are more than 5 percent fat by weight.

Most lean fish have a mild, slightly sweet flavor and a fine flake, though some (cod, for example) flake in large chunks. The most common lean fish include cod, haddock, ocean perch, pollock, sea bass, rockfish, catfish, flounder, tilefish, halibut, grouper, and snapper. They're interchangeable in most recipes.

Salmon, tuna, mackerel, sardines, and anchovies are well known for their high omega-3 content, but other fatty fish also provide these "good" fats, although not usually in the same amounts. Also explore trout (a huge family, including freshwater species such as rainbow and brook and seagoing trout such as steelhead), bluefish, swordfish, and shark (usually found as mako or blacktip steaks). Fatty fish takes well to grilling and pan searing.

IS IT DONE YET?

The speediness of preparation that makes fish such a great meal choice is also its challenge: fish and shellfish can go from tender to rubbery in a flash. Fish, unlike cows and chickens, aren't constrained by gravity—floating and swimming gives them an entirely different type of muscle. Their flesh is leaner because there's no marbling, and it cooks very quickly because it isn't as dense. Forget the rule about cooking fish until it flakes; at that point it's overcooked. A better rule is to check to see if it's done *before* the recipe specifies.

Many factors can affect cooking times, including the weight of the pan and differences in oven temperature. If you're cooking thin fillets, by the time the outside is opaque, the inside should be close to done. Using a thin sharp knife, separate the flakes in the thinnest part. If it flakes, the thicker part is done. (When the thicker part flakes, it's overdone.)

With thicker (1 inch or more) fillets, it takes about 8–10 minutes to cook through. (Fish continues to cook when you remove it from the heat, so you may wish to remove it on the early side.) Separate the flakes as above. If the fish is no longer translucent, it's done. If you're cooking thick fillets such as pollock, monkfish, snapper, bass, or orange roughy, begin checking the fish after 7 minutes per inch of thickness. If a knife goes in easily, the fish is nearly done; if it meets resistance, cook it a minute or two longer. Peek into the thickest part of the fillet. It's done when it is completely opaque, so remove it from the heat when there is a bit of translucence.

If you're cooking whole fish, begin checking after 8 or so minutes per inch of thickness. Press it with your finger. If it's mushy, cook it 2 minutes per pound longer and check again. Next, use a chopstick and press at the thickest point. If you can touch bone without much resistance, tug the fins. When they separate easily, the fish is done.

HANDLE SHELLFISH WITH CARE

Shellfish is incredibly perishable, so purchase it on the day you plan to cook it—or buy frozen shellfish and put it in the freezer immediately when you get home. Some shellfish is purchased live—lobster, clams, and mussels, for example—and they should be placed in the refrigerator and used that day. Smell shellfish to be sure it has a briny aroma, and avoid anything that smells musty or like ammonia. If you have any doubts about the shellfish, ask to see the tags that certify the shellfish came from unpolluted beds. (By law, fishmongers are required to keep these tags.) Oysters and mussels do contain some carbohydrate, so limit the size of your portions.

THE BIG FREEZE

When it comes to fish, frozen isn't necessarily bad—in fact, it's often preferable to fresh. Deep-sea fish such as swordfish and tuna is almost always frozen, since fishing boats can remain at sea for several weeks; freezing prevents the catch from spoiling. Shrimp, scallops, and lobster are often frozen at sea, too. Sometimes, but not always, it's thawed by the time you buy it. If you plan to freeze your fish when you get it home, ask the counterperson if the fish has been thawed. The store may have frozen fish in the back that you can buy instead.

In addition to the recipes that follow, you'll find more in other chapters of this book. For example, "Soups and Stews" (page 122) tempts your taste buds with Thai Coconut-Shrimp Soup, Sea Scallops Étouffée, and Gulf Oyster Stew. In "Sandwiches, Wraps, Fillings, and Pizza" (page 55), you'll find Open-Faced Fried Catfish Sandwiches with Spicy Mayonnaise, Smoked Whitefish Salad, and Mediterranean-Style Tuna Salad, among others. Also check out the numerous fish and shellfish dishes at www.atkins.com.

Batter-Fried Haddock

Phases 2, 3, 4

Serve this dish with tartar sauce—find our recipe on www.atkins.com—or with malt vinegar, which is how the Brits enjoy fish and chips. Use cod or grouper instead of haddock, depending on which looks freshest at the market.

PER SERVING:
Net Carbs: 3 grams
Total Carbs: 6 grams
Fiber: 3 grams
Protein: 34 grams
Fat: 27 grams
Calories: 400

Makes: 6 servings
Active Time: 20 minutes
Total Time: 1 hour, 20 minutes

- 1 cup Atkins Cuisine All Purpose Baking Mix, divided
- ¾ teaspoon salt
- 2 large eggs, separated
- ½ cup low-carb beer, at room temperature (see page 141)
- ¼ cup heavy cream
- 2 tablespoons water
- Canola oil, for frying (about 1½ cup)
- 1½ pounds skinless haddock fillets, cut into large strips
- Malt vinegar or lemon wedges

1. Combine ½ cup baking mix and salt in a medium bowl. Combine egg yolks, beer, cream, and water in another medium bowl; pour into dry ingredients. Stir until well combined; let batter sit at room temperature for 1 hour.
2. When ready to cook, pour oil to a depth of 3 inches into a large, heavy-bottomed saucepan or Dutch oven. Set over high heat until shimmering. Meanwhile, beat egg whites in a medium bowl with a handheld mixer on high speed until soft peaks form; gently fold into batter.
3. Working in batches, dredge fish pieces in remaining ½ cup baking mix; dip into batter, coating evenly. Shake off excess batter and slip fish pieces into oil; fry 4 or 5 at a time until golden, about 4 minutes. Drain fish on a wire rack set over a jelly roll pan or baking sheet, or on paper towels. Serve hot with vinegar or lemon wedges.

Variation: Batter-Fried Shrimp

Phases 2, 3, 4

Prepare Batter-Fried Haddock as above, substituting 1½ pounds peeled and deveined large shrimp for the fish.

Almond-Crusted Catfish Fingers

Phases 2, 3, 4

PER SERVING:
Net Carbs: 6 grams
Total Carbs: 11 grams
Fiber: 5 grams
Protein: 39 grams
Fat: 58 grams
Calories: 720

Makes: 4 servings
Active Time: 20 minutes
Total Time: 30 minutes

Fried catfish fingers are a treat typically made with a coating of cracker meal, bread crumbs, or flour, but we've given them an equally delicious and crispy treatment that's much lower in carbs.

- ¾ cup or more canola oil, for frying
- 2 large eggs
- 1 tablespoon cold water
- 1½ tablespoons Old Bay Seasoning or any Cajun spice blend
- ¾ teaspoon salt
- 1½ pounds catfish fillets, cut into 1½-inch-wide strips
- ¼ cup Atkins Cuisine All Purpose Baking Mix
- 1 cup almond meal (see page 11)
- 1 lemon, cut into wedges

1. Heat oil in a large, heavy-bottomed saucepan or Dutch oven over high heat until shimmering.
2. Lightly beat eggs in a small bowl; whisk in water and spice blend.
3. Dredge catfish in baking mix and shake off any excess. Dip into egg mixture and then dredge in almond meal. Slip catfish pieces into oil; fry 4 or 5 at a time until golden, about 2 minutes per side. Drain fish on paper towels. Serve hot with lemon wedges.

TIP TIME

AN OLD FAVORITE

A potent mix of celery seed, salt, mustard, red pepper, black pepper, bay leaves, cloves, ginger, mace, cardamom, cinnamon, and paprika, Old Bay Seasoning was developed seventy years ago. It's the perfect complement to shellfish and fish, but it can also spice up chicken, meats, veggies, and Bloody Marys. Find it in the spice aisle of your supermarket.

Herbed Flounder en Papillote*

Phases 1, 2, 3, 4

Cooked in tightly sealed parchment paper (*papillote* is French for "paper"), which puffs up as the fish steams in its own juices. Or use aluminum foil.

PER SERVING:
Net Carbs: 6 grams
Total Carbs: 6 grams
Fiber: 0 grams
Protein: 33 grams
Fat: 9 grams
Calories: 240

Makes: 4 servings
Active Time: 20 minutes
Total Time: 30 minutes

- 1 tablespoon plus 4 teaspoons butter, divided
- 4 small shallots, thinly sliced
- ½ teaspoon salt
- ⅛ teaspoon white pepper
- 4 (6-ounce) skinless flounder fillets
- ¼ cup chopped mixed fresh herbs such as basil, dill, or parsley
- 1 small lemon, cut into 8 thin slices
- 4 (12-by-20-inch) pieces of parchment paper

1. Heat oven to 475°F. Fold each sheet of paper (or foil) in half; with the fold in the center, cut into a half heart shape. Rub 1 teaspoon butter over half of each sheet; set aside.
2. Melt remaining tablespoon butter in a medium skillet over high heat. Add shallots, salt, and pepper; sauté until soft, about 3 minutes.
3. Set fillets on buttered sides of paper hearts; top with herbs, shallots, and lemon. Cover with unbuttered side of foil, taking care to align edges; crimp edges tightly shut. Transfer packets to baking sheet; bake until fish is just cooked through, about 10 minutes.
4. To serve, carefully cut open each packet and slide fish onto serving plates.

Variation: Flounder en Papillote with Vegetables

Phases 2, 3, 4

Prepare recipe as above, adding 1 cup thinly sliced zucchini, 4 thinly sliced white mushrooms, and 1 thinly sliced red bell pepper to the shallots; sauté vegetables over high heat in 2 tablespoons butter until soft, about 5 minutes. Top each fillet with vegetable mixture before baking.

*See photo on color page 20

Sole Meunière

Phases 2, 3, 4

PER SERVING:
Net Carbs: 2 grams
Total Carbs: 5 grams
Fiber: 3 grams
Protein: 39 grams
Fat: 14 grams
Calories: 300

Makes: 4 servings
Active Time: 25 minutes
Total Time: 25 minutes

WEEKDAY

Meunière is French for "miller's wife." The term refers to dusting food lightly in flour before it's sautéed in butter. Using low-carb baking mix in this update gives the dish a nuttiness that white flour cannot impart. Sole is the classic fish prepared à la meunière, but flounder or any other flat fish works well.

4 (6-ounce) skinless sole fillets
½ cup Atkins Cuisine All Purpose Baking Mix
1 tablespoon virgin olive oil
3 tablespoons butter, divided
2 tablespoons freshly squeezed lemon juice
2 tablespoons chopped fresh parsley
2 teaspoons chopped fresh tarragon
Salt
Freshly ground black pepper

1. Dredge fillets in baking mix, pressing to coat on both sides; shake off excess. Set aside.
2. Heat oil and 1 tablespoon butter in a large skillet over high heat. Add sole; sear until golden, about 3 minutes per side. Transfer to a platter; cover loosely to keep warm.
3. Wipe skillet clean; return to high heat. Add remaining 2 tablespoons butter; cook until nutty smelling and golden, about 3 minutes. Remove from heat; stir in lemon juice, parsley, tarragon, and salt and pepper to taste; spoon over sole and serve right away.

TIP TIME

KISSING COUSINS

Like sole, flounder is a flatfish with a very fine flake, pearly gray flesh, and sweet, mild flavor. The two are interchangeable in recipes. You'll usually find both sole and flounder filleted.

Salt-Crusted Whole Snapper with Lemon and Basil

Phases 1, 2, 3, 4

This succulent salt-crusted fish makes a dramatic presentation. Stuffing the cavity with citrus and herbs infuses the fish with delicate flavor as it bakes; the salt crust keeps it moist. You can substitute tilefish, Pacific perch, or sea bass for snapper.

PER SERVING:
Net Carbs: 1 gram
Total Carbs: 1 gram
Fiber: 0 grams
Protein: 49 grams
Fat: 15 grams
Calories: 340

Makes: 6 servings
Active Time: 10 minutes
Total Time: 1 hour

10 large egg whites
4 cups kosher salt
1 (3½- to 4-pound) whole red snapper, gutted and scaled, head and tail intact
1 cup fresh whole basil leaves
2 lemons, one cut into slices, one cut into wedges
¼ cup extra-virgin olive oil

1. Heat oven to 450°F.
2. Put egg whites in a large bowl; whip until foamy with a handheld mixer on high speed. Stir in salt until mixture has a sandy texture. On a baking sheet, spread half of the salt mixture in a rectangle just larger than the fish; place fish on top (trim the tail if you have difficulty fitting the fish on your pan). Insert basil and lemon slices into fish cavity. Pat remaining salt mixture over fish to cover completely. The fish should be completely encased in a good layer of salt. Bake until an instant-read thermometer inserted into thickest part of fish registers 130°F, about 45 minutes. Let stand for 5 minutes.
3. To serve, rap around the edge of the salt crust with a wooden spoon to loosen top; lift off. Drizzle fish with oil and serve with lemon wedges.

TIP TIME

USE YOUR YOLKS

Cover leftover egg yolks tightly, refrigerate, and use within 4 days. Or freeze after beating with ¼ teaspoon salt for every 4 yolks and sealing tightly in a freezerproof container. Defrost in the fridge before using.

Baked Bluefish with Garlic and Lime

Phases 1, 2, 3, 4

PER SERVING:
Net Carbs: 4 grams
Total Carbs: 6 grams
Fiber: 2 grams
Protein: 34 grams
Fat: 14 grams
Calories: 290

Makes: 4 servings
Active Time: 10 minutes
Total Time: 25 minutes

This recipe is about as easy as they come. Rich in omega-3s, bluefish stands up well to the flavors of lime and garlic. Baking the limes gives them an extra tang when squeezed over the cooked fish.

- 2 tablespoons virgin olive oil, plus more for baking dish
- 2 cloves garlic, minced
- ¼ teaspoon red pepper flakes
- 1½ pounds bluefish fillets
- Salt
- 3 limes, quartered

1. Put a 9-by-13-inch baking dish in oven and heat to 425°F.
2. Combine oil, garlic, and red pepper flakes in a small bowl. Rub fillets with garlic mixture and season generously with salt to taste.
3. Using potholders, carefully remove baking dish from oven; add fillets, skin side down, and limes. Bake until fish is opaque and flakes easily, 10–12 minutes. Serve, squeezing limes over fish once they are cool enough to handle.

TIP TIME

FISH FOR FIRST-TIMERS

Fish retains its moisture when baked, which means a few extra minutes in the oven shouldn't affect the flavor and texture. That means that baking fish is more forgiving than most other methods of cooking.

Variation: Southwestern Bluefish with Garlic and Lime

Phases 1, 2, 3, 4

Prepare Baked Bluefish with Garlic and Lime as above, adding ¼ cup chopped fresh cilantro, 1 teaspoon ground cumin, and ½ teaspoon ground coriander to the garlic mixture, and substituting ½ teaspoon chili powder for the red pepper flakes.

Roasted Ginger-Tamari Salmon Steaks*

Phases: 3, 4

In the summer, try this easy Asian-inspired salmon recipe on the grill instead of in the oven. Either way, grilled asparagus makes a perfect accompaniment.

PER SERVING:
Net Carbs: 7 grams
Total Carbs: 8 grams
Fiber: 1 gram
Protein: 39 grams
Fat: 25 grams
Calories: 420

Makes: 4 servings
Active Time: 15 minutes
Total Time: 4 hours, 15 minutes

- ¾ cup freshly squeezed orange juice
- ½ cup tamari (see page 11)
- ¼ cup peeled and minced fresh ginger
- 2 cloves garlic, chopped
- 2 teaspoons dark (toasted) sesame oil
- 4 (7-ounce) salmon steaks, about 1¼ inches thick

1. Combine orange juice, tamari, ginger, garlic, and oil in a resealable plastic bag. Add salmon and turn bag to coat. Refrigerate 4 hours, turning once.
2. Heat oven to 400°F. Transfer salmon to baking dish, reserving marinade. Roast until just cooked through, about 10 minutes.
3. Meanwhile, pour all but ½ cup of the marinade into a small saucepan; bring to a boil over high heat. Reduce heat to medium and boil until glaze slightly thickens and reduces to ½ cup, about 5 minutes. Serve with salmon.

WEEKEND

Variation: Roasted Salmon Steaks with Spicy Ginger-Tamari Sauce

Phase 3, 4

Prepare Roasted Ginger-Tamari Salmon Steaks as above, adding 2 tablespoons chopped fresh cilantro, 1 sliced scallion, and ½ teaspoon chili sauce to the glaze mixture just before serving.

*See photo on color page 21

Poached Salmon with Eggs, Onions, and Capers

Phases 1, 2, 3, 4

PER SERVING:
Net Carbs: 3 grams
Total Carbs: 4 grams
Fiber: 1 gram
Protein: 47 grams
Fat: 33 grams
Calories: 510

Makes: 6 servings
Active Time: 15 minutes
Total Time: 1 hour

Nothing is more impressive than poached salmon, and few dishes are easier—you don't even need a special fish-poaching pan. Because it doesn't brown, poaching leaves fish pale in color and with a moist, tender texture. Serve on a bed of watercress or other greens. If you wish, serve with Remoulade or the classic Dill Sauce (find both at www.atkins.com) or another sauce of your choice.

1 (2½-pound) salmon fillet
6 tablespoons salt
2 tablespoons cider vinegar
8 hard-boiled eggs, quartered
1 small red onion, finely chopped
⅓ cup capers, rinsed and drained
2 lemons, cut in wedges

1. Set a roasting pan, a disposable aluminum pan, or fish poacher over two stove burners. Add the salmon; pour in enough water to cover salmon by 1 inch. Add salt and vinegar. Bring water to a boil over high heat; turn off heat and let the salmon stand for 30 minutes.
2. Using 2 large spatulas, carefully transfer salmon to a serving platter. Sprinkle with onions and capers and arrange eggs around the fish. Serve warm, or cover with plastic wrap and refrigerate until chilled.

Baked Salmon with Mustard-Nut Crust

Phases 2, 3, 4

We've become so accustomed to grilled and pan-seared salmon that it's easy to overlook one of the easiest and tastiest methods around: baking. This recipe also works extremely well with other thick fillets such as halibut, grouper, or Chilean sea bass. You'll find the recipe for Atkins Cuisine Bread at www.atkins.com. Tear the bread in pieces and pulse in a food processor.

PER SERVING:
Net Carbs: 3 grams
Total Carbs: 5 grams
Fiber: 2 grams
Protein: 39 grams
Fat: 35 grams
Calories: 490

Makes: 4 servings
Active Time: 5 minutes
Total Time: 20 minutes

4 (6-ounce) center-cut fillets of salmon
2 tablespoons coarse-grain Dijon mustard
¼ cup fine bread crumbs made from 2 slices of Atkins Cuisine Bread (see note above)
½ cup finely ground pecans or walnuts
1 tablespoon chopped fresh parsley

1. Preheat oven to 450°F. Place the rack in the middle of the oven. Line a baking sheet with foil and place fillets on sheet. Spread ½ tablespoon mustard on each fillet, covering top evenly.
2. Combine bread crumbs, nuts, and parsley in a small bowl. Divide among fillets, pressing onto mustard to form an even crust. Bake until just cooked through, about 10–15 minutes, being careful not to burn the nuts. Serve right away.

TIP TIME

ALL IN THE FAMILY

There are six major types of salmon: pink, chum, sockeye, coho, king (sometimes called Chinook), and Atlantic. Each has a different nutrient composition, and the levels of nutrients can fluctuate throughout the year.

WEEKDAY

Sautéed Salmon Cakes

Phases 2, 3, 4

PER SERVING:
Net Carbs: 1 gram
Total Carbs: 3 grams
Fiber: 2 grams
Protein: 33 grams
Fat: 34 grams
Calories: 440

Makes: 4 servings
Active Time: 30 minutes
Total Time: 30 minutes

These salmon cakes are elegant and tasty enough to serve to company, but quick enough to make as a family meal. They're best made with leftover poached salmon (see Poached Salmon with Eggs, Onions, and Capers on page 190), but canned salmon does the trick as well. Serve with a grainy mustard, Tartar Sauce (see www.atkins.com for our recipe), or lemon wedges.

- 1½ cups leftover poached salmon, at room temperature, or 3 (6-ounce) cans red or sockeye salmon, drained
- 2 scallions, very finely chopped
- ¼ cup finely ground pecans
- ¼ cup regular (not low-fat) mayonnaise
- 3 tablespoons mixed chopped herbs, such as dill, basil, and parsley, or 1 teaspoon mixed dried herbs
- 1 teaspoon Dijon mustard
- 2 large eggs, lightly beaten
- 2 tablespoons butter or 1 tablespoon virgin olive oil and 1 tablespoon butter

1. Heat oven to 400°F.
2. Combine salmon, scallions, pecans, mayonnaise, herbs, mustard, and eggs in a medium bowl; mix well. Using your hands, form mixture into 8 patties approximately 2 inches wide and ¾ inch thick.
3. Heat butter in a large skillet over medium-high heat. Add salmon cakes; cook until golden brown, about 4 minutes per side. Serve hot with desired condiment.

TIP TIME

PRICE-CONSCIOUS PECANS

When you purchase shelled pecans or any other nuts for cooking, opt for pieces rather than whole or half nuts. They're usually significantly less expensive.

WEEKDAY

Swordfish Kebabs with Scallions

Phases 1, 2, 3, 4

Swordfish is a great choice for grilling and, thanks to its firm flesh, holds up extremely well as kebabs. Shark, halibut, and tuna also make good kebabs.

PER SERVING:
Net Carbs: 2 grams
Total Carbs: 3 grams
Fiber: 1 gram
Protein: 32 grams
Fat: 13 grams
Calories: 260

Makes: 4 servings
Active Time: 20 minutes
Total Time: 4 hours, 20 minutes

2 tablespoons virgin olive oil
3 cloves garlic, finely chopped
1 tablespoon fresh finely grated lemon zest
½ teaspoon dried thyme
⅛ teaspoon red pepper flakes
1½ pounds swordfish steaks, cut into 1½-inch chunks
8 scallions, trimmed and cut in 2-inch pieces
Salt
1 lemon, cut into wedges

4 (12-inch or 14-inch) steel skewers

1. Combine oil, garlic, zest, thyme, and pepper flakes in a large bowl or resealable plastic bag. Add swordfish and stir or turn bag to coat thoroughly. Cover bowl or seal bag; refrigerate 4 hours or overnight.
2. Shortly before removing fish from the bowl, add scallions and coat with marinade.
3. Prepare a medium-high-heat grill. Remove fish and scallions from marinade and discard marinade.
4. Thread fish onto the skewers, alternating each chunk with a piece of scallion. Season fish generously with salt to taste. Grill until fish is opaque throughout but still moist, about 10 minutes, turning frequently. Serve hot with lemon wedges.

TIP TIME

GET A GRILL BASKET

Skewers are great for grilling firm-fleshed fish such as swordfish, but most fish fillets are very fragile and will fall apart, making a grill basket a handy device. It also helps when grilling scallops and shrimp.

Mediterranean-Style Grilled Swordfish Steaks

Phases 1, 2, 3, 4

PER SERVING:
Net Carbs: 2 grams
Total Carbs: 3 grams
Fiber: 1 gram
Protein: 40 grams
Fat: 24 grams
Calories: 390

Makes: 4 servings
Active Time: 20 minutes
Total Time: 1 hour

WEEKEND

Swordfish steaks may or may not have skin on them; cut or peel it off before cooking. Steaks also come in a variety of thicknesses. Be sure all four steaks are comparable in thickness so they cook at the same rate. Try any combination of parsley, basil, chervil, chives, or thyme for seasonings.

¼ cup virgin olive oil
3 cloves garlic, finely chopped
1 tablespoon freshly squeezed lemon juice
4 (7-ounce) skinless swordfish steaks, each about ½ inch thick
Salt
Freshly ground black pepper
1 medium plum tomato, diced
⅓ cup pitted, sliced black olives
2 tablespoons fresh mixed herbs

1. Combine oil, garlic, and lemon juice in a baking dish. Transfer 1 tablespoon of the mixture to a small bowl; set aside. Add swordfish to baking dish and turn to coat. Refrigerate for 20 minutes, turning steaks once.
2. Prepare a high-heat grill, or heat a grill pan until very hot. Remove fish from marinade, season with salt and pepper to taste, and grill until just cooked through, about 4 minutes per side.
3. Meanwhile, add tomato, olives, and herbs to reserved marinade; toss gently to combine. Season with salt and pepper to taste and serve on top of fillets.

TIP TIME

OUT, OUT, LITTLE PIT

To pit olives easily, press them with the side of a chef's knife, a meat mallet, or even a small skillet to break the skin, then pull the pit away with your fingers. You can use a paring knife on harder-to-pit varieties.

Pecan-Crusted Trout with Orange-Sage Butter

Phases 2, 3, 4

To save time, you can prepare the seasoned butter for this simple, elegant dish in advance—it will keep for up to 2 months in the freezer (thaw at room temperature before using).

PER SERVING:
Net Carbs: 2 grams
Total Carbs: 4 grams
Fiber: 2 grams
Protein: 38 grams
Fat: 43 grams
Calories: 550

Makes: 4 servings
Active Time: 30 minutes
Total Time: 1 hour 10 minutes

Seasoned Butter

2 tablespoons butter, at room temperature
1 teaspoon minced shallot
1 teaspoon finely chopped fresh sage
¼ teaspoon fresh finely grated orange zest
⅛ teaspoon white wine vinegar
⅛ teaspoon salt

Trout

1 cup pecans, toasted and finely chopped
4 (6- to 8-ounce) trout fillets, skin on
¾ teaspoon salt
¼ teaspoon freshly ground black pepper
1 large egg white, lightly beaten
2 tablespoons butter
2 tablespoons olive oil

1. For the seasoned butter, combine butter, shallot, sage, orange zest, vinegar, and salt in a small bowl; blend well to distribute ingredients thoroughly. Spoon seasoned butter onto waxed paper; roll paper around butter to form a log. Twist ends to secure butter; roll gently across counter to form an even cylinder. Refrigerate while preparing trout.
2. For the trout, put pecans in a shallow bowl or on a plate. Season trout with salt and pepper on both sides; brush flesh side with egg whites. One at a time, dredge fillets, flesh side down, into nuts; press lightly to coat. Transfer to a plate, coated side up. Repeat with remaining fillets; cover and refrigerate for 30 minutes.
3. Heat butter and oil in a large nonstick skillet over medium-high heat. Add fillets, nut side down; sear until crust is golden and fish is just cooked through, about 3 minutes per side. Turn fillets carefully as crust is fragile.
4. Slice seasoned butter into 4 rounds. Top each fillet with 1 round; serve right away.

Maryland Steamed Crabs

Phases 1, 2, 3, 4

PER SERVING:
Net Carbs: 0 grams
Total Carbs: 0 grams
Fiber: 0 grams
Protein: 23 grams
Fat: 13 grams
Calories: 210

Makes: 4 servings
Active Time: 10 minutes
Total Time: 30 minutes

This dish is all about the quality of the crabs and giving them just enough seasoning to let their pure richness shine. The Eastern Shore of Maryland is famous worldwide for crabs fixed this way—it just takes a large pot and a bit of planning.

3 cups water
1 cup distilled white vinegar
24 live large male crabs (usually called jimmies)
1 cup Old Bay Seasoning or other crab seasoning blend (see page 184)
¼ cup salt
¼ cup butter, melted

1. Choose a very large pot (at least 12 quarts) with a tight-fitting lid and fit it with a steamer insert. Add water and vinegar, cover, and bring to a boil over medium-high heat.
2. Add enough crabs to form a single layer; season with a little Old Bay and salt. Continue layering and seasoning until all the crabs are in the pot and all the seasoning has been used. Cover and steam until the crabs are cooked through, about 20 minutes. Serve right away with melted butter.

WEEKDAY

Sautéed Soft-Shell Crabs*

Phases 2, 3, 4

When soft-shell season hits, it creates quite a clamor on the East Coast. These little specialties are delectable, and simple cooking keeps the true flavor alive. Soft-shell crabs are full of water, and they tend to spit as they hit the hot fat. Be careful of your hands and face, and wear an apron to protect your clothing.

PER SERVING:
Net Carbs: 5 grams
Total Carbs: 10 grams
Fiber: 5 grams
Protein: 23 grams
Fat: 30 grams
Calories: 390

Makes: 4 servings
Active Time: 15 minutes
Total Time: 25 minutes

8 soft-shell crabs, cleaned and dressed
½ teaspoon salt
¼ teaspoon freshly ground black pepper
1 cup Atkins Cuisine All Purpose Baking Mix
1 tablespoon Old Bay Seasoning or other crab seasoning blend (see page 184)
4 tablespoons (½ stick) butter
4 tablespoons canola oil
1 lemon, cut into wedges

1. Season crabs with salt and pepper. Combine baking mix and Old Bay in a shallow bowl or plate; dredge crabs in mixture, shaking off excess. Set aside.
2. Heat 2 tablespoons butter and 2 tablespoons oil in a large skillet over high heat. Add four crabs; cook until golden, about 3 minutes per side. Transfer to paper towels to drain. Repeat with remaining butter, oil, and crabs. Serve right away with lemon wedges.

*See photo on color page 23

Shrimp Diablo

Phases 1, 2, 3, 4

PER SERVING:
Net Carbs: 7 grams
Total Carbs: 9 grams
Fiber: 2 grams
Protein: 18 grams
Fat: 24 grams
Calories: 320

Makes: 6 (1¼-cup) servings
Active Time: 25 minutes
Total Time: 30 minutes

WEEKDAY

Diablo ("devil" in Spanish) refers to the spicy kick of this tomato-and-jalapeño-infused sauce. Be sure to wear gloves when working with jalapeños to prevent irritation.

4 tablespoons (½ stick) butter
1 medium yellow or white onion, chopped
1 celery rib, trimmed and chopped
1 green bell pepper, stemmed, seeds and ribs removed, and chopped
4 cloves garlic, minced
1 (14½-ounce) can diced tomatoes
¼ pound button mushrooms, sliced
1 cup heavy cream
1 pound medium shrimp, peeled and deveined
1 jalapeño, seeded and finely chopped
1 tablespoon freshly squeezed lemon juice
2 tablespoons chopped fresh basil
2 teaspoons chopped fresh thyme
Salt
Freshly ground black pepper

1. Melt butter in a large skillet over medium-high heat. Add onion, celery, and bell pepper; sauté until soft, about 4 minutes. Add garlic and sauté until fragrant, about 30 seconds. Add tomatoes and mushrooms; reduce heat to medium and simmer until sauce thickens slightly, about 5 minutes.
2. Stir in cream, shrimp, jalapeño, and lemon juice. Reduce heat to medium-low, cover, and simmer until shrimp turn pink, about 4 minutes. Stir in basil, thyme, and salt and pepper to taste; serve right away.

TIP TIME

GO GENTLE WITH GARLIC

Garlic burns easily. Cook it over low heat, or add it when other ingredients are almost done and sauté until just fragrant.

Peel-and-Eat Shrimp

Phases 1, 2, 3, 4

Shrimp is America's favorite seafood, but it's often overcooked. Following this simple method will give you tender, juicy, flavorful shrimp every time. Pickling spice is a blend of seasonings that's available in supermarkets. The ingredients can vary widely, but it may include bay leaves, ginger, mustard seeds, peppercorns, allspice, coriander, cloves, and cinnamon.

PER SERVING:
Net Carbs: 4 grams
Total Carbs: 4 grams
Fiber: 0 grams
Protein: 46 grams
Fat: 4 grams
Calories: 240

Makes: 4 servings
Active Time: 5 minutes
Total Time: 25 minutes

WEEKDAY

2 quarts (8 cups) water
¼ cup cider vinegar
2 tablespoons pickling spice
1 tablespoon salt
2 pounds medium shrimp, shell-on
1 lemon, cut into wedges

1. Combine water, vinegar, pickling spice, and salt in a 5-quart saucepan; bring to a boil over high heat. Reduce heat to medium and simmer 20 minutes.
2. Bring back to a boil over high heat. Add shrimp; turn off heat, cover and let stand until shrimp turn pink, about 4 minutes. Serve right away with lemon wedges, or refrigerate until cool, about 1 hour, before serving.

TIP TIME

DON'T SKIMP ON SHRIMP

Ignore signs about the number of shrimp to a pound—what's considered "extra-large" at one market may be "medium" at another. Instead, purchase shrimp by the pound, and don't forget that there's considerable waste with the shells. (Figure at least 1½–2 pounds with shells for four diners.) Shrimp should look firm and fill the shells.

Vietnamese Grilled Calamari Salad

Phases 2, 3, 4

PER SERVING:
Net Carbs: 11 grams
Total Carbs: 17 grams
Fiber: 6 grams
Protein: 30 grams
Fat: 4 grams
Calories: 220

Makes 4 servings
Active Time: 20 minutes
Total Time: 20 minutes

WEEKDAY

Squid is best either cooked quickly—grilled or fried at high temperatures—or simmered for several hours. Keep a close eye on it once you put it on the grill. Overcooking renders squid tough and tasteless; undercooking leaves it rubbery. Use tamari if you have no fish sauce.

Dressing
2 tablespoons fish sauce (nam pla or nuoc mam)
⅛ teaspoon red pepper flakes
2 teaspoons granular sugar substitute
1 tablespoon freshly squeezed lime juice
½ teaspoon freshly grated lime zest
1 clove garlic, minced

Salad
1 large head romaine lettuce, chopped
2 plum tomatoes, each cut into 8 wedges
1 medium cucumber, peeled, seeded, and cut into ½-inch dice
1 cup loosely packed, coarsely chopped mint leaves
1 cup loosely packed, coarsely chopped basil
Olive oil cooking spray
1½ pounds squid, cleaned
Salt
Freshly ground black pepper

1. For the dressing, whisk fish sauce, red pepper flakes, sugar substitute, lime juice and zest, and garlic in a small bowl; set aside.
2. For the salad, combine lettuce, tomatoes, cucumber, mint, and basil in a salad bowl.
3. Mist grill pan with cooking spray and set over high heat. Rinse squid; pat dry with paper towels and season with salt and pepper. Grill until just opaque, 1½–2 minutes maximum per side. Cool on cutting board for 1 minute, and then slice into ½-inch rings.
4. Toss salad with dressing, season with salt and pepper to taste, and divide among four plates. Top with squid and serve.

Chapter 12

VEGETARIAN ENTRÉES

If you're a vegetarian who's reading this book, you probably already know that it is perfectly possible to follow a low-carb lifestyle without eating meat, poultry, and fish—and without subsisting on tofu morning, noon, and night. Or perhaps your family is into "meatless Mondays," or you simply prefer a vegetarian dinner after having a burger at lunch. The recipes in this chapter are proof that low carb is not synonymous with meat—and that vegetarian food can taste great. To get started, try our Tofu in White Wine with Mustard and Dill, Tomato and Leek Gratin with Gruyère and Walnuts, Mustardy Mac 'n' Cheese, and Vegetable Curry with Seared Noodles. All are incomparably delicious in their own right.

THE LOW-CARB APPROACH

Nonetheless, it does take a bit of thought to be a low-carb vegetarian. Many traditional vegetarian meals are based on such combinations as legumes and grains, cheese and pasta, or nuts and grains. These pairings ensure sufficient protein, but they tend to push carb counts sky high. A great deal also depends on how you define "vegetarian." If you're an ovo-lacto vegetarian (you eat eggs and dairy), you should have no difficulty getting the protein you need; we recommend you start in Phase 2, Ongoing Weight Loss, at 30 grams of Net Carbs a day, so you can include nuts, all cheeses, yogurt, and legumes in your meals. If you're a vegan and don't eat dairy or eggs, you can still do Atkins, but we recommend you start in Phase 2 at 50 grams of Net Carbs a day so that legumes, nuts, and seeds provide sufficient protein. Regardless of the phase you're in, vegetarians need to be especially careful with portion sizes in order to keep carbs under control.

SOY FOODS 101

Soy foods are inherently low in carbs and are the cornerstone of a vegetarian diet. Soy contains all of the essential amino acids (the building blocks of protein). Versatile and nutritious, foods made from soybeans—including tofu, tempeh, miso, and textured vegetable protein—have made their way from natural foods stores to supermarkets and from vegetarian restaurants to mainstream menus. If you haven't cooked with soy foods, here are some of the ingredients you'll find in the recipes in this chapter:

- *Miso* is a paste made from fermented soybeans. It comes in many colors and flavors. Lighter misos are more delicate and best used as a table condiment or in soups and sauces; robustly flavored darker varieties work well in marinades. Shinshu is a good all-purpose miso. Refrigerate miso in an airtight container.

- *Soy cheese* is just what it sounds like. Be sure to read labels to avoid brands that contain hydrogenated oils. Those that contain casein (a milk protein) will melt better but are unacceptable for vegans.
- *Soy flour* is high in isoflavones, folate, and iron and contains about three times the protein of wheat flour—but no gluten, which means soy flour must be combined with whole-wheat flour when baking. (Atkins Cuisine All Purpose Baking Mix includes both soy flour and wheat gluten.)
- *Soy milk*, when fortified, is high in vitamins A, B_{12}, and D, as well as calcium, riboflavin, and zinc. Use in lieu of milk in almost any recipe. Avoid flavored and sweetened varieties.
- *Tempeh* is a tender, chunky cake made of fermented soybeans. It's higher in protein and has a more assertive flavor and texture than tofu.
- *Textured vegetable protein* (TVP) and its fraternal twin, textured soy protein (TSP), are similar to ground beef when hydrated and cooked. You'll also find it packaged as meat substitutes that can stand in for bacon, hotdogs, burgers, sausage, and more.
- *Silken tofu* has a custard-like consistency that makes it ideal in puréed soups, dips, and sauces. It comes in soft, medium, firm, and extra-firm consistencies and may be packed in aseptic packages that don't need to be refrigerated until they're opened. Use silken tofu as you would sour cream, or to give smoothies a rich, thick texture.
- *Regular tofu* takes particularly well to stir-frying and grilling. It also comes in a variety of textures, but it is denser, so it stays together better than silken tofu. You'll find it in the refrigerated section of the supermarket. Unless otherwise noted, our recipes use regular tofu.
- *Tofu shirataki noodles* are made from a high-fiber Asian yam, which contains a substance called glucomannan. When mixed with tofu, it makes a rather chewy but almost carb-free substitute for high-carb pasta. Look for it in the refrigerated area of the produce department.

USE YOUR BEAN

Soy is not the only bean you'll be relying on. Other legumes—for simplicity's sake, we're talking here about dried beans, including lentils and peas—come in a rainbow of colors, an array of sizes, and a variety of textures, from the rich and creamy butter bean to the firm and nutty chickpea. Beans are a good source of protein; they also contain carbohydrates and some fats, as well as B vitamins and fiber. Fresh beans and peas such as sugar snaps are covered in "Vegetables and Other Sides" (page 98). Dried beans need to be soaked and cooked before eating. Although they cost more, canned beans are far more convenient.

ABOUT SEITAN

Seitan is fairly chewy and rather bland. It's made from wheat gluten cooked in soy sauce, so it isn't actually a soy food. Seitan is extremely high in protein and low in Net Carbs. Its firm texture makes it ideal in stir-fries, and it can be used like tofu in many recipes. It can toughen with overcooking, so it's best to add it at the end of cooking.

A WORLD OF CHEESES

Cheese can be categorized in a variety of ways—where it's from, which animal's milk it's made from, how long it's been aged. Hard and semi-hard cheeses are aged from six to twenty-four months; soft and semisoft cheese are usually aged from three to six months; fresh cheeses obviously aren't aged at all. The aging process removes moisture and concentrates nutrients and flavors. For example, an ounce of mozzarella supplies about 150 milligrams of calcium. Aged Parmesan, on the other hand, provides more than twice that, 334 milligrams. Cheese is also an excellent source of protein, vitamins, and minerals, but it does contain carbohydrates (and calories), so limit consumption to about 4 ounces a day.

GO WITH THE GRAIN—CAREFULLY

After you've added legumes, fruits, and starchy vegetables back into your meals, so long as your weight is under control or you're close to your goal weight you should be able to add grains, too. The trick is to select grains that are high in nutrients yet comparatively low in Net Carbs, such as barley, wild rice, quinoa, and bulgur. You'll find grain recipes in "Vegetables and Other Sides" (page 98), most of which are suitable for vegetarians or can be adapted by adding a protein source to the dish or serving it with one.

Other tasty vegetarian entrées can be found in "Soups and Stews" (page 122), "Breakfast and Brunch Dishes" (page 16), "Snacks, Appetizers, and Hors d'Oeuvres" (page 37), and "Sandwiches, Wraps, Fillings, and Pizza" (page 55). Also check out the recipe database at www.atkins.com for dozens more.

The recipes in this chapter tend to include more ingredients than do the other entrées. The reality is that without the strong flavors of meat, poultry, and fish, it's all the more important to include a rich blend of tastes, textures, and seasonings to produce delectable dishes based on tofu, tempeh, or seitan—all of which are inherently bland. Still, we've made every effort to keep the recipes as simple and speedy as possible.

Scrambled Tofu Burritos

Phases 3, 4

PER SERVING:
Net Carbs: 13 grams
Total Carbs: 30 grams
Fiber: 17 grams
Protein: 28 grams
Fat: 35 grams
Calories: 490

Makes: 6 servings
Active Time: 25 minutes
Total Time: 25 minutes

WEEKDAY

Be sure to wear gloves to prevent irritation when working with jalepeños or any other hot chiles.

- ¼ cup virgin olive oil
- 1 small yellow or white onion, chopped
- ⅓ cup pine nuts
- 2 cloves garlic, chopped
- 1 jalapeño, seeded and chopped
- 1½ teaspoons ground cumin
- 1 teaspoon turmeric
- 2 (14-ounce) packages firm tofu, drained, patted dry, and mashed with a fork
- 3 plum tomatoes, chopped
- ¼ cup lime juice
- 1½ teaspoons salt
- 2 tablespoons chopped cilantro
- 6 (8- or 9-inch) low-carb tortillas (see page 66)
- 6 ounces Monterey Jack cheese, shredded (1½ cups)
- 1 small romaine heart, shredded
- ¾ cup sour cream

1. Heat oil in a large skillet over medium-high heat. Add onion and sauté until softened, about 3 minutes. Add pine nuts, garlic, jalapeño, cumin, and turmeric; sauté until fragrant, about 1 minute. Add tofu, tomatoes, lime juice, and salt; sauté to heat through, about 5 minutes. Remove from heat and stir in cilantro. Keep warm.
2. Place 1 tortilla on a plate and cover with a damp paper towel; continue, alternating tortillas and towels. Microwave for 1 minute or more, until tortillas are warm.
3. Divide tofu mixture among tortillas and top with cheese. Wrap up and serve with romaine and sour cream.

TIP TIME

TOASTY WARM TORTILLAS

To warm tortillas in the oven, wrap in a damp dishtowel, put in a casserole dish, cover tightly, and heat for 20 minutes at 250°F.

Lemon-Rosemary Baked Tofu with Mushroom Sauce

Phases 2, 3, 4

Here tofu is baked with tamari and other seasonings and then further enhanced with a savory mushroom sauce. Fresh herbs enhance the taste.

PER SERVING:
Net Carbs: 11 grams
Total Carbs: 13 grams
Fiber: 2 grams
Protein: 22 grams
Fat: 31 grams
Calories: 400

Makes: 4 servings
Active Time: 20 minutes
Total Time: 30 minutes

Tofu

2 (14-ounce) packages extra-firm tofu, drained, patted dry, and cut into 1-inch pieces
6 tablespoons freshly squeezed lemon juice
4 tablespoons tamari
4 tablespoons extra-virgin olive oil
2 tablespoons red wine vinegar
4 teaspoons finely chopped fresh rosemary
2 teaspoons freshly grated lemon zest
½ teaspoon granular sugar substitute

Sauce

2 tablespoons extra-virgin olive oil
6 ounces cremini or button mushrooms, wiped clean, trimmed, and thinly sliced
1 small yellow or white onion, finely chopped
1 clove garlic, chopped
½ cup vegetable broth
1 tablespoon tamari
2 teaspoons chopped fresh thyme
1 tablespoon chopped fresh parsley
Salt
Freshly ground black pepper

1. For the tofu, heat oven to 425°F. Combine tofu, lemon juice, tamari, oil, vinegar, rosemary, lemon zest, and sugar substitute in a glass baking dish; toss gently. Bake until tofu is golden brown, about 30 minutes.
2. For the sauce, heat oil in a large skillet over high heat. Add mushrooms and onion; sauté until soft and light golden, about 7 minutes. Add garlic and sauté until fragrant, about 30 seconds. Add broth, tamari, and thyme; reduce heat to medium-low and simmer until sauce thickens, about 4 minutes. Stir in parsley and salt and pepper to taste.
3. Top tofu with sauce and serve warm.

Le Grand Aïoli

Phases 3, 4

PER SERVING:
Net Carbs: 13 grams
Total Carbs: 21 grams
Fiber: 8 grams
Protein: 19 grams
Fat: 15 grams
Calories: 280

Makes: 4 servings
Active Time: 30 minutes
Total Time: 30 minutes

WEEKDAY

This is a great, casual party dish, particularly for the warmer months. Aïoli is a garlicky mayonnaise that is traditionally dolloped on bouillabaisse, the Provençal fish stew. It and the vegetables can be prepared a day in advance.

Aïoli
1 clove garlic, peeled
¼ teaspoon salt
1 large egg yolk
½ teaspoon Dijon mustard
¼ cup extra-virgin olive oil
¼ cup canola oil

Salad
½ head cauliflower, separated into florets (1 cup)
½ head broccoli, separated into florets (1 cup)
1 bunch asparagus, trimmed (2 cups)
¼ pound sugar snap peas
2 fennel bulbs, trimmed and cut lengthwise into eighths
1 (14-ounce) package extra-firm tofu, cut into 1-inch cubes, at room temperature
4 hard-boiled eggs, peeled and quartered

1. To make the aïoli, mince garlic on a cutting board and sprinkle with salt. With the blade of a heavy knife, mash garlic and salt into a paste. Transfer to a medium bowl. Add egg yolks and mustard; mix well. Combine olive oil and canola oil in a glass measuring cup. Slowly whisk in oil a few drops at a time until the mixture begins to thicken. Add oil slightly faster, pouring in a slow steady stream, whisking constantly, until very thick. Refrigerate until ready to use.
2. Bring a large pot of salted water to a boil over high heat. One vegetable at a time, blanch cauliflower, broccoli, asparagus, and sugar snap peas until they just soften, 2–4 minutes. Remove each batch of vegetables with a strainer or slotted spoon and bring the water back to a boil before adding the next vegetable.
3. Arrange the vegetables, tofu, and eggs on a large platter. Serve with aïoli.

Tofu in White Wine with Mustard and Dill

Phases 2, 3, 4

Serve this simple-to-prepare but savory tofu dish with a tossed salad or steamed vegetables topped with chopped nuts. To serve four, simply double the recipe.

PER SERVING:

Net Carbs: 8 grams
Total Carbs: 9 grams
Fiber: 1 gram
Protein: 25 grams
Fat: 40 grams
Calories: 500

Makes: 2 servings
Active Time: 10 minutes
Total Time: 1 hour

- ½ small red onion, thinly sliced
- 3 tablespoons extra-virgin olive oil
- 2 tablespoons white wine vinegar
- 2 tablespoons dry white wine (such as sauvignon blanc)
- 2 tablespoons finely chopped fresh dill, or 2 teaspoons dried dill
- 1 tablespoon Dijon mustard
- 1 teaspoon granular sugar substitute
- ¾ teaspoons salt
- ½ teaspoon freshly ground black pepper
- 1 (14-ounce) package extra-firm tofu, drained, patted dry, and cut into 10 (½-inch-thick) slices
- 2 ounces dill Havarti cheese, sliced into 10 pieces

1. Heat oven to 400°F.
2. Combine onion, oil, vinegar, wine, dill, mustard, sugar substitute, salt, and pepper in an 8-inch-square glass baking dish. Add tofu and toss to coat. Arrange tofu in a single snug layer; bake for 45 minutes, until almost all liquid evaporates and onions are golden brown. Remove from oven.
3. Top each slice of tofu with a slice of cheese. Return to oven and bake 5 more minutes to melt cheese. Serve hot.

TIP TIME

PRESSING THE TOFU

Pressing tofu eliminates some of the water, making it denser and firmer. Place firm tofu between two plates; weight it down with a heavy can so the sides bulge but don't crack. Let it stand for up to 1 hour, pour off water, and use or refrigerate for up to 2 days.

WEEKEND

Tempeh-Roasted Cauliflower and Peppers with Curried Cashew Sauce

Phases 3, 4

PER SERVING:
Net Carbs: 20 grams
Total Carbs: 24 grams
Fiber: 4 grams
Protein: 19 grams
Fat: 31 grams
Calories: 430

Makes: 6 (1⅔-cup) servings
Active Time: 30 minutes
Total Time: 1 hour 10 minutes

WEEKEND

Cashews make a rich and creamy dairy-free sauce you can also use on steamed green beans, asparagus, or almost any other vegetable. This three-part dish uses a lot of ingredients, but your taste buds will appreciate its complex taste. Be sure to use unsweetened rice wine and plain tempeh (without rice, other grains, or legumes).

Cauliflower and Peppers

3 tablespoons freshly squeezed lemon juice
3 tablespoons canola oil
2 teaspoons ground coriander
1½ teaspoons salt
1 teaspoon ground cumin
½ teaspoon red pepper flakes
1 medium cauliflower, cored and separated into florets
1 red bell pepper, stemmed, seeds and ribs removed, and cut into 1-inch pieces
1 yellow bell pepper, stemmed, seeds and ribs removed, and cut into 1-inch pieces

Tempeh

¼ cup canola oil
¼ cup unsweetened, unseasoned rice vinegar
¼ cup dry sherry
2 tablespoons tamari (see page 11)
1 tablespoon peeled and finely chopped fresh ginger
1 clove garlic, chopped
2 (8-ounce) packages plain tempeh, cut into 1-inch cubes

Sauce

1 tablespoon canola oil
1 small yellow or white onion, coarsely chopped
2 cloves garlic, peeled
2 teaspoons peeled and finely chopped fresh ginger
2 teaspoons curry powder
½ teaspoon turmeric
1 cup plus 2 tablespoons water
⅓ cup chopped cashews
1 teaspoon freshly squeezed lemon juice
Salt

1. For the cauliflower and peppers, heat oven to 450°F. Combine lemon juice, oil, coriander, salt, cumin, and red pepper flakes in a large bowl. Add cauliflower and bell peppers; toss well to coat. Transfer vegetables to a baking sheet and roast, stirring every 10 minutes, until golden brown, about 40 minutes.
2. Meanwhile, for the tempeh, heat oil, vinegar, sherry, tamari, ginger, and garlic in a large skillet over high heat. Add tempeh; reduce heat to low, cover, and simmer to allow flavors to blend, 20 minutes. Uncover skillet; increase heat to medium and cook until nearly dry, about 10 minutes.
3. For the sauce, heat oil in another large skillet over medium-high heat. Add onion, garlic, and ginger; sauté until onions are soft, about 3 minutes. Add curry and turmeric; cook until fragrant, about 1 minute. Transfer mixture to blender. Add water and cashews; purée until creamy. Return sauce to skillet; simmer until thickened, about 5 minutes. Stir in lemon juice; season with salt to taste.
4. Toss roasted vegetables and tempeh with sauce in a large bowl. Serve hot.

TIP TIME

PEELING GINGER

Ginger should have smooth, unpuckered skin; the root itself is quite knobby and bumpy. Peeling around the lumps can be tricky if you do it with a knife—instead, drag the side of a teaspoon along the root. The skin is thick enough that it should come off easily.

Tempeh and Vegetables in Spicy Coconut-Lemon Broth

Phases 3, 4

PER SERVING:
Net Carbs: 19 grams
Total Carbs: 4 grams
Fiber: 5 grams
Protein: 20 grams
Fat: 46 grams
Calories: 560

Makes: 4 (1¼-cup) servings
Active Time: 25 minutes
Total Time: 40 minutes

WEEKEND

Tempeh, made by fermenting cooked soybeans, is higher in protein than tofu. It also has a somewhat more pronounced flavor. Avoid tempeh products with rice or another grain, which are significantly higher in carbs.

- 3 tablespoons canola oil, divided
- 1 (8-ounce) package plain tempeh, cut into 1-inch cubes
- 1 small yellow or white onion, thinly sliced
- 2 cloves garlic, thinly sliced
- 1 tablespoon peeled and minced fresh ginger
- 1 teaspoon ground coriander
- 1 teaspoon turmeric
- 1 teaspoon paprika
- 1 teaspoon granular sugar substitute
- ½ teaspoon red pepper flakes
- 1 (13½-ounce) can unsweetened coconut milk
- 2 tablespoons tamari (see page 11)
- 2 tablespoons freshly squeezed lemon juice
- 1 teaspoon freshly grated lemon zest
- ½ small head green cabbage, cut into ½-inch slices (3 cups)
- Salt
- ¼ cup chopped fresh cilantro
- ½ cup chopped roasted peanuts (optional)

1. Heat 2 tablespoons oil in a medium skillet over medium-high heat. Add tempeh and sauté until lightly browned, about 5 minutes. Transfer to a bowl.
2. Heat remaining tablespoon oil in skillet over medium-high heat. Add onion and sauté until soft, about 4 minutes. Add garlic, ginger, coriander, turmeric, paprika, sugar substitute, and red pepper flakes; sauté until fragrant, about 30 seconds. Add coconut milk, tamari, lemon juice, and lemon zest; reduce heat to low.
3. Add tempeh and cabbage, cover, and simmer until cabbage is very soft, about 15 minutes.
4. Season with salt to taste, stir in cilantro, top with peanuts if desired, and serve hot.

Tomato and Leek Gratin with Gruyère and Walnuts

Phases 3, 4

Choose sun-dried tomatoes packed in oil for this recipe, but be sure to drain them well before using. You can find dehydrated TVP (see page 202) in a natural foods store or in most well-stocked supermarkets. It takes only 5–10 minutes to rehydrate in broth, which also adds flavor.

PER SERVING:

Net Carbs: 13 grams

Total Carbs: 20 grams

Fiber: 7 grams

Protein: 33 grams

Fat: 46 grams

Calories: 595

Makes: 4 servings

Active Time: 25 minutes

Total Time: 1 hour 25 minutes

WEEKEND

- ½ cup dehydrated TVP
- 1 cup vegetable broth, divided
- 2 tablespoons butter, plus more for pie plate
- 3 medium leeks, light green and white parts only, outer layer and roots removed
- 3 tablespoons extra-virgin olive oil, divided
- 2 teaspoons chopped fresh thyme or ¾ teaspoon dried
- 1 clove garlic, finely chopped
- ⅓ cup sour cream
- 4 ounces Gruyère, shredded (1 cup)
- 8 oil-packed sun-dried tomatoes, drained and sliced
- 2 large eggs, lightly beaten
- 2 tablespoons chopped fresh parsley, divided
- ¾ teaspoon salt
- ¼ teaspoon freshly ground black pepper
- ⅔ cup walnuts, finely chopped

1. Heat oven to 400°F. Combine TVP with ¾ cup broth and set aside. Lightly butter a 9-inch glass pie plate and set aside.
2. Cut leeks in half lengthwise and wash carefully in cold water to remove any soil. Cut into ⅛-inch slices.
3. Heat butter and 2 tablespoons oil in a large heavy skillet over medium heat. Add leeks and sauté until slightly soft, about 4 minutes. Add thyme and garlic; sauté until fragrant, about 30 seconds. Add sour cream and remaining ¼ cup broth; simmer until leeks are very soft, about 3 minutes. Transfer leeks to a bowl and let cool to room temperature.
4. Add cheese, tomatoes, eggs, TVP, 1 tablespoon parsley, salt, and pepper to leek mixture; stir to combine. Fill pie plate with mixture; smooth top with wet spatula. Spread walnuts on top; drizzle with remaining tablespoon oil.
5. Bake gratin until golden and bubbly, about 40 minutes. Sprinkle with remaining tablespoon parsley; let stand 10 minutes before serving.

Spinach-Mushroom Quiche

Phases 2, 3, 4

PER SERVING:
Net Carbs: 7 grams
Total Carbs: 11 grams
Fiber: 4 grams
Protein: 28 grams
Fat: 45 grams
Calories: 550

Makes: 6 servings
Active Time: 30 minutes
Total Time: 2 hours 10 minutes

WEEKEND

Glass bakeware heats up more slowly than metal, but glass retains heat longer. If you don't have a glass pie plate, feel free to use metal, but increase the oven temperature by 25°F. If you are in Phase 3 or 4, you can use Flaky Piecrust (page 237) instead, for a Net Carb count of 13 grams, if you prefer.

- 1 (9-inch) Atkins Basic Piecrust (page 235)
- 1 tablespoon virgin olive oil
- 10 ounces button mushrooms, wiped clean, trimmed, and thinly sliced
- ¾ cup frozen chopped spinach, thawed and well drained
- 5 large eggs
- ¾ cup heavy cream
- ½ teaspoon salt
- ¼ teaspoon freshly ground black pepper
- 6 ounces Gruyère or Emmentaler cheese, shredded (1½ cups)

1. Roll out the piecrust between two sheets of plastic wrap to an 11-inch circle. Remove top sheet of plastic; turn out into a 9-inch glass pie plate. Remove top plastic and press crust into plate. Crimp edges with fingers; pierce bottom with a fork several times. Freeze until cold, about 30 minutes.
2. Heat oven to 425°F. Line crust with aluminum foil and fill with pastry weights or dried beans; bake until light golden on edges, about 10 minutes. Remove foil and weights; bake until bottom is light golden, about 5 minutes. Set aside to cool slightly. Leave oven on.
3. Meanwhile, heat oil in a large skillet over high heat. Add mushrooms and sauté until browned, about 7 minutes. Transfer to a bowl; mix in spinach. Whisk eggs, cream, salt, and pepper in another bowl; stir in cheese. Spread mushroom mixture evenly on bottom of crust; pour in egg mixture. Bake until filling is puffy and deep golden brown on top and a knife inserted in the center comes out clean, about 25 minutes.
4. Let stand at room temperature 30 minutes before serving.

Artichoke, Roasted Pepper, and Goat Cheese Frittata

Phases 2, 3, 4

Having certain staples on hand makes it easy to get a meal on the table fast. With a cylinder of goat cheese in the fridge, artichoke hearts in the freezer, and a jar of marinated roasted red peppers in the pantry, you could have this colorful frittata in the oven in about the time it would take you to make a shopping list and find your car keys.

PER SERVING:
Net Carbs: 8 grams
Total Carbs: 9 grams
Fiber: 1 gram
Protein: 24 grams
Fat: 35 grams
Calories: 450

Makes: 4 servings
Active Time: 15 minutes
Total Time: 40 minutes

- 8 large eggs
- ¼ teaspoon salt
- ⅛ teaspoon red pepper flakes
- 8 ounces fresh goat cheese, crumbled
- 1 cup defrosted, drained, and coarsely chopped artichoke hearts
- 1 jarred roasted red pepper, patted dry and thinly sliced
- ¼ cup virgin olive oil
- 1 medium yellow or white onion, thinly sliced

1. Heat oven to 400°F.
2. Whisk eggs, salt, and red pepper flakes in a large bowl. Stir in goat cheese, artichoke hearts, and roasted red pepper.
3. Heat oil in a 10-inch ovenproof skillet over high heat. Add onion and sauté until soft and light brown, about 3 minutes. Pour in egg mixture. Transfer pan to oven and bake until firm and slightly puffed, about 15 minutes. Serve right away.

TIP TIME

A GIFT FROM THE GOATS

Chèvre, French for "goat," is also the name of fresh cheese made from goat milk. Tart with a texture ranging from moist to dry, creamy to semi-firm, the cheese may also have herbs blended into it. Although chèvre is usually cylinder-shaped, it also comes in disks, cones, and pyramids.

Mustardy Mac 'n' Cheese*

Phases 3, 4

PER SERVING:
Net Carbs: 20 grams
Total Carbs: 32 grams
Fiber: 12 grams
Protein: 31 grams
Fat: 43 grams
Calories: 600

Makes: 4 (1¼-cup) servings
Active Time: 15 minutes
Total Time: 30 minutes

Take our simple, basic recipe and dress it up as much or as little as you please. To shave 5 minutes off the time—or if you simply prefer a creamy dish—omit Steps 4 and 5 and serve directly from the saucepan. Feel free to add more mustard if you like.

- 4 ounces Atkins Cuisine Penne Pasta**
- I medium head cauliflower, cut into florets
- ¾ cup plain unsweetened soy milk
- ¼ cup heavy cream
- 2 large eggs
- ½ teaspoon salt
- ¼ teaspoon cayenne
- 12 ounces sharp Cheddar cheese, shredded (3 cups)
- 2 tablespoons Dijon mustard
- 2 tablespoons (¼ stick) butter, at room temperature

1. Prepare penne according to package directions. Drain and set aside.
2. Meanwhile, steam cauliflower in a steamer basket set in a large covered saucepan over boiling water for 5 minutes. Drain and set aside.
3. Whisk soy milk, cream, eggs, salt, and cayenne in a large heavy-bottomed saucepan; stir in cheese and mustard. Set over medium heat. Add pasta, cauliflower, and butter; cook, stirring constantly, until sauce becomes smooth and thick, about 5 minutes.
4. Meanwhile, heat broiler and arrange oven rack in the middle of the oven.
5. Transfer the pasta mix from the saucepan to an 8-inch-square or 9-inch-round ovenproof casserole dish. Broil for 2–3 minutes, just until a crust develops. Serve right away.

*See photo on color page 27
**Order from www.atkins.com.

Protein-Powered Eggplant Parmesan

Phase: 3, 4

The eggplant in this casserole is baked instead of fried, letting its subtle flavor shine through—and making it less of a calorie bomb. Hunt's and Muir's Glen are two readily available brands of tomato purée.

PER SERVING:
Net Carbs: 15 grams
Total Carbs: 23 grams
Fiber: 8 grams
Protein: 33 grams
Fat: 19 grams
Calories: 360

Makes: 6 servings
Active Time: 30 minutes
Total Time: 1 hour 20 minutes

- 1 large eggplant, cut into ½-inch-thick slices
- 4 tablespoons virgin olive oil, divided
- 1 small yellow or white onion, chopped
- ¼ pound button mushrooms, wiped clean, trimmed, and sliced
- 1 clove garlic, chopped
- 1 (15-ounce) can tomato purée
- 1¼ cups vegetable broth
- 1 cup TVP (see page 202)
- 1 teaspoon dried basil
- ¾ teaspoon dried oregano
- ½ teaspoon salt
- ¼ teaspoon freshly ground black pepper
- 12 ounces shredded whole-milk mozzarella (1½ cups)
- ½ cup grated Parmesan cheese

1. Heat oven to 450°F. Line a baking sheet with foil.
2. Brush eggplant with 3 tablespoons oil and arrange in a single layer on baking sheet. Bake until golden brown and soft, about 25 minutes.
3. Meanwhile, heat remaining tablespoon oil in a large skillet over high heat. Add onion and mushrooms; cook until vegetables are soft, about 5 minutes. Add garlic and cook until fragrant, about 30 seconds. Add tomato purée, broth, TVP, basil, oregano, salt, and pepper; simmer until sauce thickens, about 10 minutes. If eggplant is not done, remove sauce from heat and cover to keep warm.
4. To assemble, reduce oven temperature to 350°F. Arrange half of the eggplant in a 2-quart glass baking dish; top with half of the sauce, half of the mozzarella, and half of the Parmesan. Repeat layers. Bake until hot and bubbling, about 25 minutes. Cool slightly and serve warm.

Tofu Pad Thai*

Phases 3, 4

PER SERVING:
Net Carbs: 14 grams
Total Carbs: 21 grams
Fiber: 7 grams
Protein: 22 grams
Fat: 29 grams
Calories: 410

Makes: 4 servings
Active Time: 30 minutes
Total Time: 30 minutes

WEEKDAY

The classic Thai dish is usually made with chicken or shrimp, but tofu takes to the seasonings equally well.

- 3 (8-ounce) packages spaghetti-style tofu shirataki noodles
- ¼ cup fish sauce (nam pla or nuoc mam)
- ⅓ cup freshly squeezed lime juice
- 2 tablespoons granular sugar substitute
- ¼ teaspoon red pepper flakes
- 3 tablespoons canola oil, divided
- 1 (14-ounce) package firm tofu, drained, patted dry, and cut in 1-inch cubes
- 3 large eggs, lightly beaten
- 8 scallions, cut into 1-inch pieces
- 2 cloves garlic, finely chopped
- 2 cups mung bean sprouts, rinsed and patted dry
- ½ cup chopped fresh cilantro
- ½ cup unsalted dry-roasted peanuts, chopped
- 1 lime, cut into wedges

1. Drain and rinse noodles well. Parboil in water to cover for 2–3 minutes, drain, and set aside.
2. Combine fish sauce, lime juice, sugar substitute, and red pepper flakes in a small bowl; set aside.
3. Heat 2 tablespoons oil in a large nonstick skillet or wok over high heat. Add tofu and sauté until just browned on all sides, about 6 minutes. Transfer to a plate.
4. Add eggs to skillet; cook, stirring, until just scrambled, about 1 minute. Transfer to plate with tofu. Wipe out skillet and add remaining tablespoon oil; return to high heat. Add scallions and garlic; sauté until garlic just begins to brown, about 1 minute. Remove and set aside.
5. Pour the fish sauce mixture into the skillet and boil, about 5 minutes, until reduced to half. Add reserved pasta, eggs, and tofu; and bean sprouts; cook to heat through, about 1 minute. Transfer to plates; sprinkle with cilantro and peanuts. Serve right away with lime wedges.

*See photo on color page 28

Vegetable Curry with Seared Noodles

Phases 3, 4

If you've never had seared noodles before, you're in for a real treat. Here we've combined low-carb spaghetti with curry powder and vegetables, but you'll probably find numerous variations of your own. Make sure the spaghetti contains no more than 5 grams of Net Carbs per serving. You should be able to find low-carb spaghetti in most well-stocked supermarkets.

PER SERVING:
Net Carbs: 15 grams
Total Carbs: 39 grams
Fiber: 24 grams
Protein: 18 grams
Fat: 26 grams
Calories: 440

Makes: 4 (2-cup) servings
Active Time: 25 minutes
Total Time: 55 minutes

WEEKEND

- 6 ounces low-carb spaghetti (see note above)
- 4 tablespoons virgin olive oil, divided
- ½ medium yellow or white onion, chopped
- 2 tablespoons peeled and grated fresh ginger
- 2 tablespoons curry powder
- 2 medium zucchini, cut in half lengthwise, then cut into ¼-inch half-moons
- 1 medium yellow or orange bell pepper, stemmed, seeds and ribs removed, cut into 1-inch squares
- 1 medium tomato, seeded and chopped
- 1 (14-ounce) package firm tofu, drained, patted dry, and cut in ½-inch dice
- 1 cup vegetable broth
- 2 teaspoons granular sugar substitute
- 1 teaspoon salt, divided
- ¼ teaspoon freshly ground black pepper, divided
- ¼ cup chopped fresh mint
- ½ cup sliced, blanched almonds
- 1 tablespoon tamari (see page 11)

1. Bring a large pot of lightly salted water to a boil over high heat. Add spaghetti and cook according to package directions; drain thoroughly.
2. Meanwhile, heat 2 tablespoons oil in a large nonstick skillet over medium-high heat. Add onion and sauté until it starts to soften, 3–4 minutes. Add ginger and curry; sauté until fragrant, 1 minute. Stir in zucchini and bell pepper; cook, stirring occasionally, until the vegetables begin to soften, 2–3 minutes.

3. Add tomato, tofu, broth, sugar substitute, ¾ teaspoon salt, and ⅛ teaspoon pepper. Bring to a boil, reduce the heat to medium-low and simmer until vegetables are tender, 18–20 minutes. Transfer to a bowl and stir in mint and almonds; cover to keep warm.
4. Add remaining 2 tablespoons oil to skillet and set over medium-high heat. Add noodles and cook, stirring often, until they begin to brown and crisp, 2–3 minutes.
5. Stir in tamari and remaining ¼ teaspoon salt and ⅛ teaspoon pepper; cook 30 seconds and serve hot.
6. To serve, divide noodles among 4 shallow bowls and top each with 1½ cups of vegetable curry mixture.

TIP TIME

PICKING PEPPERS

Select bell peppers with smooth, glossy skins and fresh-looking stems. If color doesn't matter in your recipe, choose red rather than green peppers; they supply more than twice the vitamin C.

Seitan Shepherd's Pie with Tofu Topping

Phases 3, 4

Mirin, sometimes called rice wine, is more traditional than dry sherry in Japanese cooking, but it contains sugar, so we used sherry instead. If you prefer to avoid alcohol, use unseasoned rice vinegar in place of the sherry.

PER SERVING:
Net Carbs: 20 grams
Total Carbs: 23 grams
Fiber: 3 grams
Protein: 24 grams
Fat: 20 grams
Calories: 360

Makes: 6 servings
Active Time: 30 minutes
Total Time: 1 hour 40 minutes

WEEKEND

Filling
3 tablespoons virgin olive oil
2 small yellow or white onions, chopped
2 medium carrots, peeled and cut into ½-inch slices
¾ pound button mushrooms, wiped clean, trimmed, and sliced
6 ounces green beans, cut into 1-inch lengths
2 (8-ounce) packages seitan, cut into ½-inch chunks
1 (14-ounce) can diced tomatoes
½ cup vegetable broth
2 tablespoons dry sherry
1 tablespoon tamari (see page 11)
2 teaspoons chopped fresh thyme, or ¾ teaspoon dried
2 teaspoons chopped fresh sage, or ¾ teaspoon dried
Salt
Freshly ground black pepper

Topping
1 (14-ounce) package firm tofu, cut into 1-inch cubes
3 tablespoons cider vinegar
¼ cup virgin olive oil
2 cloves garlic, chopped
1 tablespoon fresh thyme, or 1 teaspoon dried
1 teaspoon salt
¼ teaspoon freshly ground black pepper

1. Heat oven to 350°F.
2. For the filling, heat oil in large skillet over medium-high heat; add onion and sauté until soft, about 5 minutes. Add carrots, mushrooms, and green beans; sauté until vegetables begin to soften. Add seitan, tomatoes, broth, sherry, tamari, thyme, and sage; cover and simmer until vegetables are tender, 10–15 minutes. Uncover and simmer until liquid thickens

slightly, about 10 minutes. Season with salt and pepper to taste. Pour into a 2- to 3-quart glass baking or casserole dish or 10-inch glass pie plate.

3. Meanwhile, for the topping, combine tofu, vinegar, oil, garlic, thyme, salt, and pepper in a food processor and purée.
4. Spread topping evenly over filling; bake until the topping is golden brown, about 50 minutes. Let stand 5 minutes before serving.

TIP TIME

MUSHROOM MAGIC

Mushrooms are an excellent way to add flavor to many foods: They contain glutamic acid, a natural compound on which the flavor enhancer monosodium glutamate is based. Leave packaged mushrooms in their wrapping and refrigerate for up to a week. Bulk mushrooms should be placed in a paper bag; fold it over loosely before refrigerating and store for up to 5 days.

Seitan and Black Bean Chili

Phases 3, 4

This dish cooks fast and is as hearty as chili made with meat. If you can find canned black soybeans to replace the black beans, you can cut out some carbs. If you don't use tomato paste often, look for it in tubes, which are resealable and last for months in the fridge. Read the label, though, as some tubed pastes are twice as concentrated as canned pastes; if so, use only half the amount called for.

PER SERVING:
Net Carbs: 26 grams
Total Carbs: 34 grams
Fiber: 8 grams
Protein: 20 grams
Fat: 11 grams
Calories: 270

Makes: 4 (1-cup) servings
Active Time: 20 minutes
Total Time: 30 minutes

WEEKDAY

- 1 tablespoon virgin olive oil
- 1 small yellow or white onion, chopped
- 1 green or red bell pepper, stemmed, seeds and ribs removed, and chopped
- 1 jalapeño, finely chopped
- 2 cloves garlic, chopped
- 1 tablespoon tomato paste
- 1 tablespoon chili powder
- ½ teaspoon dried oregano
- 1 (14-ounce) can diced tomatoes
- 1 (14-ounce) can black beans, with liquid
- 1 (8-ounce) package seitan, very finely chopped
- Salt
- Freshly ground black pepper
- ¼ cup sour cream
- 1 ounce sharp Cheddar cheese, shredded (¼ cup)
- 1 scallion, thinly sliced

1. Heat oil in a large heavy-bottomed pot over high heat. Add onion, bell pepper, and jalapeño; sauté until soft, about 3 minutes. Add garlic and sauté until fragrant, about 30 seconds. Add tomato paste, chili powder, and oregano; cook to heat tomato paste, about 1 minute. Add tomatoes, beans, and seitan; bring to a boil.
2. Reduce heat to low and simmer until vegetables are very tender and chili has thickened, about 10 minutes.
3. Season with salt and pepper to taste. Ladle into bowls and garnish with sour cream, cheese, and scallion.

Warm Lentil Salad with Smoked Mozzarella and Arugula

Phases 3, 4

PER SERVING:
Net Carbs: 16 grams
Total Carbs: 25 grams
Fiber: 9 grams
Protein: 23 grams
Fat: 19 grams
Calories: 350

Makes: 4 (1-cup) servings
Active Time: 25 minutes
Total Time: 25 minutes

WEEKDAY

French lentils (sometimes called Le Puy lentils) hold their shape well, making them a better choice for salads than brown lentils.

- 5 tablespoons virgin olive oil
- 1 medium red onion, chopped
- 2 small fennel bulbs, trimmed and thinly sliced
- 2 cloves garlic, finely chopped
- 2 teaspoons dried tarragon
- ½ teaspoon red pepper flakes
- ¼ cup vegetable broth
- 1 cup canned, drained French lentils (see note above)
- 8 ounces smoked mozzarella, cut into ½-inch dice
- 8 oil-packed sun-dried tomatoes, drained and thinly sliced
- ¼ cup red wine vinegar
- ½ teaspoon salt
- 4 cups arugula
- 4 tablespoons finely chopped fresh parsley

1. Heat oil in a large skillet over high heat. Add onion and cook until slightly soft, about 2 minutes. Add fennel, garlic, tarragon, and pepper flakes; cook until fragrant, about 30 seconds. Add broth, cover, and simmer until fennel is crisp-tender, about 2 minutes.
2. Uncover pan and remove from heat; stir in lentils, mozzarella, tomatoes, vinegar, and salt. Divide arugula among four plates; top each with one-fourth of the lentil mixture and 1 tablespoon parsley. Serve warm.

Variation: Greek Lentil Salad with Feta and Spinach

Phases 3, 4

Prepare as above, substituting 2 chopped large tomatoes for the fennel (and broth). Substitute 4 ounces feta for the mozzarella, ⅓ cup sliced black olives for the sun-dried tomatoes, and baby spinach leaves for the arugula.

Braised Red Lentils with Eggplant and Ricotta Salata

Phases 3, 4

Ricotta salata is a dry salted ricotta, made from the whey of Pecorino Romano. If you can't find it, substitute a mild feta or fresh goat cheese instead. Garam masala is a classic Indian spice mix; it can be found in the spice or Indian food section of most supermarkets.

PER SERVING:
Net Carbs: 25 grams
Total Carbs: 31 grams
Fiber: 6 grams
Protein: 16 grams
Fat: 16 grams
Calories: 320

Makes: 6 (1⅔-cup) servings
Active Time: 20 minutes
Total Time: 1 hour 10 minutes

WEEKEND

- 2 tablespoons butter
- 1 medium yellow or white onion, chopped
- 1 tablespoon peeled and grated fresh ginger
- 1 clove garlic, chopped
- 1½ teaspoons garam masala (see note above)
- 1 teaspoon turmeric
- 1 medium eggplant, cut into ½-inch dice
- 1 (14 ½-ounce) can diced tomatoes
- 4 cups water
- 1 cup red lentils
- 2 bay leaves
- 1 medium zucchini or summer squash, cut into ½-inch dice
- 1 teaspoon salt
- ½ teaspoon freshly ground black pepper
- 16 ounces ricotta salata, crumbled
- ¾ cup sliced blanched almonds
- 2 tablespoons chopped fresh cilantro

1. Melt butter in a large saucepan over medium-high heat. Add onion and sauté until soft, about 3 minutes. Add ginger, garlic, garam masala, and turmeric; sauté until fragrant, about 30 seconds. Add eggplant and tomatoes; cook until eggplant begins to soften, about 3 minutes. Add water, lentils, and bay leaves; increase heat to high and bring to a boil.
2. Cover, reduce heat to low and simmer until lentils have absorbed almost all the water, about 35 minutes. Remove bay leaves.
3. Add zucchini, salt, and pepper; simmer until zucchini and lentils are soft, about 5–7 minutes. Stir in ricotta salata, almonds, and cilantro just before serving.

Chapter 13

DELECTABLE DESSERTS

One of the beauties of the low-carb lifestyle is that desserts are on the menu from day one. Even in Phase 1 of the Atkins Diet you can enjoy Chocolate Truffles, Coconut Meringues, and Chocolate-Orange Soufflés. The field opens up significantly in Phase 2, and by the time you're close to or maintaining your goal weight, you could be savoring Almond-Plum Tart, Pineapple Upside-Down Cake, and a delicious variety of cakes, tarts, cookies, and other sweets. Our recipes include seven piecrust recipes you can pair with fruit, pudding, or ice cream fillings to come up with your own pies. Plus you'll find hundreds more dessert recipes suitable for all phases of the program at www.atkins.com.

Most desserts need to bake or chill, meaning that the majority of the following recipes are coded for the weekend. A few scrumptious exceptions include Cranberry-Orange Fool, Chocolate-Orange Soufflés, and Mini-Muffin-Tin Chocolate Brownies. But, as always, the active time for all recipes is 30 minutes or less. If you plan ahead—by making a piecrust on the weekend, for example—you'll be able to enjoy some of these treats during the week.

ART AND SCIENCE

It's often said that cooking is an art but baking is a science—and indeed, the alchemy between eggs, flour, butter, and sweetener can be downright mystifying to the uninitiated. A host of variables, from the metal or glass of the pan you use to the weather, can affect whether your cake rises or your soufflé falls.

The good news is making desserts and baked goods with low-carb ingredients is no more difficult than when using conventional ingredients. Several of the techniques are exactly the same. Sorting the wheat from the chaff is important in selecting ingredients for low-carb baked goods. Refined (white) flour and sugar are very high in carbs (and lacking in much nutritional value), but fortunately there are several lower-carb and far more nutritious alternatives. Some of these are naturally lower in carbohydrates; others are specially formulated. They give nuts, berries and other fruits, and real cream starring roles—their rich textures and sweet flavors are often lost among sugar-saturated treats.

FLOUR POWER

Flour provides structure to baked goods: A high-protein flour helps to create the large holes prized in artisanal bread; low-protein flours are used in cakes, cookies, and piecrusts to produce tenderness and a delicate crumb. That said, even whole-wheat flour is too high in carbs for use in the initial weight-loss phases of Atkins.

Flours made from soy, nuts, or grains other than wheat cannot completely replace wheat flour in most cake or cookie recipes. A cake made only of soy flour will be dense and flat, not light and airy. Many of our Phase 3 and 4 recipes, therefore, use some combination of whole-wheat flour and/or soy or another "flour," such as almond meal. Atkins Cuisine All Purpose Baking Mix, which contains wheat gluten (a form of protein), bran, and modified starch, along with soy flour, is a boon to low-carb bakers. Phase 2 baked goods rely wholly on the baking mix, sometimes in combination with almond meal. (For more on low-carb baking, see page 16.)

Once you've used the Atkins baking mix in some of these recipes, you might be inspired to adapt some of your favorite conventional baked goods recipes. It's denser than flour, so you generally need to use less of it. For example, a recipe that calls for 1½ cups of flour may need only about 1 cup of baking mix. There's no leavening agent (baking soda or baking powder) in the baking mix, so keep those measurements the same as in the original recipe. Using lemon, vanilla, almond, and maple extracts helps mute the flavor of soy, as do such spices as cinnamon, cardamom, ginger, nutmeg, and allspice. We also often use almond (or another nut) meal to replace wheat flour.

THE RIGHT (SWEET) STUFF

Although moderate amounts of whole-grain flours are acceptable in later phases of Atkins, sugar in any form, including honey or molasses, should be avoided. Sucralose is a sugar substitute sold under the brand name Splenda, and can be used in baking with excellent results. We used granular sucralose in all of these recipes, and we strongly suggest that you do, too. Sugar substitutes can vary tremendously in sweetening power. If you opt to use a different sugar substitute, your dessert may be far too sweet or off-puttingly sour or bitter. Unlike many sugar substitutes, sucralose doesn't lose its sweetness when heated, so cooked and baked foods made with it taste better than those made with other sugar substitutes.

THE RIGHT CHOCOLATE

Chocolate may not be synonymous with dessert, but show me a restaurant menu without at least one chocolate treat on it! Likewise, on the following pages you'll find many chocolate delectables, from Pistachio-Chocolate Truffles to Chocolate Piecrust. Some of them call for unsweetened cocoa, but others include sugar-free low-carb chocolate. Such products rely for sweetness on sugar alcohols such as maltitol, mannitol, xylitol, sorbitol, and glycerin, which are non-nutritive sugar substitutes. Most sugar alcohols behave similarly in the body, but some people can experience gastric distress when they consume them in excess. (You'll note that recipes that use chocolate as an ingredient also list the number of grams of sugar alcohol in the nutritional data. Sugar alcohols have no impact on blood sugar levels and are therefore subtracted, along with fiber, from total carbs to yield the Net Carb gram count.)

You can also use baker's chocolate, which is unsweetened chocolate. Note that it is not the same as the bittersweet and semisweet kinds. The latter two supply almost *three times* the grams of Net Carbs than does unsweetened chocolate. If your recipe requires sweetened low-carb chocolate, you can make it yourself. To make 1 ounce of semisweet chocolate, add 1½–2 teaspoons sucralose to ½ ounce of unsweetened chocolate.

FAT IS FLAVOR'S FRIEND

If you've ever followed a low-fat eating plan, you've probably eaten an alarming number of fat-free cookies yet still felt hungry. Fat, as you've probably since learned, is indispensable to the Atkins program, but it is also essential to good taste and texture. It provides what food chemists call "mouth feel"—it imparts a creamy richness to foods, making them palatable. It also helps to create the feeling of satiety.

When it comes to baked goods, fat helps to tenderize them: it coats the proteins in flour and prevents gluten from overdeveloping. Although you can use oils in baked goods, they can give a somewhat greasy texture. The best fat for baking is unsalted butter, which provides a mix of saturated and unsaturated fats, and its flavor is inimitable. Unsalted butter is often fresher than salted butter—salt is a preservative, so salted butter may stay on warehouse or refrigerator shelves longer. The amount of salt in butter can vary from one manufacturer to another, and salt also muddies the flavor of butter. You'll get better and more consistent flavor by adding salt to unsalted butter.

One more important point about butter: use only stick form for baking. The air mixed into whipped butter means it has less fat by volume and won't give the same results.

THE ESSENTIAL EGG

In addition to being an excellent source of protein and a fine food in their own right, eggs play a crucial role in baking. Egg whites have leavening properties, and egg yolks help to emulsify and provide a moist texture. Whether beaten together or separately, both yolks and whites trap air bubbles, making foods light and airy and helping to leaven cakes (they lack the leavening power of yeast or baking powder, however). When beating egg whites, be sure that your bowl and beaters are scrupulously clean. Any fat will prevent the whites from foaming properly. Fat can adhere to plastic, so use a metal, glass, or ceramic bowl, and spotless beaters or whisk. A large balloon whisk or oscillating beaters will incorporate air much faster than a smaller whisk or a stationary mixer.

When you're frying eggs for breakfast, it doesn't really matter what size eggs you buy, but size definitely matters when you use them in recipes! It takes 5 large eggs to measure one cup, but only 4 extra-large or jumbo eggs or 6 medium eggs. But because recipes call for eggs by quantity and size rather than volume, choosing a different size can spell the difference between success and failure. Our recipes always call for large eggs.

Now that we've covered the basics, let's get down to the fun part: making and eating dessert—without the guilt!

Coconut Custard

Phases 2, 3, 4

Unsweetened coconut milk is often used in Thai or Indian cooking and can be found in the Asian and/or Caribbean section of the grocery store.

PER SERVING:
Net Carbs: 6 grams
Total Carbs: 6 grams
Fiber: 0 grams
Protein: 5 grams
Fat: 36 grams
Calories: 360

Makes: 4 (½-cup) servings
Active Time: 10 minutes
Total Time: 4 hours 45 minutes

1 cup heavy cream
¾ cup unsweetened coconut milk
⅛ teaspoon salt
1 large egg
2 large egg yolks
2 tablespoons granular sugar substitute
1½ teaspoons coconut extract

4 (6-ounce) ramekins

1. Heat oven to 350°F.
2. Combine cream, coconut milk, and salt in a small saucepan; bring to a simmer over medium heat.
3. Meanwhile, combine egg, egg yolks, and sugar substitute in a medium bowl. Slowly whisk hot cream into egg mixture; stir in coconut extract. Strain custard through a fine-mesh sieve; divide among the ramekins.
4. Set ramekins in a roasting pan; fill pan with hot water to halfway up the sides of ramekins. Bake until just set, about 35 minutes. Remove custards; cover and refrigerate to chill, about 4 hours or overnight.
5. To serve, run a sharp knife around inner rim of each ramekin to loosen. Dip bottom of each ramekin into hot water for a few seconds; invert onto dessert plates.

TIP TIME

SIMMER AND STRAIN

Heating cream to a simmer and then whisking it slowly into eggs increases the temperature of the eggs gradually—it's called tempering—which liquefies the yolks and sugar substitute. Straining the mixture removes the bands of tissue that hold the egg yolk in place.

WEEKEND

Creamy Vanilla Pudding

Phase 2, 3, 4

PER SERVING:
Net Carbs: 4 grams
Total Carbs: 4 grams
Fiber: 0 grams
Protein: 6 grams
Fat: 31 grams
Calories: 320

Servings 4 (½-cup) servings
Active Time: 10 minutes
Total Time: 2 hours 10 minutes

Boost the vanilla flavor by dropping the vanilla bean into the simmering cream after you've added the seeds, but fish it out before you transfer the pudding to dishes. If you prefer, substitute pure vanilla extract.

1 cup heavy cream
½ cup water
8 large egg yolks
¼ cup granular sugar substitute
⅛ teaspoon salt
1 (4-inch-long) vanilla bean (or 2 teaspoons pure vanilla extract)

1. Bring 2 inches water to a boil in the bottom of a double boiler over high heat. In the top of the double boiler, combine the cream, water, egg yolks, sugar substitute, and salt. Using a paring knife, slit open the vanilla bean and scrape out the seeds. Add seeds to liquid. Set over simmering water and cook, stirring constantly, until mixture thickens enough to coat the back of a wooden spoon, about 4 minutes.
2. Transfer to dessert bowls; cover surface of puddings with plastic wrap and refrigerate until set, about 2 hours.

Variations: Creamy Chocolate Pudding

Phase 2, 3, 4

Prepare Creamy Vanilla Pudding as above, substituting 3 tablespoons cocoa powder for the vanilla bean, adding 1 teaspoon pure vanilla extract, and using only 7 large egg yolks.

Creamy Coffee Pudding

Phase 2, 3, 4

Prepare Vanilla Pudding as above, substituting 2 teaspoons instant coffee granules for the vanilla bean.

Chocolate-Orange Soufflés

Phases 1, 2, 3, 4

The orange flavor in these warm chocolate souffés comes from orange extract, making them perfectly acceptable for Phase 1. We used Hershey's sugar-free chocolate, but there are numerous other brands available.

PER SERVING:
Net Carbs: 3 grams
Total Carbs: 11 grams
Fiber: 1 gram
Sugar Alcohols: 7 grams
Protein: 5 grams
Fat:18 grams
Calories: 210

Makes: 6 servings
Active Time: 10 minutes
Total Time: 25 minutes

- 5 tablespoons butter, plus more for ramekins
- ⅓ cup granular sugar substitute, plus more for ramekins
- 6½ ounces low-carb or sugar-free chocolate bars (see note above)
- 1 teaspoon orange extract
- 5 large eggs, separated
- ¼ teaspoon cream of tartar
- 6 (6-ounce) ramekins

1. Heat oven to 425°F. Lightly butter ramekins; coat the insides with sugar substitute. Set on a baking sheet.
2. Melt chocolate, butter, and orange extract in a small saucepan over low heat. (Or microwave as explained in tip below.) Transfer to a medium bowl. Whisk in egg yolks; set aside.
3. Combine egg whites and cream of tartar in another medium bowl; whip with an electric mixer on high speed until frothy. Slowly add sugar substitute; whip until soft peaks form, about 3 minutes. Fold one-third of the egg whites into chocolate mixture; gently fold in remaining whites. Divide batter among ramekins; bake until puffed and set, about 13 minutes. Serve right away.

TIP TIME

PUT THE MICROWAVE TO WORK

To melt chocolate, simply chop it, place it in a large bowl, and microwave on medium for 1½ minutes. Stir, then microwave on medium at 30-second intervals until it's melted before adding other ingredients.

WEEKDAY

Tangy Lemon Gelatin

Phase 2, 3, 4

PER SERVING:
Net Carbs: 4 grams
Total Carbs: 5 grams
Fiber: 1 gram
Protein: 2 grams
Fat: 0 grams
Calories: 25

Makes: 4 (½-cup) servings
Active Time: 15 minutes
Total Time: 2 hours, 15 minutes

WEEKEND

If you've only had gelatin made from an artificially flavored mix, you'll be surprised at how delightfully tart it is when made with real fruit. Serve this with slightly sweetened whipped cream if desired. If you plan to invert the gelatin onto a serving platter, mist the mold with cooking spray before pouring in the gelatin in Step 3.

1⅔ cups water, divided
1 packet powdered unflavored gelatin
½ cup granular sugar substitute
3 tablespoons freshly grated lemon zest
⅓ cup freshly squeezed lemon juice

1. Combine ⅓ cup water and gelatin in a medium bowl; let stand 5 minutes to allow gelatin to bloom.
2. Meanwhile, combine remaining 1⅓ cups water, sugar substitute, and lemon zest in a medium saucepan with lid; bring to a boil over high heat. Remove from heat; cover and steep 5 minutes.
3. Strain zest-water mixture into bowl with gelatin, discarding solids; stir until gelatin dissolves. Stir in lemon juice; divide among four dessert dishes or pour into a 4-cup gelatin mold. Cover with plastic wrap; refrigerate until set, 2–4 hours.

Variations: Creamy Lemon Gelatin

Phases 2, 3, 4

Prepare Lemon Gelatin as above, replacing ½ cup of the water in Step 2 with heavy cream.

Lime-Mint Gelatin

Phase 2, 3, 4

Prepare Lemon Gelatin as above, substituting lime zest for lemon zest and lime juice for lemon juice. Stir in ¾ cup chopped mint leaves with the sugar substitute.

Lickety-Split Vanilla Ice Cream

Phases 2, 3, 4

This ice cream takes only four ingredients and 10 minutes to prepare; the hard part is waiting for it to chill! (Also check out Basic Custard Ice Cream at www.atkins.com.) To jazz it up, before freezing stir in 2 teaspoons pure maple extract, 1½ teaspoons pure lemon extract, 1½ teaspoons pure almond extract, or an additional 1 teaspoon pure vanilla extract. Or, in the last few minutes of processing, slowly incorporate ½–1 cup toasted nuts, crumbled low-carb candy or granola bars, or fresh chopped berries.

PER SERVING:
Net Carbs: 4 grams
Total Carbs: 4 grams
Fiber: 0 grams
Protein: 2 grams
Fat: 36 grams
Calories: 340

Makes: 8 (½-cup) servings
Active Time: 10 minutes
Total Time: 1½ hours

3¼ cups heavy cream
½ cup plus 1 tablespoon granular sugar substitute
Pinch salt
½ teaspoon pure vanilla extract

1. Combine cream, sugar substitute, salt, and vanilla in a medium bowl and refrigerate until very well chilled, at least 1 hour.
2. Process according to the instructions for your ice cream maker.
3. Transfer to a container and freeze until ready to serve. Scoop into dessert dishes.

TIP TIME

REALITY CHECK

Opt for pure flavoring extracts, not artificial ones. You'll be astonished at the difference pure vanilla and pure almond extracts make compared to their artificial counterparts.

Mint Granita

Phases 2, 3, 4

PER SERVING:
Net Carbs: 6 grams
Total Carbs: 7 grams
Fiber: 1 gram
Protein: 1 gram
Fat: 0 grams
Calories: 25

Makes: 4 servings
Active Time: 20 minutes
Total Time: 2 hours 40 minutes

Granita is the Italian word for refreshing dessert ices with a pleasingly granular texture. The key to obtaining the proper consistency is frequent stirring as the ice freezes, which prevents it from forming large clumps of ice.

2 cups water
2 cups mint leaves, coarsely chopped
⅔ cup granular sugar substitute
2 tablespoons freshly squeezed lemon juice

1. Combine water, mint, and sugar substitute in a medium saucepan; bring to a boil over high heat. Reduce heat to medium-low and simmer 3 minutes. Remove from heat, stir in lemon juice, and cool 15 minutes.
2. Strain mixture into an 8-inch-square baking dish. Place in freezer until ice crystals begin to form, about 30 minutes. Using a fork, break up ice and return to freezer. Continue breaking up ice crystals every 30 minutes, until mixture is granular and completely frozen, about 2 hours. Once the mixture is frozen, cover pan with plastic wrap.
3. To serve, remove granita from freezer and thaw for 2–3 minutes, breaking up any large ice crystals. Scoop into dessert bowls.

Lemon-Lime Semifreddo

Phases 2, 3, 4

The tangy citrus flavor of this semifreddo ("half-cold" in Italian) makes it a warm-weather delight. The presentation is also spectacular, even more so when garnished with sliced strawberries and shaved low-carb chocolate.

PER SERVING:
Net Carbs: 5 grams
Total Carbs: 6 grams
Fiber: 1 gram
Protein: 5 grams
Fat: 38 grams
Calories: 380

Makes: 8 servings
Active Time: 20 minutes
Total Time: 8 hours 30 minutes

- Olive oil cooking spray
- 3 large egg yolks
- ½ cup granular sugar substitute, divided
- ¾ teaspoon pure vanilla extract
- 2 teaspoons freshly grated lemon zest
- 3 tablespoons freshly squeezed lemon juice
- 2 teaspoons grated fresh lime zest
- 2 tablespoons freshly squeezed lime juice
- 1 (8-ounce) package cream cheese
- 2 cups heavy cream
- ½ cup walnut halves, toasted and chopped

1. Line a 5-by-9-inch loaf pan with plastic wrap; mist with cooking spray.
2. Combine egg yolks, ¼ cup sugar substitute, and vanilla in the bowl of an electric mixer. Beat on high speed, stopping to scrape down sides of bowl once or twice, until light yellow and stiff, 2–3 minutes; stop machine. Add lemon zest and juice and lime zest and juice; beat until well combined. Scrape down bowl and add cream cheese; beat until smooth. Transfer to a large bowl.
3. Wipe out bowl of mixer and add remaining ¼ cup sugar substitute and cream. Beat on high speed until stiff peaks form, 2–3 minutes. Gently fold one-third of whipped cream into egg yolk mixture until just combined; repeat twice. Spoon half of mixture into pan, then scatter walnuts on top. Spoon remaining mixture over nuts, smoothing top, and then cover with plastic wrap. Freeze for 8 hours.
4. To serve, unwrap plastic over semifreddo and invert it onto a serving plate; remove plastic wrap. Let stand 10 minutes to soften slightly. With a knife dipped in hot water, cut into 8 slices and set on dessert plates.

Cranberry-Orange Fool

Phases 2, 3, 4

PER SERVING:
Net Carbs: 4 grams
Total Carbs: 5 grams
Fiber: 1 gram
Protein: 1 gram
Fat: 22 grams
Calories: 220

Makes: 4 (½-cup) servings
Active Time: 10 minutes
Total Time: 20 minutes

WEEKDAY

Fools are old-fashioned desserts that deserve rediscovery—the name comes from the French *fouler,* meaning to "purée" or "mash." Made of cooked, puréed fruit that's folded into whipped cream, fools are light yet rich, and they're tasty warm or chilled. Cranberry Fool is a perfect dessert for Thanksgiving dinner.

1 cup fresh or frozen cranberries
⅓ cup water
2 teaspoons freshly grated orange zest
1 cup heavy cream, chilled
2 tablespoons granular sugar substitute
½ teaspoon pure vanilla extract

1. Simmer cranberries and water over medium-high heat until mixture thickens and cranberries pop, 5–10 minutes. Transfer to food processor or blender and purée. Pour into medium bowl. Add orange zest and stir to blend.
2. Meanwhile, whip cream, sugar substitute, and vanilla with an electric mixer on medium-high speed until soft peaks form.
3. Fold one-third of the whipped cream into cranberries; fold in remaining cream. Scoop into dessert bowls and serve, or refrigerate for up to 4 hours.

Variation: Mixed Berry Fool

Phases 2, 3, 4

Follow the recipe for Cranberry-Orange Fool above, but omit the orange zest. Instead of cranberries, purée 1½ cups of a combination of blueberries, raspberries, and strawberries; combine with the water but don't cook. Proceed from Step 2.

Atkins Basic Piecrust

Phases 2, 3, 4

This versatile recipe gives you enough dough for a single crust; however, it doubles easily if your recipe calls for both top and bottom crusts. Like all piecrusts, this can be made ahead of time and frozen for up to a month.

- 1¼ cups Atkins Cuisine All Purpose Baking Mix
- ¼ teaspoon salt
- 1 teaspoon granular sugar substitute
- ½ cup (1 stick) cold unsalted butter, cut into small pieces
- 2–3 tablespoons ice water

1. Pulse baking mix, salt, and sugar substitute in a food processor to incorporate; add butter and pulse until mixture resembles a coarse meal, about 30 seconds. Pulse in water until dough just comes together, about 30 seconds.
2. Transfer dough to a sheet of plastic wrap; form into a disk about 6 inches in diameter. Wrap tightly in plastic; refrigerate until firm, about 30 minutes.
3. Roll and bake as directed in pie recipe.

PER SERVING:
Net Carbs: 2 grams
Total Carbs: 5 grams
Fiber: 3 grams
Protein: 10 grams
Fat: 14 grams
Calories: 170

Makes: 8 servings (one 9-inch crust)
Active Time: 5 minutes
Total Time: 35 minutes

Variations: Almond Piecrust

Phases 2, 3, 4

Prepare Atkins Basic Piecrust as above, adding 1 teaspoon pure almond extract with the water.

Cinnamon Piecrust

Phases 2, 3, 4

Prepare Atkins Basic Piecrust as above, adding 1 teaspoon cinnamon with the sugar substitute.

Nutty Piecrust

Phases 2, 3, 4

PER SERVING:
Net Carbs: 2 grams
Total Carbs: 4 grams
Fiber: 2 grams
Protein: 3 grams
Fat: 24 grams
Calories: 230

Makes: 8 servings (one 9-inch crust)
Active Time: 10 minutes
Total Time: 25 minutes

This flourless crust is ideal for almost any filling, from Cranberry Fool to Lickety-Split Vanilla Ice Cream. We used pecans, but you could use any nut. Depending on the type of filling used, you may want to add 1 teaspoon cinnamon or another spice to the crust. To save time, make ahead of time and freeze for up to 3 months before filling it.

2 cups pecans, ground (see tip)
4 tablespoons unsalted butter, melted
1 large egg white
2 tablespoons granular sugar substitute
½ teaspoon salt

1. Heat oven to 350°F.
2. Combine ground nuts and melted butter in a small bowl.
3. Beat egg white with granulated sugar substitute and salt in a medium bowl until frothy.
4. With a fork, combine the nut and butter mixture with the egg white mixture. Place in a greased 9-inch pie pan, evenly distributing the mixture on the bottom and the sides of the pan; pat gently but firmly.
5. Bake 15 minutes, until nuts are toasted and crust is set. Allow to cool completely on a wire rack before filling. Or wrap tightly with plastic wrap and freeze up to 3 months before filling.

TIP TIME

DON'T OVERDO IT

The best way to finely grind pecans is to pulse them in a food processor, but be careful not to overprocess them or you'll wind up with pecan butter!

Flaky Piecrust

Phases 3, 4

This all-purpose dough lives up to its name and is great for both sweet dessert pies and tarts and savory ones like quiches. (Omit the sugar substitute for savory dishes.) Using half whole-wheat pastry flour—if your supermarket doesn't have it, try a natural foods store—produces a lighter crust than in Atkins Basic Piecrust (page 235), but it's higher in carbs.

PER SERVING:
Net Carbs: 6 grams
Total Carbs: 8 grams
Fiber: 2 grams
Protein: 5 grams
Fat: 12 grams
Calories: 160

Makes: 8 servings (one 9-inch crust)
Active Time: 5 minutes
Total Time: 35 minutes

½ cup whole-wheat pastry flour
½ cup Atkins Cuisine All Purpose Baking Mix
1 teaspoon granular sugar substitute (optional)
¼ teaspoon salt
½ cup (1 stick) cold unsalted butter, cut into small pieces
3 tablespoons ice water, plus more if needed

1. Pulse flour, baking mix, sugar substitute, and salt in a food processor to incorporate.
2. Add butter and pulse until mixture resembles coarse meal, about 30 seconds. Pulse in water until dough just comes together, about 30 seconds, adding additional tablespoons of water if needed.
3. Transfer dough to a sheet of plastic wrap; form into a disk about 6 inches in diameter. Wrap tightly in plastic; refrigerate until firm, about 30 minutes.
4. Roll and bake as directed in pie recipe. The piecrust can be stored in the refrigerator for up to 3 days or in the freezer for up to 1 month.

Crumbly Piecrust

Phases 3, 4

PER SERVING:
Net Carbs: 5 grams
Total Carbs: 7 grams
Fiber: 2 grams
Protein: 4 grams
Fat: 13 grams
Calories: 160

Makes: 8-servings (one 9-inch piecrust)
Active Time: 20 minutes
Total Time: 1 hour 35 minutes

WEEKEND

Adding almond meal makes this piecrust more crumbly than our other piecrusts. Fill this cookie-like crust with pastry cream or whipped cream and fresh fruit for a quick, fresh dessert.

½ cup whole-wheat flour
¼ cup almond meal (see page 11)
¼ cup Atkins Cuisine All Purpose Baking Mix
⅛ teaspoon salt
1 tablespoon granular sugar substitute
7 tablespoons cold unsalted butter, cut into small pieces
1 large egg, lightly beaten
½ teaspoon almond extract

1. Pulse whole-wheat flour, almond meal, baking mix, salt, and sugar substitute in a food processor to incorporate; add butter and pulse until mixture resembles coarse meal, about 30 seconds. Pulse in egg and extract. Pulse until dough just comes together, about 30 seconds.
2. Transfer dough to a sheet of plastic wrap; form into a disk about 6 inches in diameter. Wrap tightly in plastic; refrigerate until firm, about 30 minutes.
3. Meanwhile, heat oven to 375°F. Roll out dough between two sheets of plastic wrap to a 10-inch disk. Remove top sheet of plastic; invert dough into a 9-inch tart pan with removable bottom. Carefully remove remaining plastic as you press dough into pan; trim any excess.
4. Bake piecrust until lightly browned and set, about 15 minutes. Cool completely before filling.

Variation: Chocolate Piecrust

Phases 3, 4

Prepare Crumbly Piecrust as above, substituting 2 tablespoons cocoa powder for 2 tablespoons of the whole-wheat flour, and add an additional 2 teaspoons granular sugar substitute.

Sweet Cherry Pie

Phases 3, 4

Cinnamon adds a wonderful flavor and aroma to the single crust on this deep-dish-style pie. You can adapt this recipe to many other fruits or fruit combos (see variations that follow). Make the piecrust dough ahead of time to speed this dessert along.

PER SERVING:
Net Carbs: 13 grams
Total Carbs: 32 grams
Fiber: 19 grams
Protein: 13 grams
Fat: 17

Makes: 8 servings (one 9-inch pie)
Active Time: 10 minutes
Total Time: 1 hour, 15 minutes

4 cups fresh or frozen cherries, pitted
1½ teaspoons Dixie Carb Counters Thick-It-Up thickener*
2 tablespoons granular sugar substitute
1 tablespoon butter, cut into cubes
1 Cinnamon Piecrust (page 235)
1 large egg, lightly beaten

1. Combine cherries, thickener, and sugar substitute in a medium bowl; transfer to a 9-inch glass pie plate. Dot top of cherry mixture with butter; set aside.
2. Roll piecrust dough between two sheets of plastic wrap to a 10-inch diameter circle. Remove top sheet of plastic wrap; invert dough onto fruit and carefully remove remaining sheet of plastic wrap. Fold overhanging dough under and pinch or press with the tines of a fork to create a decorative edge; cut a 1-inch slit in the center of the pie. Chill pie until dough is firm, about 30 minutes.
3. About 10 minutes before removing pie from refrigerator, heat oven to 375°F.
4. Brush dough with beaten egg. Bake until crust is golden brown and juices are bubbling, about 35 minutes. Serve warm.

WEEKEND

*Order from www.dixiediner.com.

Variations: Blueberry Pie

Phases 2, 3, 4

Follow recipe for Sweet Cherry Pie as on the preceding page, substituting 4 cups fresh or frozen blueberries for the cherries.

Apple-Strawberry Pie

Phases 3, 4

Follow recipe for Sweet Cherry Pie as on the preceding page, omitting the cherries and replacing with 4 medium Granny Smith apples (peeled, cored, and cut into ½-inch chunks) and 1 cup strawberries, halved. Also add 1 teaspoon freshly grated lemon zest to the fruit mixture.

Apple-Cranberry Pie

Phases 3, 4

Follow recipe for Sweet Cherry Pie as on the preceding page, substituting 4 medium Granny Smith apples (peeled, cored, and cut into ½-inch chunks) and 1 cup fresh or frozen cranberries for the cherries. Also add 2 more tablespoons of sugar substitute and 1 teaspoon freshly grated orange zest to the fruit mixture.

Almond-Plum Tart

Phases 3, 4

Made from butter and almonds, frangipane is a classic base for fruit tarts. This recipe uses a wonderful low-carb version that works very well with a number of seasonal fruits—try it with peaches, nectarines, pears, or sweet cherries. Be sure the butter is at room temperature. Cold butter doesn't combine properly with sugar substitute and other ingredients.

PER SERVING:

Net Carbs: 10 grams
Total Carbs: 14 grams
Fiber: 4 grams
Protein: 8 grams
Fat: 30 grams
Calories: 350

Makes: 8 servings (one 9-inch pie)
Active Time: 30 minutes
Total Time: 2 hours 10 minutes

½ cup (1 stick) unsalted butter, at room temperature
⅓ cup granular sugar substitute
1 large egg
1 cup almond meal (see page 11)
1 tablespoon Atkins Cuisine All Purpose Baking Mix
1 teaspoon pure almond extract
1 Crumbly Piecrust, unbaked (page 238)
4 small plums, pitted and quartered

1. Combine butter and sugar substitute in a medium bowl; beat with an electric mixer on medium-high speed until light and fluffy. Add egg; mix on low speed until just combined. Add almond meal, baking mix, and almond extract; mix on low speed until just until combined. Set aside.
2. Roll out piecrust dough between two sheets of plastic wrap to a 10-inch circle. Remove top sheet of plastic; invert dough into a 9-inch tart pan with a removable bottom. Carefully remove remaining plastic as you press dough into pan; trim excess.
3. Spread almond mixture evenly in crust; refrigerate until filling and crust are firm, about 30 minutes.
4. Heat oven to 350°F.
5. While oven is warming, press plums into filling to cover evenly; bake until filling is lightly brown and plums are tender, about 40 minutes. Let stand for 30 minutes at room temperature before serving.

Pineapple Upside-Down Cake*

Phases 3, 4

PER SERVING:
Net Carbs: 12 grams
Total Carbs: 15 grams
Fiber: 3 grams
Protein: 6 grams
Fat: 17 grams
Calories: 220

Makes: 8 servings
Active Time: 15 minutes
Total Time: 50 minutes

WEEKEND

An old-fashioned favorite, but minus the sugar, white flour, and canned pineapple swimming in corn syrup, this dish will please young and old. Pineapples are tricky to core and tough to peel; look for cored and peeled fruit in the produce department (it may be near the cut-up melon). Serve with whipped cream if desired.

Topping
1 tablespoon unsalted butter
½ medium pineapple, cut into 6 slices

Cake
½ cup whole-wheat flour
¼ cup Atkins Cuisine All Purpose Baking Mix
½ cup almond meal (see page 11)
¾ teaspoon ground cardamom
⅛ teaspoon ground cloves
½ teaspoon ground ginger
½ teaspoon baking powder
½ teaspoon baking soda
¼ teaspoon salt
6 tablespoons unsalted butter, at room temperature
⅓ cup granular sugar substitute
½ teaspoon pure vanilla extract
½ cup sour cream
1 large egg, lightly beaten

1. Heat oven to 350°F. Melt butter in an 8-inch ovenproof cast-iron or nonstick skillet over medium-high heat. Add pineapple slices; cook until golden, about 4 minutes per side. Arrange slices evenly in pan; set aside.
2. Combine whole-wheat flour, baking mix, almond meal, cardamom, cloves, ginger, baking powder, baking soda, and salt in a small bowl.
3. Combine butter, sugar substitute, and vanilla in a large bowl; beat with an electric mixer on medium speed until fluffy. Add sour cream and egg; beat on low speed until just combined, scraping sides of bowl if necessary. Add flour mixture; beat on low speed until just combined.
4. Spread batter evenly over pineapple slices. Bake until a toothpick inserted in center comes out clean, about 25 minutes. (Do not overbake or the cake will dry out.) Loosen edges of cake with knife; invert onto serving plate. Serve warm or room temperature.

*See photo on color page 31

Toasted Pecan Cake

Phases 3, 4

This cake is delicious without frosting, but our variation gilds the lily. Wait until the cake is cool to frost it.

PER SERVING:
Net Carbs: 9 grams
Total Carbs: 12 grams
Fiber: 3 grams
Protein: 5 grams
Fat: 17 grams
Calories: 220

Makes: 8 servings
Active Time: 25 minutes
Total Time: 55 minutes

- Olive oil cooking spray
- ½ cup pecans, toasted and finely ground (see page 236)
- ¾ cup whole-wheat flour
- ¼ cup Atkins Cuisine All Purpose Baking Mix
- ½ teaspoon baking powder
- ½ teaspoon baking soda
- ¼ teaspoon salt
- 6 tablespoons unsalted butter, at room temperature
- ½ cup granular sugar substitute
- 1 teaspoon pure vanilla extract
- 1 large egg
- 1 large egg yolk
- ½ cup sour cream

1. Heat oven to 350°F. Mist an 8-inch round cake pan with cooking spray; set aside.
2. Combine pecans, whole-wheat flour, baking mix, baking powder, baking soda, and salt in a medium bowl.
3. Cream butter, sugar substitute, and vanilla in medium bowl with an electric mixer on medium speed until fluffy. Add egg and yolk; beat until incorporated, scraping down sides of bowl. Add sour cream; beat until incorporated. Add flour mixture; mix on low speed until just combined.
4. Spread batter into pan; bake until a toothpick inserted in center comes out clean, about 20 minutes. Invert cake on a wire rack to cool. Wrap in plastic wrap until ready to serve; transfer to a plate and cut into wedges.

Variation: Toasted Pecan Cake with Maple Frosting

Phases 3, 4

Cream 3 sticks (1½ cups) unsalted butter, ¼ cup sugar-free pancake syrup, 1 teaspoon pure vanilla extract, and a pinch of salt in a medium bowl with an electric mixer on medium speed until fluffy. Spread frosting on the top and sides, using a spatula.

Mini-Muffin-Tin Chocolate Brownies

Phases 2, 3, 4

PER SERVING:
Net Carbs: 2 grams
Total Carbs: 17 grams
Fiber: 2 grams
Sugar Alcohols: 13 grams
Protein: 4 grams
Fat: 17 grams
Calories: 190

Makes: 8 (3 muffin) servings
Active Time: 10 minutes
Total Time: 20 minutes

WEEKDAY

Baking these melt-in-your-mouth brownies in small mini-muffin tins ensures portion control—and means less time in the oven. We used Hershey's sugar-free chocolate bars, but any sugar-free chocolate is fine. Don't worry if the batter doesn't fill the muffin cups; the eggs make the muffins rise.

- 4 tablespoons (½ stick) butter, plus more for muffin tin
- 8½ ounces sugar-free or low-carb dark chocolate
- 3 large eggs
- ⅛ teaspoon salt
- 1 tablespoon Atkins Cuisine All Purpose Baking Mix

1. Heat oven to 375°F. Lightly butter two 12-cup mini-muffin tins; set aside.
2. Melt butter and chocolate in a small heavy-bottomed saucepan over low heat; set aside to cool slightly.
3. Beat eggs and salt in a medium bowl with an electric mixer on high speed. Add baking mix; beat on low speed just to combine. Add cooled chocolate; whisk on low speed to combine.
4. Divide batter among muffin cups (it will not fill them). Bake until tops are puffed and cracked, about 8–10 minutes. Cool in tin for 5 minutes; transfer to a wire rack to cool completely, about 20 minutes. Store in an airtight container for up to 4 days.

Variations: Mini-Muffin-Tin Mocha Brownies

Phases 2, 3, 4

Prepare Mini-Muffin-Tin Chocolate Brownies as above, adding 1 tablespoon instant coffee granules to chocolate-butter mixture.

Mini-Muffin-Tin Mexican Chocolate Brownies

Phases 2, 3, 4

Prepare Mini-Muffin-Tin Chocolate Brownies as above, adding 1 teaspoon cinnamon and ½ teaspoon pure almond extract to chocolate-butter mixture.

Vanilla Meringues

Phases 1, 2, 3, 4

Baking meringues at very low heat keeps them snow-white and maintains their light-as-air texture. If they're browning, turn the temperature down to 175°F. Find parchment paper in the baking aisle.

PER SERVING:
Net Carbs: 1 gram
Total Carbs: 1 gram
Fiber: 0 grams
Protein: 1 gram
Fat: 0 grams
Calories: 10

4 large egg whites
½ cup granular sugar substitute
1 teaspoon pure vanilla extract
¼ teaspoon cream of tartar
⅛ teaspoon salt

Makes: 24 (2-meringue) servings
Active Time: 15 minutes
Total Time: 1 hour 15 minutes

1. Heat oven to 200°F. Line two baking sheets with parchment paper; set aside.
2. Combine egg whites, sugar substitute, vanilla, cream of tartar, and salt in a large bowl; beat with an electric mixer on medium-high speed until medium peaks form. Dollop generous tablespoonfuls of meringue onto baking sheets; bake until dry and crisp, about 1 hour. Cool completely on the baking sheet.
3. Store in an airtight container for up to 5 days.

WEEKEND

TIP TIME

WHEN TO STOP BEATING

Beaten egg whites with soft peaks flop over in a gentle curve when you lift the whisk or eggbeater. Stiff peaks remain upright. Medium peaks are somewhere in the middle.

Variation: Coconut Meringues

Phases 2, 3, 4

Prepare Vanilla Meringues as above, adding 1 teaspoon pure coconut extract and carefully folding in 3 tablespoons toasted unsweetened coconut after the beaten egg whites form medium peaks.

No-Bake Cheesecake with Toasted Nut Crust

Phases 2, 3, 4

PER SERVING:
Net Carbs: 4 grams
Total Carbs: 7 grams
Fiber: 3 grams
Protein: 10 grams
Fat: 44 grams
Calories: 440

This eggless recipe relies on cream cheese, which must be very soft or the mixture will be difficult to whisk smooth. Pop it in the microwave on medium for 2 minutes if you're pressed for time. Or mix the filling in a food processor to remove any lumps. To make this recipe suitable for the first two weeks of Phase 1, omit the crust and simply pour the filling into the pie plate. Torani Sugar Free Vanilla syrup is sold at Shop-Rite, Food Emporium, and other supermarkets. Go to www.torani.com to find a store near you.

Makes: 10 servings
Active Time: 20 minutes
Total Time: 4 hours, 35 minutes

WEEKEND

Crust

Olive oil cooking spray
1¾ cups almonds, hazelnuts, macadamias, or pecans, toasted (see page 247)
5 tablespoons unsalted butter, melted
4 teaspoons granular sugar substitute
¼ teaspoon salt

Filling

⅓ cup plus 2 tablespoons sugar-free vanilla syrup
1 packet powdered unflavored gelatin
1 cup heavy cream
1 teaspoon freshly grated lemon zest
2 (8-ounce) packages cream cheese, very soft
2 tablespoons freshly squeezed lemon juice

1. Mist a 9-inch pie plate with cooking spray.
2. For the crust, pulse nuts in a food processor until finely chopped. Add butter, sugar substitute, and salt; pulse until combined. Transfer mixture to pie plate; spread evenly and press to cover bottom. Refrigerate while preparing filling.
3. For the filling, combine syrup and gelatin in a medium bowl; let stand 5 minutes to allow gelatin to bloom.
4. Meanwhile, combine cream and lemon zest in a small saucepan over high heat; bring just to a boil. Add to gelatin; whisk to dissolve gelatin.

Add cream cheese and lemon juice; whisk or beat with an electric mixer until smooth.

5. Pour filling into crust. Cover with plastic wrap; refrigerate until set, about 4 hours. Slice and serve.

Variations: Almond No-Bake Cheesecake

Phases 2, 3, 4

Prepare No-Bake Cheesecake with Toasted Nut Crust as on the preceding page, using almonds for the crust and substituting 1 teaspoon pure almond extract for the lemon juice.

Blueberry Swirl No-Bake Cheesecake

Phases 2, 3, 4

Prepare No-Bake Cheesecake with Toasted Nut Crust as on the preceding page through Step 4. Divide batter in half. Stir ¾ cup low-carb (no added sugar) blueberry jam into one half, and ½ cup fresh blueberries into the other. Dollop half cupfuls of both batters randomly into pie plate; using a butter knife, gently swirl batter.

TIP TIME

ROAST, DON'T TOAST

Roasting nuts enhances their flavor. Preheat the oven to 350°F. Place the nuts on a shallow baking pan and roast until golden, stirring once. Begin to check them at the 5-minute point, and cook them no longer than 10 minutes. Nuts burn easily, so be vigilant.

Crustless Ginger Cheesecake with Lime–Sour Cream Topping*

Phase 2, 3, 4

PER SERVING:
Net Carbs: 4 grams
Total Carbs: 4 grams
Fiber: 0 grams
Protein: 7 grams
Fat: 24 grams
Calories: 250

Makes: 12 servings
Active Time: 20 minutes
Total Time: 2 hours 45 minutes

Cold temperatures can mute flavors. Let the chilled cheesecake come to room temperature before serving to bring out the most flavor. Baking the cheesecake in a pan of water insulates it and helps to diffuse the heat, so it cooks evenly. If you don't have a springform pan, use a pie plate—it's easier to remove cheesecake from a pan with sloping sides than one with straight sides.

Cheesecake

20 ounces (2½ eight-ounce packages) cream cheese, at room temperature
⅓ cup granular sugar substitute
½ teaspoon pure vanilla extract
1 teaspoon ground ginger
3 large eggs
3 large egg yolks

Topping

1¼ cups sour cream
2 tablespoons granular sugar substitute
2 teaspoons freshly grated lime zest

1. Heat oven to 350°F. Line bottom of a 10-inch springform pan with parchment or wax paper. Wrap outside of pan tightly with aluminum foil.
2. For the cheesecake, combine cream cheese, sugar substitute, vanilla, and ginger in a bowl; beat with an electric mixer on medium speed until fluffy. One at a time, add eggs and egg yolks, beating on low speed until combined. Transfer to springform pan. Set springform pan into a roasting pan; carefully pour in hot water to reach 1 inch up the side of the springform pan. Bake until just set in the center, about 20 minutes.
3. Meanwhile, for the topping: combine sour cream, sugar substitute, and lime zest in a bowl; set aside.

*See photo on color page 32

WEEKEND

4. When cheesecake is just set, spread sour cream mixture evenly on top. Bake 5 minutes longer. Cool on a wire rack for 30 minutes. Cover with plastic wrap; refrigerate at least 1½ hours before serving.

TIP TIME

SAVE THOSE EGG WHITES

If your recipe requires more yolks than whites, store the leftover whites in an airtight container in the refrigerator for up to 4 days or in the freezer for up to 6 months. You can also freeze them in ice cube trays—one egg white per compartment—and then store in a resealable freezer bag or container. Remove them the day before you'll use them and thaw overnight in the fridge.

Cardamom Butter Cookies

Phases 2, 3, 4

PER SERVING:
Net Carbs: 3 grams
Total Carbs: 6 grams
Fiber: 3 grams
Protein: 9 grams
Fat: 14 grams
Calories: 180

Makes: 12 (2-cookie) servings
Active Time: 10 minutes
Total Time: 22 minutes

WEEKDAY

Keep these treats on hand for coffee breaks or after-school snacks. Cardamom is used in many Scandinavian desserts.

- 1½ cups Atkins Cuisine All Purpose Baking Mix
- ½ cup almond meal (see page 11)
- ¼ teaspoon baking powder
- ½ teaspoon salt
- 10 tablespoons (1¼ sticks) unsalted butter, at room temperature
- ½ cup granular sugar substitute
- 1 large egg
- 1 tablespoon water
- 2 teaspoons pure vanilla extract
- ¾ teaspoon ground cardamom

1. Heat oven to 350°F. Line 2 baking sheets with parchment paper; set aside.
2. Combine baking mix, almond meal, baking powder, and salt in a medium bowl. Combine butter and sugar substitute in a large bowl; cream with an electric mixer on high speed until light and fluffy. Add egg, water, vanilla, and cardamom; beat on medium speed until combined, scraping down sides of bowl as necessary (mixture may look watery). Add flour mixture; mix on low speed until dough comes together.
3. Divide dough in half, and then in half again. Make 6 equal balls from each quarter portion of dough. Place 12 balls on each baking sheet. Press each gently with the tines of a fork in a crisscross pattern; bake until lightly browned on the edges, about 10 minutes. Transfer cookies to a wire rack to cool completely. Store in an airtight container for up to 1 week.

Variation: Lemon Butter Cookies

Phases 2, 3, 4

Follow the recipe above for Cardamom Butter Cookies, substituting 2 teaspoons freshly grated lemon zest for the ground cardamom.

Chocolate Truffles

Phases 1, 2, 3, 4

These rich little mouthfuls make a perfect hostess gift, particularly set in mini cupcake liners in a gift box. In addition to the Pistachio-Chocolate Truffles and Peppermint-Chocolate Truffles variations on the following page, you can roll the truffles in other finely chopped nuts or in toasted shredded coconut. We used Hershey's sugar-free chocolate, but there are many other brands of low-carb chocolate available.

PER SERVING:
Net Carbs: 2 grams
Total Carbs: 12 grams
Fiber: 2 grams
Sugar Alcohols: 8 grams
Protein: 1 gram
Fat: 10 grams
Calories: 110

Makes: 6 (2-truffle) servings
Active Time: 10 minutes
Total Time: 1 hour 20 minutes

4 ounces low-carb or sugar-free milk or dark chocolate, finely chopped
2 tablespoons heavy cream
1 tablespoon unsalted butter, at room temperature
1 tablespoon brandy or pure vanilla extract
1 tablespoon unsweetened cocoa powder

1. Place chocolate in a small microwavable bowl; set aside. Place cream and butter in another small microwavable bowl; set aside.
2. Microwave chocolate for 30 seconds on medium; repeat for another 30 seconds. Microwave the bowl of chocolate a third time, along with the bowl of cream and butter, for another 30 seconds. Remove and pour the hot cream and butter mixture over the partially melted chocolate; let sit 1 minute. Stir to completely melt the chocolate and smooth the mixture. Add brandy or vanilla and thoroughly mix. If the chocolate isn't completely melted, return to the microwave for an additional 20 seconds.
3. Place the bowl in the refrigerator, covered with plastic wrap, for about 1 hour or until firm.
4. Sift cocoa onto a plate. Working quickly to avoid melting, form 12 equal-size balls of the chocolate mixture with your fingers, immediately rolling each in cocoa to coat evenly. Set on a serving plate. Serve right away or refrigerate in an airtight container for up to 5 days.

Variations: Pistachio-Chocolate Truffles*

Phases 2, 3, 4

Follow the recipe on the preceding page for Chocolate Truffles, but omit brandy and replace with pure vanilla extract; instead of cocoa, roll truffles in ¼ cup finely chopped pistachios.

Peppermint-Chocolate Truffles

Phases 2, 3, 4

Follow the recipe on the preceding page for Chocolate Truffles, but omit brandy and replace with pure vanilla or peppermint extract; instead of cocoa, roll truffles in ¼ cup crushed sugar-free striped peppermint hard candies.

WEEKEND

*See photo on color page 30

GLOSSARY

Not sure about the difference between barbecue and grill? Or between chopping and mincing? Don't know a batter from a dough? If you're unfamiliar with any of the terms in the recipes, check them out on this list:

Bake. The generic term for cooking foods in an oven, usually at a moderate temperature (around 350°F). Because the heat comes from all sides, baked foods don't usually need to be turned over. Baking is usually done in an open pan; otherwise, trapped moisture would steam the food, although dishes that might dry out or become too brown before they cook through might be covered for all or part of the baking time.

Baking pan. A low (usually 2- to 3-inch-deep) aluminum or other metal pan for baking or roasting that comes in an extensive range of sizes. The term can also include specialty pans such as muffin tins, cake pans, pie pans, and loaf pans. Nonstick pans are useful, but cooking spray or oil also keeps foods from sticking.

Baking dish. A low pan made from tempered glass (Pyrex) or ceramic (but not metal). Baking dishes come in many shapes and sizes. We most often use 8-inch square and 9-by-13-inch ones.

Baking sheet (or tin). A flat pan measuring about 10 by 15 inches with a lip on one short side. Lining it with aluminum foil or parchment paper simplifies cleanup.

Barbecue. Not to be confused with grill, barbecue is neither a verb nor an appliance. Barbecue is pork, beef, chicken, or other meat that's seasoned with a rub, cooked over low heat, and sometimes served with a sauce. (The appliance is a grill, as is the cooking method.)

Batter. A somewhat thin mixture of flour (or a flour substitute), eggs, milk, and flavorings that can be spooned or poured before cooking. Batters can be used to coat foods before frying (as in tempura) or used to make cakes, pancakes, waffles, and the like.

Beat. To combine two or more foods at high speed, usually in a circular movement.

Blanch. To briefly plunge vegetables (or fruits) into boiling water (sometimes only a few seconds) and then into ice water to stop the cooking. Blanching helps to set the color, soften the texture, or loosen skins on tomatoes or fruit such as peaches. Blanching may also used to make foods palatable and brighter—such as broccoli for crudités.

Blind-bake. To cook a piecrust before filling it with a custard or other filling. The crust is usually pricked with a fork to allow steam to escape, and is often covered with foil and weighted with pie weights or dried beans, which are removed before the filling is added.

Boil. To submerge in vigorously bubbling (212°F at sea level) water or another liquid. Most vegetable recipes instruct you to bring the liquid to a boil and then reduce the heat so that it simmers. If you use a marinade as a sauce, it must be cooked at a rolling boil for at least 3 minutes—start timing when the boil begins, not when you put it on the stove—to kill any pathogens.

Braise. To slow cook in a small amount of liquid and sometimes with vegetables in a covered dish. Tougher cuts, such as beef brisket, become tender when they're braised, and are often referred to as pot roasts. Braised dishes usually involve larger cuts on the bone, in contrast to stews.

Broil. To cook fairly flat and tender cuts such as steaks and chops directly under a heating element at high heat and close range. This sears the surface quickly, browning the exterior and sealing in juices. Most foods need to be turned over to brown on both sides, although fish fillets are so thin that they cook through before they brown. Sliced zucchini, eggplant, bell peppers, asparagus, and other vegetables can also be broiled.

Brown. To cook food until the surface is browned. Ground meat and sausage will have no pink remaining and other foods may develop a brown crust.

Chiffonade. To cut leaves into very thin ribbons. The easiest way to accomplish this is to stack a few leaves, roll them into a cylinder, and then cut across it at ⅛-inch intervals.

Chop. To cut food into small pieces; the size may be specified, but the shape doesn't usually matter.

Combine. To mix two or more foods until they become a unified mixture.

Cream. To combine two or more ingredients, typically butter and sugar substitute, until they become smooth and creamy.

Deep-fat thermometer. A thermometer that registers much higher temperatures than instant-read ones; used to ascertain the temperature of the oil.

Deep-fry. To quickly cook small pieces of food submerged in a deep pan in fat heated to a temperature of roughly 365°F—the exact temperature depends upon the food. As long as the fat is at the proper temperature, the exterior of the food seals upon contact, becoming crisp, and the interior stays moist. The cooking fat is discarded after use. When deep-frying broccoli, zucchini, okra, mushrooms, or cauliflower, the food must be very dry. Wet or high-moisture foods will spatter violently when they hit the hot fat unless breaded or coated in batter.

Dice. To cut food into ⅛–¼-inch cubes.

Double boiler. A saucepan with an insert that allows you to melt chocolate or make custards at very low temperature. You can fashion a double boiler out of a saucepan and metal bowl.

Dough. A stiff mixture of flour and liquid like eggs or milk and flavorings. Dough is much thicker than batter and cannot be poured.

Drain. To pour off liquid from a food. The liquid is usually discarded and only the food used.

Dredge. To coat food before cooking, usually with crumbs, flour, or meal (as opposed to a

batter). The coating protects food from cooking too quickly and adds flavor and crunch.
Drippings. Fat and juices that collect when meat or poultry is roasted. Drippings are used to make pan sauces and gravy.
Dutch oven. See page 15.

Emulsion. A mixture in which any water-based liquid is suspended in a fat.

Fold. To combine a light or delicate substance with a heavier, denser one. The lighter mixture (such as beaten egg whites or whipped cream) is always spooned over the heavier mixture so it isn't crushed. Use a rubber or silicone spatula to combine the two, scooping the heavier mixture from the bottom and allowing it to gently fall over the lighter one.
Fork-tender. A degree of doneness: a fork stuck into the food (usually a meat) can pierce it easily. If you try to lift the food, it falls off the fork.

Grill. Similar to broiling, but the direct source of heat, whether hot coals or a heating element, is below rather than above the food. The fuel used to fire the grill can add flavor. Grilling is often done on a grate that gives foods appealing crosshatch marks. You can also grill on the cook top on special ridged pans.

Instant-read thermometer. A thermometer with a very thin shaft (so it won't allow much juice to escape) that's inserted at the end of cooking meat, poultry, or fish. (For more, see page 13.)

Jelly roll pan. Similar to a baking sheet, with a ¾-to-1-inch rim on all four sides, which catches spills and drips. Lining it with aluminum foil or parchment paper simplifies cleanup.
Julienne. To cut food into matchstick-size pieces. Simply slice the food ¼ inch thick, and then lay each slice on its side and cut into ¼-inch thick strips. Or use a mandoline.

Loaf pan. These are made of glass, aluminum, or steel and usually come in 4-by-8-inch or 5-by-9-inch sizes; the larger size is more versatile. They're ideal for making bread and meatloaves, but you can also make either on a jelly roll pan or in another baking dish.

Mandoline. Not be confused with the stringed instrument, which is spelled differently. A hand-operated tool with a variety of adjustable blades for cutting firm vegetables or fruit into slices of even thickness and for julienne and other configurations.
Mince. To cut food into minuscule pieces. Like chopping, the shape isn't usually important.
Muffin tin. Metal or Silpat (made from a form of silicone) tins come in an array of sizes and configurations, from mini to jumbo, as well as those just for making muffin tops. Those with cups that are about 2¼ inches across are most versatile. Nonstick tins make it easy to remove muffins.

Nonreactive. Referring to cookware or dishes made from a material that won't cause a chemical reaction with acidic ingredients, such as tomatoes, vinegar, yogurt, buttermilk, or citrus fruits. Nonreactive materials include well-seasoned cast iron, enamel-coated cast iron, most anodized aluminum, lined copper pots, stainless steel, glass, ceramic and pottery, and plastic.

Pan-fry. To cook food in hot fat over moderate to high heat. Unlike deep-frying, which covers the food completely, the fat is only about ½ inch deep. It is discarded after cooking, unlike sautéing.

Pan-sear. This cooking method involves a hot pan, hot fat, and food of uniform size, but no stirring. The food is cooked on one side, and then the other. The surface of the food sears upon contact so it doesn't stick to the pan. Burgers, cube (minute) steaks, and chops also take well to pan-searing..

Parboil. To partially cook food by boiling it briefly in water, so it can be added to other quick-cooking foods later in a recipe. This prevents the faster cooking foods from being overcooked and ensures all ingredients will be done at the same time. (Also see Blanch.)

Parchment paper. A heavy grease- and moisture-resistant paper that can be used to tightly wrap and cook fish, chicken, vegetables, and other foods in the oven or to line baking pans. Most supermarkets sell parchment paper. Look for it near the foil and waxed paper or in the baking aisle.

Pie plate. A round, slope-sided dish made of aluminum, glass, or ceramic, usually 9 or 10 inches in diameter; our recipes call for 9-inch ones. Pie plates often have scalloped rims to make shaping the edging of the pie a bit easier.

Poach. To cook delicate foods such as eggs or chicken breasts in liquid that's at more than a simmer, but not quite at a boil.

Purée. To turn foods (usually solids) into a smooth, thick consistency, using either a blender or a food processor. You can also press the food through a sieve or strainer.

Reduce. To cook so that liquid evaporates, thickening the mixture, which is called a reduction.

Roast. To cook in an (usually) uncovered pan in the oven at 350°F (for large, well marbled cuts of meat or poultry) to 425°F (for vegetables and smaller cuts such as pork tenderloin). The (usually) shallow pan should be big enough for air to circulate around the food (if it's too small the food may steam), but not so big that any drippings evaporate or burn. Meat, poultry, or fish is elevated on a rack or layer of vegetables so the roast doesn't stew in its juices. Roasting isn't suitable for tough cuts of meat, which only become tougher.

Rolling boil. A vigorous boil that doesn't dissipate when stirred. (See Boil.)

Saucepan. See page 15.

Sauté. To cook small, uniformly sized pieces in hot fat in a hot pan, while stirring frequently, to quickly sear the surface of the food so it doesn't stick to the pan. The stirring helps to minimize browning. Meat and poultry should be patted dry, and vegetables should be added carefully, as moisture causes the hot fat to spatter. You can sauté foods in just about any pan, but you'll find it easier to stir if your pan has 2- to 3-inch sloping sides. Unlike in frying, the fat is consumed as part of the dish.

Sear. To cook food (usually cuts of meat, poultry, or fish) in a skillet over fairly high heat to brown it and seal in the juices. Frequent movement inhibits browning, so it's best to turn food only once. Although broiling and grilling can sear foods, we use the term to describing pan-searing, which is done in a skillet with a small amount of fat.

Sift. To shake fine-textured foods such as flour, baking powder, or spices through a fine-mesh sieve or a special sifter. This increases the food's volume by incorporating air.
Simmer. A slow, gentle cooking method that keeps food tender and allows flavors to blend. The liquid is heated just until small bubbles begin to break the surface (185°F at sea level).
Springform pan. A high, round metal pan with a clamp that loosens so the sides of the pan can be separated from the bottom. Springform pans are ideal for cheesecake.
Steam. To cook above, not in, simmering liquid in a covered pan. The vapor cooks the food, which is elevated in a collapsible, perforated steamer basket. Tiered bamboo Chinese steamers operate on the same principle. You can also fashion a steamer from a plate set on top of a tuna fish can with the top and bottom removed. Almost any vegetable can be steamed; it's also a great way to cook fish.
Stew. To cook together several foods in a small amount of simmering liquid in a covered saucepan so the juices condense on the lid and fall back over the food, keeping it moist and flavorful. In addition to meat-, poultry-, and fish-based stews, leeks, celery, cabbage, collards, fennel, tomatoes, and summer squash take well to stewing. Stewing is similar to braising—it tenderizes tough foods—but stewed foods aren't always browned before the liquid is added, and are usually cut into small pieces.
Stir-fry. To cook bite-size pieces of food in oil a wok or skillet while stirring constantly. This method relies on two principles: the hotter the fat is, the less likely food is to stick to the pan, and the more you stir the food, the less likely it is to stick. (The pan and oil are typically much hotter than in sautéing.) Stir-frying is extremely fast, so you need to cut foods into small pieces of uniform size. Denser foods (such as meat or broccoli stems) should be added before less dense foods (such as bell peppers or snow peas). And because you should stir constantly, all the foods, including any sauce ingredients, should be measured and ready to go before you put pan to heat.
Strain. To pour off liquid from a food. Unlike draining, when you strain, the liquid is reserved and the food is usually discarded.

Temper. To stabilize eggs by mixing in a small amount of hot liquid before cooking them. This increases their temperature gradually so they remain tender and smooth; if heated too quickly, eggs will curdle or scramble.

Water bath. A method of cooking delicate mixtures, such as cheesecake batters or custards. The pan with the batter is set into a larger pan, which is filled with water, before the entire setup is transferred to the oven. The water diffuses the heat so the batter cooks very gently.
Whip. To beat ingredients so that air is incorporated into them, making them fluffy. Egg whites and heavy cream are most often whipped.
Wok. This utensil is designed to sit in, not on, a heat source, so unless you have a specially configured stove they are not the best choice, even for stir-frying. On most stoves only the bottom of the pan gets heated; the sloping sides remain too cool. Unless you have a special wok element, a large skillet will often give you better results.

ACKNOWLEDGMENTS

All cookbooks, but especially illustrated cookbooks such as this one, require a team effort. I was fortunate that Olivia Bell Buehl, of Editorial Strategies, headed up the team that developed *The New Atkins for a New You Cookbook*. In that role, she coordinated recipe developers, recipe testers, and nutritionists who made sure the recipes fit the Atkins guidelines (a process that can involve several iterations), edited the recipes, and worked closely with me on the accompanying text. Christine Senft Callahan and Martha Schueneman also provided valuable editorial assistance. Olivia also worked closely with photographer Mark Ferri, who created the beautiful images, assisted by Brian Smith; food stylist A. J. Battifarano, assisted by Christine Langfeld, who prepared the food and then made it look mouthwatering for photography; and prop stylist Francine Matalon-Degni, who enlivened the table settings, always finding the perfect plate, serving dish, or napkin.

Without a team of other talented freelancers, this book would not have been possible. My thanks to the team of recipe developers who patiently followed my long list of instructions about which ingredients were acceptable and which were not, and then made luscious sweet and savory dishes that prove that there's no need to compromise taste for healthful meals on Atkins. Thank you, Annie Bailey, Peter Berley, David Bonam, Mindy Fox, Robin Kline, Kelly Kochendorfer, Paul Picciuto, Sarah Reynolds, Wendy Sidewater, Alice Thompson, Fred Thompson, and Alison Tozzi. Amanda Dorato and Nancy Hughes tested all the recipes in their own kitchens to duplicate the results you can expect. Recipe developer Jennifer Knollenberg also tested many of the recipes by other developers, and ran some of the nutritionals, as did dietician Kelly Beneduce.

Thanks also to Monty Sharma, Scott Parker, and Chip Bellamy of Atkins Nutritionals, who green-lighted this follow-up to *The New Atkins for a New You*—and understood that the Atkins Diet is always about the food! Lindsay Ostenson and Lisa Wells played valuable roles in coordinating the project in house. Joy Tutela of the David Black Literary Agency provided valuable insights.

Finally, I'd like to thank another team: the editorial, graphic, and production team at Touchstone. Thanks to Michelle Howry, Stacy Creamer, David Falk, Sally Kim, Allegra Ben-Amotz, Marcia Burch, Jessica Roth, Josh Karpf, Cherlynne Li, Ruth Lee-Mui, Kevin McCahill, and Marcella Berger.

RECIPE PHASE CHART

	Phase 1	Phase 2	Phases 3 & 4	Weekday	Weekend	Comments
Breakfast and Brunch Dishes						
French Toast		X	X	X		
Baked French Toast		X	X	X		
Spicy Pecan Pancakes		X	X		X	
Ginger-Spice Muffins		*	X	X		*Omit whole-wheat flour for Phase 2
Lemon–Poppy Seed Bread		*	X		X	*Omit whole-wheat flour for Phase 2
Cheddar-Dill Scones		*	X	X		*Omit whole-wheat flour for Phase 2
Whole-Wheat Currant Scones			X	X		
Peanut-Strawberry Breakfast Bars			X		X	
Crunchy Tropical Berry and Almond Breakfast Parfait		X	X	X		
Atkins Basic Muesli			X	X		
Cinnamon Granola			X		X	
Coconut-Orange Granola			X		X	
Hot Wheat Cereal with Cherry-Walnut Butter			X		X	
Hot Wheat Cereal with Cherry-Almond Butter			X		X	
Western Omelet	X	X	X	X		
Steak and Scrambled Eggs	X	X	X		X	
Sausage and Bell Pepper Frittata	X	X	X	X		
Frittata Lorraine	X	X	X	X		
Turkey-Cauliflower Hash	X	X	X	X		
Ricotta with Melon and Pistachios		X	X	X		
Strawberry-Vanilla Protein Shake		X	X	X		
Mocha Smoothie		X	X	X		
Snacks, Appetizers, and Hors d'Oeuvres						
Sun-Dried Tomato Dip	X	X	X	X		
Sun-Dried Tomato Dip with Walnuts	*	X	X	X		*After 2 weeks in Phase 1
Speedy Spinach Dip	X	X	X	X		
Curried Spinach Dip	X	X	X	X		
Olive Tapenade	X	X	X	X		

	Phase 1	Phase 2	Phases 3 & 4	Weekday	Weekend	Comments
Classic Tapenade	X	X	X	X		
Baba Ghanoush		X	X		X	
Roasted Garlic Hummus		X	X		X	
Avocado Hummus		X	X	X		
Spicy Black Bean Dip		X	X	X		
Creamy Black Bean Dip		X	X	X		
Garlicky White Bean Dip		X	X	X		
Zucchini Crisps	X	X	X	X		
Chili-Cheese Crisps		X	X		X	
Italian Cheese Crisps		X	X		X	
Cheese-Stuffed Cherry Tomatoes	X	X	X	X		
Smoky Cheese Log	X	X	X		X	
Nut-Rolled Salmon-Cheese Ball	*	X	X		X	*After 2 weeks in Phase 1
Lime-Chili Grilled Wings	X	X	X		X	
Summer Rolls		*	X		X	*Adaptable to Phase 2
Shrimp Satay with Nuoc Cham	*	X	X		X	*Smaller portion in Phase 1
Mild Mushroom-Lentil Pâté			X	X		
Roasted Spiced Pecans	*	X	X	X		*After 2 weeks in Phase 1
Tamari-Roasted Pecans	*	X	X	X		*After 2 weeks in Phase 1
Sweet and Salty Almonds	*	X	X	X		*After 2 weeks in Phase 1
Sandwiches, Wraps, Fillings, and Pizza						
Grown-Up Grilled Cheese		X	X	X		
Grilled Cheese with Tomato		X	X	X		
Grilled Cheese with Ham		X	X	X		
Tuna Melt		X	X	X		
Atkins Hamburger Buns			X		X	
Open-Faced Fried Catfish Sandwiches with Spicy Mayonnaise		X	X	X		
Sloppy Joes			X		X	
Chicken Teriyaki Burgers	X	X	X	X		
Lamb Gyros	*	X	X	X		*Adaptable to Phase 1
Portobello Burgers with Blue Cheese Sauce (without bun)		X	X		X	
Portobello Burgers with Blue Cheese Sauce (with bun)			X		X	
Chicken Caesar Wraps	*	X	X	X		*Adaptable to Phase 1
Chicken-Pesto Salad	*	X	X	X		*After 2 weeks in Phase 1
Deviled Ham Salad	X	X	X	X		
Cheddar-Deviled Ham Salad	X	X	X	X		
Curried Egg Salad	X	X	X	X		

	Phase 1	Phase 2	Phases 3 & 4	Weekday	Weekend	Comments
Spicy Shrimp-Egg Salad	X	X	X	X		
Tofu “Egg” Salad	X	X	X	X		
Spicy Tofu “Egg” Salad	X	X	X	X		
Mediterranean-Style Tuna Salad	X	X	X	X		
Smoked Whitefish Salad	X	X	X	X		
Mozzarella, Kalamata, and Tomato Panini		X	X	X		
Smoked Mozzarella, Kalamata, and Prosciutto Panini		X	X	X		
Sautéed Onion, Black Olive, and Goat Cheese Pizza		*	X		X	*Adaptable to Phase 2
Zucchini and Roasted Red Pepper Pizza		*	X		X	*Adaptable to Phase 2
Salads and Dressings						
Athenian Salad	*	X	X	X		*Adaptable to Phase 1
Caprese Salad	X	X	X	X		
Mexican Avocado Salad	X	X	X		X	
Endive and Almond Salad	*	X	X	X		*After 2 weeks in Phase 1
Endive and Avocado Salad	*	X	X	X		*After 2 weeks in Phase 1
Shaved Fennel Salad with Lemon Dressing	*	X	X		X	*Half portion in Phase 1
Fennel-Mushroom Salad with Parmesan		X	X		X	*Half portion in Phase 1
Cucumber-Dill Salad	*	X	X		X	*Smaller portion in Phase 1
Creamy Cucumber Salad	*	X	X		X	*Smaller portion in Phase 1
Tomato and Red Onion Salad	X	X	X	X		
Tomato Salad with Cucumbers and Olives	X	X	X	X		
Mushrooms and Greens with Sherry Vinaigrette	*	X	X	X		*Half portion in Phase 1
Mushrooms and Greens with Bacon and Eggs	X	X	X	X		
Orange and Goat Cheese Salad			X	X		
Orange and Avocado Salad with Mint			X	X		
Slaw with Vinegar Dressing	X	X	X		X	
Lemony Slaw with Capers	X	X	X		X	
Broccoli and Jicama Slaw		*	X		X	*Smaller portion in Phase 2
Tabbouleh Salad			X	X		
Green Tabbouleh Salad			X	X		
Curried Quinoa with Snow Peas			X	X		
Wheat Berries with Sun-Dried Tomatoes and Feta			X		X	
Wheat Berries with Olives and Feta			X		X	
Creamy Potato and Cauliflower Salad			X		X	
Curried Potato and Cauliflower Salad			X		X	
Brown Rice Salad with Toasted Almonds			X		X	
Garlicky Spinach and Feta Salad in Tomato Halves	*	X	X	X		*Adaptable to Phase 1

	Phase 1	Phase 2	Phases 3 & 4	Weekday	Weekend	Comments
Mung Bean Sprout, Mint, and Basil Salad	*	X	X	X		*Smaller portion in Phase 1
New York Strip Steak Salad	X	X	X	X		
Chopped Salad with Bacon and Blue Cheese		X	X	X		
Vegetables and Other Sides						
Roasted Asparagus and Red Peppers with Dijon and Thyme	*	X	X	X		*Smaller portion in Phase 1
Sautéed Greens with Pecans	*	X	X	X		*After 2 weeks in Phase 1
Sautéed Greens with Balsamic Vinaigrette	X	X	X	X		
Stir-Fried Broccolini with Cashews	*	X	X	X		*Half portion after 2 weeks in Phase 1
Roasted Lemon-Garlic Brussels Sprouts		X	X	X		
Sautéed Baby Boy Choy with Garlic and Lemon Zest	X	X	X	X		
Kale with Sweet-and-Sour Vinaigrette		X	X	X		
Creamy Red Cabbage with Dill		*	X	X		*Smaller portion in Phase 2
Sautéed Escarole, Cannellini Beans, and Tomatoes		X	X	X		
Swiss Chard with Pine Nuts	*	X	X	X		*After 2 weeks in Phase 1
Swiss Chard with Pine Nuts and Golden Raisins			X	X		
Braised Lettuce	X	X	X	X		
Braised Lettuce with Peas			X	X		
Green Beans with Lemon and Cumin	X	X	X	X		
Roasted Cauliflower		X	X		X	
Spicy Roasted Cauliflower		X	X		X	
Cauliflower-Garlic Purée		X	X	X		
Spaghetti Squash with Cinnamon-Spice Butter		X	X		X	
Spaghetti Squash with Garlic-Herb-Cheese Butter		X	X		X	
Sautéed Sugar Snap Peas with Mint	*	X	X	X		*Smaller portion in Phase 1
Summer Snap Pea Medley			X	X		
Sautéed Sugar Snap Peas with Bacon	*	X	X	X		*Smaller portion in Phase 1
Edamame Succotash			X	X		
Butternut Squash Purée			X		X	
Lime-Cumin Butternut Squash Purée			X		X	
Sweet Potato Pancakes			X	X		
Orange-Spiced Sweet Potato Pancakes			X	X		
Maple-Citrus Glazed Carrots			X	X		
Roasted Root Vegetables			X		X	
Curried Root Vegetables			X		X	
Mushroom-Barley Pilaf			X		X	
Sausage, Fennel, and Leek Wild Rice Pilaf			X		X	

	Phase 1	Phase 2	Phases 3 & 4	Weekday	Weekend	Comments
Soups and Stews						
Chicken Chowder	X	X	X	X		
Chicken-Corn Chowder			X	X		
Pork and Bok Choy Soba Soup			X	X		
Vegetarian Ginger-Tofu Soba Soup			X	X		
Thai Coconut-Shrimp Soup	X	X	X	X		
Thai Coconut-Vegetable Soup	X	X	X	X		
Chinese Hot-and-Sour Soup	X	X	X	X		
Creamy Cheddar Cheese Soup	X	X	X	X		
Jalapeño-Cheddar Soup	X	X	X	X		
Versatile Vegetable Soup	*	X	X	X		*Adaptable to Phase 1
Creamy Wild Mushroom Soup		X	X	X		
Cream of Broccoli Soup	X	X	X	X		
Tomato Bisque		*	X		X	*Smaller portion in Phase 2
Cold Roasted Tomato Soup		X	X		X	
Classic Chili con Carne		X	X		X	
Hungarian Goulash	X	X	X		X	
Green Chile Pork Stew	X	X	X		X	
Sea Scallops Étouffée	*	X	X		X	*Smaller portion in Phase 1
Gulf Oyster Stew		X	X		X	
Chicken and Turkey Entrées						
Beer-Can Grilled Chicken	X	X	X		X	
Tarragon Braised Chicken	X	X	X		X	
Chicken Paprikash	X	X	X		X	
Poached Chicken Breasts in Mornay Sauce	X	X	X	X		
Mushroom-Herb-Stuffed Chicken Breasts	X	X	X		X	
Jerk Chicken	X	X	X		X	
Chicken Cutlets Milanese		X	X	X		
Chicken Cutlets with Lemon-Caper Sauce		X	X	X		
Chicken Cutlets Parmesan		X	X	X		
Green Goddess Grilled Chicken	X	X	X		X	
Classic Chicken Fricassee	X	X	X		X	
Lemon-and-Basil Chicken-Veggie Kebabs	X	X	X		X	
Thai Chicken Curry	X	X	X	X		
Chicken and Apple Sausage Patties			X	X		
Grilled Turkey Cutlets with Thyme	X	X	X	X		
Pan-Seared Turkey Cutlets	X	X	X	X		
Mexican-Style Turkey Meatloaf	*	X	X		X	*After 2 weeks in Phase 1

	Phase 1	Phase 2	Phases 3 & 4	Weekday	Weekend	Comments
Beef, Pork, Lamb, and Veal Entrées						
Florentine-Style Porterhouse Steak	X	X	X	X		
Skirt Steak with Chimichurri Sauce	X	X	X	X		
Bistro Flank Steak	X	X	X		X	
Mushroom-Smothered Minute Steak	X	X	X	X		
Chicken-Fried Steak		X	X	X		
Chicken-Fried Steak with Cream Sauce		X	X	X		
Beef and Asian Vegetable Stir-Fry		X	X		X	
Greek Meatballs	*	X	X	X		*After 2 weeks in Phase 1
Sautéed Cocktail Meatballs	*	X	X	X		*After 2 weeks in Phase 1
Roasted Pork Tenderloin with Maple-Mustard Sauce	X	X	X		X	
Cheese-Stuffed Pork Roast	*	X	X		X	*After 2 weeks in Phase 1
Sausage-Stuffed Pork Roast	X	X	X		X	
Sweet-and-Sour Pork Chops with Cabbage	*	*	X	X		*Adaptable to Phases 1 and 2
Sweet-and-Sour Bratwurst with Cabbage	*	*	X	X		*Adaptable to Phases 1 and 2
Peppery-Spicy Baby Back Ribs	X	X	X		X	
Chinese Sweet-and-Sour Pork			X	X		
Slow-Cooked Pork Shoulder	X	X	X		X	
Sautéed Italian Sausage with Fennel	X	X	X	X		
Mustard-Bourbon Glazed Ham			X		X	
Lamb, Zucchini, Mushroom, and Tomato Kebabs	*	X	X		X	*Adaptable to Phase 1
Roast Rack of Lamb with Mustard-Nut Crust	*	X	X		X	*After 2 weeks in Phase 1
Yogurt-Marinated Butterflied Leg of Lamb	*	X	X		X	*Adaptable to Phase 1
Butterflied Leg of Lamb with Moroccan Herb Paste	X	X	X		X	
Veal Provençal	*	X	X	X		*Adaptable to Phase 1
Veal Marsala	X	X	X	X		
Fontina-and-Prosciutto-Stuffed Veal Chops	X	X	X	X		
Fish and Shellfish Entrées						
Batter-Fried Haddock		X	X		X	
Batter-Fried Shrimp		X	X		X	
Almond-Crusted Catfish Fingers	*	X	X	X		*After 2 weeks in Phase 1
Herbed Flounder en Papillote	X	X	X	X		
Flounder en Papillote with Vegetables		X	X	X		
Sole Meunière		X	X	X		
Salt-Crusted Whole Snapper with Lemon and Basil	X	X	X		X	
Baked Bluefish with Garlic and Lime	X	X	X	X		
Southwestern Bluefish with Garlic and Lime	X	X	X	X		
Roasted Ginger-Tamari Salmon Steaks			X		X	

	Phase 1	Phase 2	Phases 3 & 4	Weekday	Weekend	Comments
Roasted Salmon Steaks with Spicy Ginger-Tamari Sauce			X		X	
Poached Salmon with Eggs, Onions, and Capers	X	X	X		X	
Baked Salmon with Mustard-Nut Crust	*	X	X	X		*After 2 weeks in Phase 1
Sautéed Salmon Cakes	*	X	X	X		*After 2 weeks in Phase 1
Swordfish Kebabs with Scallions	X	X	X		X	
Mediterranean-Style Grilled Swordfish Steaks	X	X	X		X	
Pecan-Crusted Trout with Orange-Sage Butter	*	X	X		X	*After 2 weeks in Phase 1
Maryland Steamed Crabs	X	X	X	X		
Sautéed Soft-Shell Crabs		X	X	X		
Shrimp Diablo	X	X	X	X		
Peel-and-Eat Shrimp	X	X	X	X		
Vietnamese Grilled Calamari Salad		X	X	X		
Vegetarian Entrées						
Scrambled Tofu Burritos		X	X	X		
Lemon-Rosemary Baked Tofu with Mushroom Sauce		X	X	X		
Le Grand Aïoli		*	X	X		*Smaller portion in Phase 2
Tofu in White Wine with Mustard and Dill	*	X	X		X	*Slightly smaller portion in Phase 1
Tempeh-Roasted Cauliflower and Peppers with Curried Cashew Sauce			X		X	
Tempeh and Vegetables in Spicy Coconut-Lemon Broth			X		X	
Tomato and Leek Gratin with Gruyère and Walnuts		*	X		X	*Slightly smaller portion in Phase 2
Spinach-Mushroom Quiche		X	X		X	
Artichoke, Roasted Pepper, and Goat Cheese Frittata	*	X	X		X	*Slightly smaller portion in Phase 1
Mustardy Mac 'n' Cheese			X	X		
Protein-Powered Eggplant Parmesan			X		X	
Tofu Pad Thai			X	X		
Vegetable Curry with Seared Noodles			X		X	
Seitan Shepherd's Pie with Tofu Topping			X		X	
Seitan and Black Bean Chili			X	X		
Warm Lentil Salad with Smoked Mozzarella and Arugula			X	X		
Greek Lentil Salad with Feta and Spinach			X	X		
Braised Red Lentils with Eggplant and Ricotta Salata			X		X	
Delectable Desserts						
Coconut Custard		X	X		X	
Creamy Vanilla Pudding		X	X		X	
Creamy Chocolate Pudding		X	X		X	
Creamy Coffee Pudding		X	X		X	
Chocolate-Orange Soufflés	X	X	X	X		
Tangy Lemon Gelatin		X	X		X	

	Phase 1	Phase 2	Phases 3 & 4	Weekday	Weekend	Comments
Creamy Lemon Gelatin		X	X		X	
Lime-Mint Gelatin		X	X		X	
Lickety-Split Vanilla Ice Cream		X	X		X	
Mint Granita		X	X		X	
Lemon-Lime Semifreddo		X	X		X	
Cranberry-Orange Fool		X	X	X		
Mixed Berry Fool		X	X	X		
Atkins Basic Piecrust		X	X		X	
Almond Piecrust		X	X		X	
Cinnamon Piecrust		X	X		X	
Nutty Piecrust	*	X	X	X		*After 2 weeks in Phase 1
Flaky Piecrust			X		X	
Crumbly Piecrust			X		X	
Chocolate Piecrust			X		X	
Sweet Cherry Pie			X		X	
Blueberry Pie		X	X		X	
Apple-Strawberry Pie			X		X	
Apple-Cranberry Pie			X		X	
Almond-Plum Tart			X		X	
Pineapple Upside-Down Cake			X		X	
Toasted Pecan Cake			X		X	
Toasted Pecan Cake with Maple Frosting			X		X	
Mini-Muffin-Tin Chocolate Brownies		X	X	X		
Mini-Muffin-Tin Mocha Brownies		X	X	X		
Mini-Muffin-Tin Mexican Chocolate Brownies		X	X	X		
Vanilla Meringues	X	X	X		X	
Coconut Meringues	*	X	X		X	*After 2 weeks in Phase 1
No-Bake Cheesecake with Toasted Nut Crust		X	X		X	
Almond No-Bake Cheesecake		X	X		X	
Blueberry Swirl No-Bake Cheesecake		X	X		X	
Crustless Ginger Cheesecake with Lime–Sour Cream Topping		X	X		X	
Cardamom Butter Cookies		X	X	X		
Lemon Butter Cookies		X	X	X		
Chocolate Truffles	X	X	X		X	
Pistachio-Chocolate Truffles	*	X	X		X	*After 2 weeks in Phase 1
Peppermint-Chocolate Truffles		X	X		X	

INDEX

ABOUT THE AUTHOR

As Vice President of Nutrition and Education, Colette Heimowitz is the driving force for nutrition information at Atkins Nutritionals, Inc. Among her responsibilities is keeping current with emerging research on human nutrition and specifically the Atkins Diet. She then "translates" that information for the general population on the Atkins website and in Atkins books. Colette is the nutritionist face to the Atkins Community, which is dedicated to helping people reach their weight-loss goals. As part of this initiative, she publishes a weekly Nutritionist Blog. She is also responsible for content devoted to educating new members about the program, including introductory videos, phase-specific courses, and interactive FAQs.

Colette has been a guest on radio programs nationwide, as well as on television networks including CNN, Fox News Channel, and MSNBC. She has more than twenty-five years of experience as a nutritionist, which includes her time working with Dr. Robert C. Atkins as Director of Nutrition at The Atkins Center for Complementary Medicine in New York City. Colette received her M.Sc. in clinical nutrition from Hunter College of the City University of New York.

In addition to her daily exercise routine, which includes walking her dog, Colette relaxes by enjoying the fruits of her profession: namely, cooking and eating.